The Edgar Cayce Plant Encyclopedia

VOLUME ONE

Jeanette M. Thomas

ISBN-13: 978-1543191035
ISBN-10: 1543191037

Photograph by
Lead photographer F. Michael (Mike) Pinkava, USA
Contributing photographers
William (Bill) Lott, USA
Mylen James (Mike) Mundt, Czech Republic
Gunnar Olsson, Sweden
Collin J. Thomas, USA

Dr. Carol Haenni - Editor

The CD of the entire Edgar Cayce Readings is available for sale through the Association for Research and Enlightenment, 215 67th Street, Virginia Beach, Virginia 23451 - 2061 http://www.edgarcayce.org/

Disclaimer
This study is presented for historical and educational purposes only. It is not intended as, nor should it be considered as, a source of prescriptive information - - or as a guide to self-diagnosis or self-treatment. Due to the possibility of unknown allergies no plant in this study should be used without first consulting a physician. It is not intended for nor should it be used as a substitute for professional medical advice and care.

This research is dedicated to friend and mentor Gladys who taught me how to research the readings and how to keep the records; to Mike who stayed the course; to my son Collin for being who he is; and to my daughter Rachel who has always given the most.

Contents

Cayce Plants

About The Author

Jeanette M. Thomas, former Administrator of Records for the Edgar Cayce Foundation in Virginia Beach, Virginia joined the Cayce organizations in the fall of 1979 as assistant to Gladys Davis Turner, serving in this capacity until Mrs. Turner's death on February 12, 1986.

Trained by Harold J. Reilly in 1980 she is one of the four founders of the Cayce Reilly School of Massotherapy and the originator of the Edgar Cayce Home Remedies program.

Her introduction to record keeping began with preparing Edgar Cayce's personal correspondence collection with nearly 6,000 people covering a 44 year time span for microfilming. She also designed a unique research methodology for the health readings published as Research Bulletins. In 1984 she began preparing the Cayce readings for computerization and managed the project which was completed in 1991.

Jeanette shares her scholarship in the Cayce material through speaking, teaching, consulting and writing. She can be contacted at: CaycePlants@info-1.com

FOREWORD

This project was born in the Philippines many years ago during a holistic health program. I was speaking about the Cayce formulas when a physician raised his hand and asked "Excuse me Jeanette, but what is poke?" When I answered *Phytolacca americana* he nodded in understanding. At that moment I realized the Cayce plants were essentially hidden within the collection and my research began. Well before the Cayce information was computerized, I turned page after page of the archival transcripts recording the names used by Cayce. They are shown here alphabetically according to the names he used.

The evolution of the long history of botanical pharmacology has also been very briefly traced and similarities to the health practices of some pre-historic civilizations are also referenced if mention of them is made by Cayce.

Wherever possible official or traditional folk usage has been documented from original translations and other sources listed in the bibliography in an effort to place each plant within its own individual historical context. The reader will soon discover the Cayce system is somewhat unique as the information sometimes deviates from both traditional herbal methods and acceptable medical practices, past and present.

Each plant is further identified as being official or unofficial in the American or British pharmacopeias at the time the Cayce information was being given.

Thank you to: Rick and Elsie Pinard and Renate Werner for being family in dark times. Roman Prochazka who carried me when I couldn't walk. Dr. Harold J. Reilly for his friendship, training, guidance and wisdom. Peter Newman who gave. Erik and Lorraine Jensen for telling me not to give up. Vic, Les, Josh and Nicholas [Nicky] Reiffer who opened their home and their hearts more than once. Ed Edwards for his special knowledge, loyal support and hundreds of books. Robert Adriance for lighting a candle in the darkness. Dr. Martyn Richardson who, as a teenage knew Edgar Cayce and retired as Dean of the New England School of Osteopathy who shared his knowledge of pharmacology and ancient medical systems. Ruth Montgomery for her encouragement in the early days of the project. Mildred N. Latimer for her hard work, loyalty and love. Olga Worrall who touched my life so deeply and inspired me to dare so long ago. Dr. John O.A. Pagano a dear friend who patiently answered hundreds of questions and who serves as an unwavering standard of excellence. John Walsh for the 1934 British Pharmacopeia. Joseph W. [Joe] Dunn for the writing formula, many plants and sage advice. Oscar and Robbert Schrover for their intelligence, advice and countless hours. Georgeann Barden, Ailene and Larry Radcliffe. Paul Mazza, Kevin McCormac and Dallas Block for kind hearts and carrying heavy things. Pulitzer Prize nominee Sidney Kirkpatrick, author of EDGAR CAYCE – An American Prophet who said the research should not be lost. Per and Ruth Madsen for sharing their almond tree. Dr. Eleonora von Wallenstern and Cammie for specialized knowledge of all things Egyptian.

A Touch of History

Four old-world river valley cultures have given rise to the earliest organized human civilizations known to date. They are the Nile River in Egypt, the Tigris and Euphrates Rivers in Mesopotamia, the Yellow and Yangtze Rivers in China and the Indus and Ganges Rivers in India. Each of these societies developed complex social structures which included participation in extensive trade networks, sustainable agriculture, the development of metallurgy and chemistry, centrally organized production of textiles and pottery and early forms of writing and mathematics. Ancient peoples in these valleys had well established religious beliefs, practiced medicine and pharmacology, and the earliest practice of modern day surgery and dentistry can be traced to these early groups. Temples and other surviving structures are clear evidence of the organized management of stable, large-scale populations over long periods of time. It is impossible to determine how long it took for these different groups to reach the apex of their accomplishments. Those familiar with the Cayce information are aware that it provides additional insights, in hundreds of individual transcripts, to many pre-historic cultures, among them Egypt, Mesopotamia, Greece, ancient Persia and India. Records of the earliest use of plants in healing begin with these early cultures.

Archeologically the early Chinese, Egyptian, Greek and Islamic civilizations are to a certain extent documented, but science has yet to discover many of the contributions of pre-historic India which is one of the most culturally, linguistically, and ethnically diverse regions yet to be definitively explored.

Researchers interested in tracing the earliest use of plants in healing must of necessity work with translations. Unfortunately even the "purest" translations have been obscured by the simple and natural changes in the meaning of words over time. Texts have also been erroneously represented because information has been taken out of context or incorrectly quoted, or excerpts have been added to or deleted. These corruptions, having entered into multiple publications, have all too often been accepted as factual.

Ancient trade practices between early cultures also contributed to confusion and questions as to where certain plants originated. Ancient traders have effectively spread the knowledge of new medicinal or food plants providing for the dissemination of seeds, roots and cuttings. Modern researchers will find that as traders plied their trade they often gave different common names to the same species in different countries and even from region to region within the same country. Other challenges include the spelling of names as they vary from translation to translation and by country, language and era, and the possibility of phonetic corruption among various languages. Each of these variants must be traced and carefully analyzed when documenting the history of a given species. While the use of plants can be traced through voluminous written records at least as far back as 5,000 years, the early history of botanical pharmacology remains far from exact or complete.

Anyone interested in the study of any early system of medicine should also not be too quick to dismiss certain practices as ignorant superstition, belief in magic, evil spirits, or simply the product of "primitive minds." Researchers should withhold such quick judgments and respect and appreciate the level of empirical knowledge attained and the philosophical and collective world-view of these civilizations. Belief systems, even in modern times, evolve as a way to explain the unknown and to ameliorate unpleasant negative emotions such as fear, anger, helplessness, resentment and anxiety. Belief systems can increase comfort levels thereby promoting health by decreasing the deleterious chemical changes powerful negative emotions produce. Eons before the nervous system of the human body came to be understood to the extent it is today, these civilizations had begun a rudimentary exploration of energy medicine. Well before the work of Carl Jung many early peoples had grasped the basic concepts of emotional and attitudinal influences on health and the importance of faith in healing, something that only began to gain mainstream recognition in the United States in the 1920's.

MESOPOTAMIAN MEDICINE

The bedrock of western, monotheistic civilization is Mesopotamia, the area between the Euphrates and Tigris Rivers, a land of ever changing borders. This region has been known by many names over the past 10,000 years. This land of the "fertile crescent" is also called Uruk, Ur, Shinar, or Akkadia, Sumer or the land of the Chaldeans. It is in this general area that the Old Testament of the Judeo-Christian Bible[1] records the building of the famous Tower of Babel. Present day Christians, Jews and Muslims refer to this geographical region as the Garden of Eden and it is often referred to as the cradle of civilization.

Archeological remains of one Sumerian civilization in southern Mesopotamia recently yielded evidence of a fairly sophisticated society organized as early as 8,000 B.C, and this individual culture may be even older. In September 2006 scientists excavating a Neolithic site at Tell Aswad at Jaidet al-Khass [a village located 22 miles outside of Damascus] found five decorated human skulls dating to as far back as 9,500 years ago.[2] The degree of sophistication in the execution of these artifacts is clear evidence they were produced by a very advanced culture.

The Mesopotamian civilization itself may even be older. Cayce refers to this region as Ur or the Ur of the Chaldeans or the land of the Hittites, and describes one pre-historic culture called The City in the Hills and the Plains which pre-dates the Sumerians by perhaps 3,000 to 5,000 years, *"when there was the building of a place for the ill, the badly treated, they that were without home, without friend." [1463-2].* A significant amount of material is provided on this early civilization founded on the humanitarian principles of healing, ministry and teaching, located near what is today Shushtar, Iran. [Also seen as Shustar] Cayce mentions the use of electrotherapy and hydrotherapy [289-9] in this early period and furthermore that men were taught a philanthropic philosophy, which was then quite rare, the humane care and treatment of the injured, the elderly and the mentally ill. It is also of interest that modern science finds some of the healing techniques from this ancient time, such as topical applications and various poultices, were actually quite effective.[3] It is further worthy of note that some of the methods in the present Cayce system are similar to those used by Mesopotamian therapeutic practitioners called "asuu."

The Babylonians enjoyed a well organized system of medicine in which there were two distinct medical practitioners. The therapeutic practitioner [these were both male and female] called asuu [sometimes seen as asu] and the aszipu [only males became aszipu] sometimes erroneously referred to as sorcerers, who focused on diagnosing psychosomatic illnesses and treating them by psychological means. The asuu are sometimes referred to as physicians as they dealt with prescribing medication and performed surgery. Early Mesopotamians further understood some diseases were contagious and had developed soap, cataract surgery and gained renowned for their ability to treat abscessed teeth.[4]

Little is yet known about the earliest people of this region although every school child knows of the world famous Babylonian Code of Hammurabi, dating to 1700 B.C., which includes among its many legal rulings the medical liability of surgeons [asuu] who make a mistake with *"the use of the knife."* French scholar René Labat [1904-1974] made a significant contribution to understanding the accomplishments of this civilization by translating 40 clay tablets to publish the <u>Treatise of Medical Diagnosis and</u>

1 Genesis 11:1-6
2 Times of Oman, Tuesday, September 26, 2006
3 Stroke in Babylonia Reynolds and Kinnier Wilson *Archeological Neurology.*2004; 61: 597-601.
4 HISTORY OF MEDICINE. Hajar A. Hajar Al BinAli, MD, FACC. Heart Views. The Official Journal of the Gulf Heart Association. Volume 2 No 4 December 2001-February 2002

<u>Prognoses</u>. These treaties, well worth a thoughtful review even today, date to roughly 1600 B.C., but their content is clearly from a much earlier time.

Syrian physicians also left important records which illustrate great similarities between the very early Egyptians and the later Assyrians, both in the practice of medicine and pharmacology. These similarities are historically indicative of a common source linking these early cultures in education and training. Among the largest links is a medical work entitled The <u>Book of Medicines</u> translated in April of 1913 by Sir Ernest Alfred Thompson Wallis Budge [1857-1934], an English Egyptologist, Orientalist, and Philologist who worked for the British Museum and who published numerous works on the ancient Near East. Budge believed the manuscript to have been originally translated from Greek into Syriac. The work quotes the actual words of Hippocrates and contains records of 400 prescriptions for various ointments and medicines including formulas ascribed to the Greek physician Galen. The manuscript, attributed to an unknown Syrian physician living in the early centuries of the Christian era, is *"written in a fine, bold Nestorian hand..."*

The pre-historic cultures that have risen to ascendancy in this part of the world may yet have significant contributions to make to the history of medicine and pharmacology. Since there is still too little known of their achievements so it is fortunate that there is a significant body of well preserved, original clay tablets yet to be translated and published. And other discoveries may lie ahead as Cayce speaks further, in transcript 870-1, of an area in what later came to be known as Chaldea where *"the third city under that in Ur"* remains to be uncovered. While it is true that in some civilizations commonalities in medicine and botanical pharmacology have developed in isolation, it is still exciting to await the discovery of the benefits this ancient center of human activity may have conveyed upon succeeding civilizations. Extensive archaeological exploration and many more scholarly translations are needed before this early period in human history can be more fully brought to light.

INDIA AND AYURVEDIC MEDICINE

Ayurvedic medicine is the oldest of the surviving healing systems being mentioned in the Vedas. The Vedas are the oldest surviving literature in the world originating somewhere between 5,000 to 10,000 years ago in India, though some scholars today actually believe the Rig Veda is closer to 12,000 years old.

Some scholars posit the Vedas as originally being revealed information transmitted for the purpose of improving the quality of physical and spiritual human life, similar to the way Judeo-Christian revealed information established dietary and hygienic practices to benefit the early Israelites, and similar to the way the Cayce model addresses health and healing. According to the texts themselves the Ayurvedic model was conceived by enlightened and wise sages as a system of living harmoniously and maintaining the body so that mental and spiritual awareness could be possible. In Sanskrit, ayur means life or living, and Veda means knowledge, so Ayurveda is defined as the "knowledge of living" or the "science of longevity." It has been said that if the Buddha, born in 560 B.C., did not know of the age or origins of these texts then they must indeed be from antiquity.

Some researchers further speculate that Ayurvedic medicine may have had its roots in even earlier times in Tibet. Cayce lends some credence to this in describing pre-history connections between what is today called Tibet, China and present day Iraq. Some medical historians believe that Ayurvedic concepts were also transported from ancient India to China and were instrumental in the early development of Chinese medicine.

Cayce has left behind over 100 transcripts in which there is information referring to pre-historic India, including an interesting group who lived around the time of the reign of Ahasuerus 405-485 B.C. [Xerxes]. One transcript states *that now would be called Persia, Arabia, portions of Turkey, all of Palestine, all of Hindustan, all of now Tibet, India - were under that rule." 1096-3.* Cayce makes only one minor reference to the Vedas in 315-4 but does make mention in transcript 364-3 of very early pre-history activity *"some ninety eight thousand years before the entry of Ram into India."* Ram was the so-called mythological hero of the Ramayana Epic, which may yet prove to be as real as what was once the "mythical" city of Troy.

In Ayurveda there are five basic elements that contain prana or universal energy. They are: earth, water, fire, air, and ether. These elements co-exist, interact and are further organized in the human body into three main categories or basic physiological principles that govern all bodily functions. These are known as the Tridosha [three humours] or doshas. The three doshas are vata, pitta, and kapha. Each person has a unique blend of the three doshas, known as the person's prakriti, which is why Ayurvedic treatment is always individualized. In Ayurveda disease is viewed as a state of imbalance in one or more of a person's doshas, and an Ayurvedic physician strives to adjust and balance them, using a variety of modalities including diet, detoxification and purification techniques, utilizing herbal, animal kingdom and mineral remedies, yoga, breathing exercises, surgery, meditation, and massage. Of all treatments, as in the Cayce model, diet is the most basic and widely used modality.

CHINA AND THE YELLOW EMPEROR

China is not the subject of significant historical focus in the Cayce collection, but it cannot be ignored in any study of plants in healing. Among the thousands of ancient Chinese medical records available only two of the oldest have been chosen for mention in this study. The basic principles of Chinese medicine were first laid down in a work entitled Huang Di Nei Ching or The Yellow Emperor's Medicine Classic. Dated to between 400 B.C. and 200 B.C. it consists of 18 volumes written as an alleged dialogue between The Yellow Emperor Huang Di and court physician Chi-Po. The Emperor asks health related questions and Chi-Po answers in detail. Actually written over a number of dynasties it is believed to have been presented this way to preserve older oral traditions of medicine and to give it official status by attributing authorship to The Yellow Emperor. The Yellow Emperor or Huang Di is regarded by many as the Mythical Father of Chinese Medicine - comparable to the legendary Thoth in Egypt. He is one of the earliest known ancestors of the Chinese culture, and it is commonly held that he lived to the age of 110 years.

The Fire Emperor Shen Nong, sometimes seen written as Shennong, is credited with original authorship of the oldest known Chinese *materia medica*, Ben Cao Jing [Classic of Herbal Medicine][5]. The actual information recorded in the Ben Cao Jing is thought to date from 2800 B.C. although some scholars feel that due to the nature of its content it is from an oral tradition dating to a much earlier time in Chinese history. It may have originally been revealed information or translated through oral traditions from a foreign culture. Shen Nong is actually credited with teaching the early Chinese people how to farm, teaching them new and improved food gathering and production methods thereby ending their precarious hunter gatherer existence. This could also suggest that Shen Nong himself may not have been a native of the region.

The original Shen Nong materia medica listed only 365 plants categorized into 3 classes: superior, middle, and inferior, whereas today there are nearly 5,000 plants in use in modern Chinese medicine. The earliest reference to a connection between Shen Nong and Chinese herbal medicine is found in the Huai Nan Zi [The South of the Huai Master] written by Liu An, who died in 122 B.C.:

"Ancient people ate grasses and drank water. They gathered the fruit from trees and ate the meat of clams. They frequently suffered from disease and poisoning. Then Shen Nong taught people for the first time how to sow the five grains, to observe whether the land was dry or wet, fertile or rocky, located in the hills or in the lowlands. He tasted the flavors of all the herbs and springs, [determining] whether they were bitter or sweet. Thus he taught people what to avoid and where they could go. At that time, [Shen Nong] encountered 70 [herbs] in one day, [determining which were] medicines and [which were] poisons."

Traditional Chinese medicine is comprised of a great many modalities including acupuncture, [contrasted with osteopathic and chiropractic in the Cayce model] moxibustion, and those therapies used in the Cayce system including massage, various types of hydrotherapy, specific and general exercises, meditation, diet and a critically objective consideration of attitudes, emotions and lifestyle. Herbalism may be the oldest modality but, like the Cayce model, it is not practiced as a separate discipline.

Chinese medicine is a reflection of centuries of observation of nature and of the natural rhythms of life. As with Ayurvedic and the much later Hippocratic schools, it centers on viewing the body as a

---

5 It is sometimes found as *Shen-nung pen ts'ao ching* or the Divine Husbandman's Materia Medica

whole organism encompassing body, mind and spirit. The physiological condition of the body is seen as a reflection of the state of both mental and spiritual at the time of diagnosis. This tradition views the natural elements within the body as fire, [heat or nervous energy] water, earth, wood and metal, all constantly vacillating. A particular herb or combination of herbs shares these elementary qualities, [categorized by their nature, taste, affinity, and primary action] and need to be matched to the individual patient at the time of diagnosis. It follows that the correct compounding of internal medicines is highly individualized. Moreover, prescribing treatments considers the cosmic balance of yin and yang, or the dual nature of creation, which is seen as positive or negative, male or female. Chinese medicine employs eight guiding principles of diagnosis found in what are called the following four primary polar opposites: Yin/yang; cold/heat; deficiency [xu] excess [shi] and interior/exterior.

The ancient healing art of Feng Shui is predicated upon all reality as energy and that the electromagnetic influences of the movement of energies have an influence on the quality of human life. Feng Shui is known and marketed today primarily to increase material wealth whereas it is actually a rather sophisticated energy modification art form. True Feng Shui addresses all aspects of existence in order to create a more harmonious life.

Egypt and The Ebers Papyrus

From the many surviving medical records of the Egyptian civilization only two have been selected for mention here due to some interesting similarities to the Cayce model. They are the Kahun Medical Papyrus, and the Ebers.

Discovered among many other ancient papyri, the Kahun Medical Papyrus was found in April of 1889 at the el-Fayium site of Lahun by Flinders Petrie. An English translation was published in 1898 and the original is now housed in the University College, London.

The date of the papyrus has been established by a note within the text itself that states: *"the 29th year of the reign of Amenenhat III" [1825 B.C.].* Much of the Kahun papyrus is unintelligible due to its poor condition and archaic language. Its content deals primarily with the health of women and with instructions for treating problems related to conception, prenatal care, the birthing process and the delivery of children. It is mentioned here because fumigation treatment techniques described in the Kahun are still known and practiced today as "steam sitz" treatments. This technique is also recommended in the Cayce system for a number of conditions, among them the successful treatment of female sterility. The Egyptians used fumigation additives such as crocodile dung, honey and sour milk whereas Cayce usually calls for the use of sweet gum resin. It is interesting that despite the differences in ingredients the concept of a fumigation technique itself remains unchanged.

The Ebers is of the greatest value to those interested in the use of plants in healing. Purchased in 1862 by an American named Edwin Smith, from a still unidentified source in Luxor, Egypt, it was sold again in 1873 for a reported $8,000.00 to German Egyptologist George Moritz Ebers for whom it is named. It is said to have been originally found in a tomb and is generally dated to 1500 B.C., however its content is thought by most scholars to be dated to 3000 B.C. or even earlier. The original is now housed in the University of Leipzig in Germany.

The papyrus is dated at 1500 B.C. from a reference within the text which reads: the *"9th year of the reign of Amenhotep I* [c. 1534 B.C.]. Yet another note within the document states *"the book of driving wekhedu[6] from all the limbs of a man was found in writings under the two feet of Anubis in Letopolis and was brought to the majesty of the king of Upper and Lower Egypt Den."* The use of the term "Lower Egypt Den" suggests the document may be dated closer to the First Dynasty period of around 3000 B.C.[7] [Den was the fifth king of the First Dynasty[8]] and many believe it to be a copy of the even more ancient books of Thoth, reputed to be the father of Egyptian medicine, pharmacy and alchemy.

The Ebers Papyrus is approximately 65 feet in length, organized into 877 paragraphs and consisting of 108 columns. Also appended to some of the paragraphs are glosses[9] shedding light on the meaning of some obsolete terms. These explanations are thought by many scholars to have been originally written into the main body of the text as "editorial updates." They often constitute the most valuable parts of the documents for present day researchers. There are two excellent English translations: <u>Papyrus Ebers: The</u>

---

6 Wekhedu, also seen as wxd, has not been definitively translated but is loosely translated as some sort of trouble, malaise, sickness or "suffering."

7 The list of kings in the 1st Dynasty include Narmer, Aha, Dier, Diet, Den, Anendijb, Semerkhat and Oa'a. however recent texts list Narmer as belonging to Dynasty O — the period before unification,

8 Alternative names in modern literature: Horus-Den, Dewen, Horus-Dewen, Udimu, Oudimou

9 A gloss is a brief explanatory note or translation of a difficult or technical expression usually inserted in the margin or between lines of a text or manuscript.

<u>Greatest Egyptian Medical Document</u> translated by Bendix Ebbell,[10] and <u>The Ebers Papyrus – A New English Translation, Commentaries and Glossaries</u> translated by Paul Ghalioungui.[11]

The Ebers is a compilation of a great many different medical texts on a variety of subjects organized into paragraphs on diseases of the skin, the heart, stomach ailments and the rectum, all with prescriptions to treat the ailments. Clearly described are five methods of administration of drugs: oral, rectal, vaginal, external applications and vapor/inhalation/fumigation. Also found are directives for the practitioner and the patient to repeat specific statements which are all too often dismissed by modern scholars as merely spells or magic incantations. As stated earlier, modern day researchers should consider these as a method or means of addressing the role of the mind and emotions in healing on the part of both the practitioner and the patient. They should be viewed from a psychological standpoint in the same category as the modern day use of prayer, meditation and affirmations and not merely dismissed as primitive superstition. The Cayce system also makes extensive use of affirmations emphasizing the critical element of the power of the mind in healing. Modern science has come a long way in recent years in admitting to the efficacy of prayer and the importance of the state of mind in health and healing. Clearly the Egyptians had an understanding of the role of the mind and emotions in the successful treatment of various diseases, also recognizing that some conditions were incurable, some the result of trauma, and some were psychosomatically induced.

Of great interest to those familiar with the Cayce information, are clues to a much more ancient medical tradition preceding the generally accepted date of the Ebers and incorporated within its text giving further evidence to its antiquity if indeed it was *"brought to the majesty of the king of Upper and Lower Egypt Den."* as recorded in the document. These are found in paragraphs 242 through 247 where remedies are referenced as having been made and used personally by various "gods," specifically Ra [also seen as Rê], Shu, Tephnis [Tefnout], Nut, and Isis.

Paragraph 247 for example, references Isis' creation of a remedy for an illness in Ra's head. *"A sixth remedy that Isis made for Ra himself to eliminate the disease that is in his head: fruit of coriander [unknown word] made into a mass, honey is mixed with it, the head is bandaged therewith so that it goes immediately well with him."* The fact that these remedies for "the gods" is mentioned in the text in such a matter of fact way indicates to some scholars that loss of biographical identity has occurred over time suggesting these "deities" may have been real people and that what was once history has passed into legend. This would date the information in the Ebers to the very foundation of Egyptian civilization.

Accurate identification of many of the plants used in Egypt without the benefit of original illustrations is problematic; however a few well documented plants in the Ebers are still used in botanical pharmacology today, including the Cayce model. Among them are almonds, senna, juniper, colocynth, pine tar, aloe, cedar, elderberry, fennel, garlic, onion, peppermint, linseed, opium or the poppy-plant, saffron, castor and watermelon. Many plants in every day use in ancient Egypt were used as "simples." Grown in home gardens they were in such common use that they were never listed in their official records. There are still many plants used by the Egyptians that have not been identified and many of the words used to name or describe the plants may never be translated.

---

10 Copenhagen Levin & Munksgaard, 1937
11 Academy of Scientific Research and Technology, Cairo, Egypt, 1987

Egypt is the subject of extensive historical focus in the Cayce collection being mentioned in well over 500 individual transcripts. It was first mentioned in 1923, on November 16 in transcript 583-1, requested by a 31 year old young lady born in Copenhagen, Denmark. Ten years later in 1933 in transcript 328-1 Cayce volunteered the name by which Egypt was known some 10,000 years ago: *"... in that land now known as the Egyptian, then Aar..."* Egypt continued to be of special interest until the end of Cayce's career in 1944 when transcript 5392-1 was recorded on August 29. For over 20 years consistent and coherent descriptions emerged transcript by transcript of social, religious, scientific and political life from the earliest pre-historic period to the time of Moses and Cleopatra.

GREECE AND ITS EGYPTIAN ROOTS

In the early days of the Greek civilization the world center of knowledge, science and culture was in Egypt. An Egyptian center of learning was called a "House of Life" and the curriculum included the study of medicine. It is interesting to note that there seem to be no records of pharmacists in ancient Egypt, as the term is understood today. It appears that physicians compounded their own prescriptions and learned the art and methods more or less through individual apprenticeships. Egyptians doctors were called *swnw*, pronounced "sewnew" in English. The practice of medicine was regulated through the temples and there were severe penalties for any deviation from what was acceptable medical practice. A "House of Life was a center of hope and help and attracted many patients, visitors and students from the then civilized world. Early Greek scholars naturally turned to Egypt for the study of metallurgy, mathematics, and medicine. Among the most notable of these scholars were the well traveled, well educated Herodotus, Pliny and Galen - who each in their time - availed themselves of the best of Egyptian medical and pharmaceutical knowledge. Through an examination of their surviving medical records it appears that Egyptian knowledge attained a certain plateau and then, for hundreds of years, advanced no further. The translation of their knowledge into the early Greek culture allowed the best of Egyptian accomplishments to be infused with new life where it subsequently inspired Graeco-Roman, Persian and other civilizations for generations to come.

Extant Greek Records
The early Greeks greatly influence both the present day organization of plants and our terminology. The word botany itself, for example, comes from the Greek language; the original meaning is "pasture," "grass" or "fodder." With the Greeks botany and plant pharmacology gradually begins to be seen as two distinct areas of scientific inquiry. Over 100 transcripts in the Cayce collection reference the Greek civilization ranging from pre-history to the time of recorded history. Greek scholars preserved, built upon and advanced the work of the Egyptians making the science of pharmacology and medicine their own. Only four of the hundreds of Grecian contributors to the subject of botanical pharmacology are mentioned in this study.

Theophrastus of Eresus, [372-287 B.C.] a philosopher and pupil of Plato, later an associate of Aristotle, is considered the father of modern botany. During his lifetime he authored 10 books on the subject of plants. Two of his largest works, On the History of Plants, and On the Causes of Plants have remained as definitive botanical references for over 1,800 years. He also described approximately 500 medicinal plants detailing how they were used. He is still cited as an authoritative source today.

Pliny the Elder [AD 23-79] descended from a prosperous family and began a military career at the age of 23 serving in what is today Germany. He rose to the rank of cavalry commander, returned to Rome and studied law finally becoming procurator in Spain where he eventually lived in semiretirement, studying and writing. His devotion to his studies and his research techniques were described by his nephew, Pliny the Younger. He described roughly 1000 plants in his 37 volume Historia Naturalis, which includes the works of many earlier authors whose writings do not survive, among them an important early Greek herbalist named Krateus [100 B.C.]. Krateus is thought to be the first to use illustrations of plants, and, while his work did not survive, Pliny references it and scholars believe some of Krateus' original illustrations were copied and have survived in other works. Pliny remains an invaluable resource for the use of plants in ancient medicine.

Pedanius Dioscorides [c. 40 A.D. - 90 A.D.] was born Anazarbus, Cilicia. He compiled and wrote <u>De Materia Medica</u> in 77 A.D. wherein he gathered together all the known medicinal substances of his time describing their properties and actions. Dioscorides included a number of the same formulas listed in the Egyptian Papyrus Ebers, prescribing them for the same ailment as the Egyptians and for this reason he is considered a definitive authority in Egyptian medicine. One of his significant achievements was making an "anaesthetic wine" from Mandragora which enabled early physicians to perform surgery or to cauterize wounds with a greater degree of comfort to the patient. A military physician under Emperor Nero of Rome, he traveled widely and his Codex was in official use throughout Europe until the 16th century.

Claudius Galen [131-201 A.D.] was the son of a wealthy architect, educated as a philosopher and a man of letters. At the age of 16 he changed his course of study to medicine. He studied in Pergamum, Smyrna, Corinth and Alexandria in Egypt. He began practicing medicine in Alexandria, which was the greatest medical centre of his day, and was later appointed personal physician to the Emperor Marcus Aurelius and his son Commodus. Galen's extensive writings were first translated into Syriac and stored at the University of Jundi Shapur in Persia where Muslim scholars later translated them into Arabic. Because of this Galen is largely credited with establishing the Hippocratic influence within early Islamic medicine. There is some uncertainty about when he died as his final works were written after 207 A.D. suggesting that his Arab biographers were correct in claiming that the great man died at the age of 87, in 216 or 217 A.D. He was among the first to emphasize the critical necessity for precise measurements in compounding internal medications. The term Galenic pharmacy is still used today in describing that branch of pharmacy which relates to the preparation of medicines by infusion or decoction as distinguished from those which are chemically prepared. The Cayce model is predominantly Galenic.

A Fusion of Cultures through Persian and Islamic Conquests

The Persians [Arabs - present day Iran] waged war against neighboring countries [including the Greeks] during a long period of invasion and conquest until they themselves were finally conquered by Alexander the Great in 332 B.C. They invaded and ruled Egypt during the 27th Dynasty and again for a ten-year period during the 31st Dynasty. During their occupations of Egypt a "scala" or systematized vocabulary was developed recording the Coptic words for plant names which were based upon ancient Egyptian and their Persian or Arabic equivalents. Coptic is a form of the ancient Egyptian language that began developing through Greek influence as early as 200 B.C. First century Egyptian Christians were named for this language. It was the predominant language of Egypt until, through the influence of continual occupation by the Persians, the Arabic language became dominant. While Coptic occasionally draws from the Greek language these scala are a critical bridge between ancient Egyptian and present day Arabic and Greek.

The rise of Islam, beginning in 630 AD, brought yet another period of invasion and conquest to the region but under the Muslims an unusual renaissance occurred. Between approximately 700 A.D. and 1300 A.D an extraordinary flowering took place in the fields of philosophy, science and the arts. The 9th century represents the height of intellectual accomplishment in Islamic science and is generally referred to as the apex of what was the 500-year long "Abbasid Golden Age." What is even more remarkable is that it was their cultural view that all knowledge was to be freely shared.

Caliph Al-Mansur [712-775 A.D.] consolidated the power of the great Islamic Abbasid Caliphate and built a new capital in 750 A.D. on the site of an ancient Persian village named Baghdad. Originally named the City of Peace it became popularly known as the Round City. Very little, if anything remains of the site today but it was here in 830 AD that the Bayt al-Hikmah or "House of Wisdom" was founded as an Arabic translation bureau, library, cultural institute and scientific academy. At first scientific and philosophical documents of other cultures were only copied and brought back to the House of Wisdom but eventually scientific research and cultural development exploded within the Islamic culture. Drawing on Babylonian, Syrian, Uruk, Persian, Indian, and Greek texts authored by Aristotle, Plato, Hippocrates, Euclid, Pythagoras and many others, Islamic scholars accumulated the greatest collection of knowledge in the world, subsequently refining and advancing it through their own discoveries. The House of Wisdom became the intellectual and scientific center of the known world, and Arabic became the language of international scholarship.

In 751 A.D., the Chinese helped pave the way for this multi-cultural, multi-lingual dissemination through their development of the technique of making paper from linen, thus ending the expensive use of parchment in book publishing. When the first paper mill was built in Baghdad in 793 A.D. the new and cheaper paper combined with the sophisticated Muslim bookbinding techniques completing the elements necessary for the practical dissemination of translations in a great variety of European languages.

The seventh Abbasid caliph, al Ma'mun [813-833 A.D.] spent his entire reign actively and vigorously encouraging scholars of all kinds in the application of their skills in matters of science and began an even greater effort in the systematic, widespread acquisition and translation of Greek, Indian, Chinese and Egyptian manuscripts, an activity that continued for a century or more.

Islamic scholars wrote and published great numbers of encyclopedias and summaries of the vast collections of the Greeks and Romans, organizing and systematizing the often inconsistent and sometimes contradictory writings. They introduced experimental investigation which gradually transformed alchemy into modern chemistry and in 750 AD the first public pharmacy opened in Baghdad, soon to be followed by 800 registered pharmacists in Baghdad alone. They established hospitals, perfected algebra and the astrolabe, produced alcohol, developed the pointed arch [known later in Europe as the Gothic arch], provided a system of free health care for the poor, wrote the first text book of ophthalmology,[12] invented the science and method of distillation, perfected the use of anesthetic for surgery, including the "Anaesthetic sponge" or "Sleeping sponge," and wrote the first pharmacopeias.

---

12 Al-Ashr Maqalat fi al-Ayn [The Ten Treaties of the Eye] by Ibn-Masawayh

CIVILIZATION MOVES WEST

The great Catholic monasteries of Europe are also given credit for the preservation of certain fields of knowledge during the so-called dark ages;[13] however, the scientific disciplines of medicine and pharmacology were largely absent from the European landscape. The preparation and administration of even the simplest of herbal remedies was often in the hands of the priests who had the only working knowledge of their use. Not to ignore or diminish the continuing role of the local herbalist in village life, it is still a fact that a paucity of European medical schools meant that "physick" gardens maintained by some monasteries were the only source of "medicine" available to the working classes of Medieval Europe.

There is much scholarly debate as to where, when and what signaled the end of the dark ages. Most scholars agree that it began in 409 A.D. when the Romans left what is now the British Isles. Pockets of darkness remained throughout Europe until roughly 1450 A.D. when the invention of the printing press by Johannes Gutenberg in Germany made the written word readily available. Most agree it was William Caxton [1422-1491] who first began lifting the darkness in England. Caxton published the first English language book, The History of Troy, while he was in Bruges, Belgium in 1476 and a year later established the first English language printing press at Westminster,[14] all less than 30 years after the printing press had been invented.

Caxton is also famous for publishing two editions of Chaucer's Canterbury Tales, Gower's Confession Amantics and Malory's Morte d'Arthur. Medical historians find it of some significance that Geoffrey Chaucer, in the General Prologue of the Canterbury Tales, identifies the authorities used by his "Doctour of Phisik:

Wel knew he the olde Esculapius,
And Deyscorides and eek Rufus,
Olde Ypocras, Haly, and Galyen,
Serapioun, Razis, and Avycen,
Averrois, Damascien, and Constantyn,
Bernard, and Gatesden, and Gilbertyn.

The list includes four Arab physicians: Jesu Jaly [Ibn 'Isa], Razi [Al-Razi, or Rhazes], Avycen [Ibn Sina, or Avicenna] and Averrois [Ibn Rushd, or Averroes]. They are included by Chaucer because they would be called today "household names." In Chaucer's day they were as famous as any of the greatest medical authorities of modern times. These four world-renowned physicians produced textbooks, methods and techniques which were published in many languages and used in medical schools throughout Europe for hundreds of years. The Persian born Avicenna [Abu Ali al-Husayn Ibn Sina 980-1037 A.D.] for example, codified Greek and Arabic medical knowledge into two volumes entitled the Book of Healing and The Canon of Medicine known as the Qanun. The Qanun was the standard medical textbook in Europe for over five hundred years.

The Islamic effort begun in the House of Wisdom in Baghdad preserved much of the knowledge of the ancient world. By collecting, copying, translating, codifying and augmenting the classical Graeco-Roman heritage that Europe had lost during the dark ages Arab mathematicians, scientists and physicians of the

---

13 476 AD to 1000 AD

14 The first English book published in England was Dictes or Sayengis of the Philosophres. It was printed by Caxton in 1477

8th to the 10th century both preserved knowledge and laid the foundations of the institutions and the science of modern mathematics, engineering, pharmacy, surgery and medicine.

HERBALISM IN THE MIDDLE AGES

During the Middle Ages a great many herbals were published. Most were written between 1470 and 1670 and were especially popular in England and Germany. During this time many herbalists made significant contributions in crude classifications and descriptions of plants alleged to have curative powers. All are worthy of study but only a few will be mentioned here.

Among the giants of the time was Otto Brunfels [1464-1534] a Carthusian Monk who later became a Lutheran school teacher and physician who published his Herbarum Vivae Eicones in about 1530. The plant genus *Solanaceae* is named in his honor and he is considered one of the early fathers of botany.

Hieronymus Bock [Jerome Bock -1498-1554] was a Lutheran minister who wrote and published Kreuterbach in 1539. He was a physician and a colleague of Brunfels. The grass genus *Tragus* and the spurge genus *Tragia* are named after him. An illustrated edition of his work was published in 1546 containing 500 exquisitely crafted woodcuts by David Kandel of Strasburg. The accuracy of the illustrations in Kreuterbach set the standards for botanical art for centuries.

Leonhard Fuchs [1501-1566] a German medical doctor and botanist was a compassionate and intelligent man who despaired at the terrible state of the practice of medicine in his time. In an effort to remedy the situation he compiled a pharmacopoeia entitled De historia stirpium, or Concerning the Description of Plants which was written, not in scholarly Latin, but in German. This meant the information was, for the first time, available to the general reading public. Fuchs was fanatical in his attention to detail and wanted no mistakes in the identification of plants, because just as in Galen's time, mistakes led to poisonings. His work was meticulously illustrated with woodcuts by Heinrich Füllmaurer and Albrecht Meyer and cut by German artist Veit Rudolf Speckle. Fuchs realized, as did Nicholas Culpepper fifty odd years later, that physicians of his day were ignorant of their medicines and often placed complete reliance on illiterate apothecaries who were in turn totally dependent upon the peasants who gathered roots and herbs. These Rhizotomoi, or root cutters, gathered plants and prepared them for drug vendors in the same fashion as Wildcrafters provide crude drug plants and plant products for the modern pharmaceutical industry and the holistic health and home remedy markets of today. A few early Rhizotomoi were talented, trustworthy, of good reputation and held in high esteem, but these were sadly in the minority. Fuchs drew on the earlier works of Dioscorides, Pliny and Galen but added at least 100 plants - accurately portrayed - to his body of work. The genus "Fuchsia" is named in his honor.

Valerius Cordus [1515-1544], author of the first German pharmacopoeia, described roughly 450 plants based on direct observation during his many field trips to produce his Historia Plantarum. His herbal treatise is of great significance because it described for the first time not only plants but also woods, barks and fruits which were being imported for medicinal use from other countries. Cordus described the structure of flowers in meticulous detail contributing the first truly scientific treatment of the subject since Theophrastus, and in the process he gained increased respect for his chosen profession from the scientific community. He received his degree in medicine from the University of Wittenberg in 1531 and was widely traveled and gifted in many languages and scientific methods. He shares credit for the discovery of ether with Paracelsus, a Swiss physician and chemist. Cordus died of malaria at the age of 29 but had by then completed five books of his Historia Plantarium.

Venetian physician and botanist Prospero Alpini[15] traveled to Egypt in 1580 where he served under the Venetian consul in Cairo, George Hemi. During his three year tenure managing date palm plantings he discovered the sexual differences in plants and published his findings. His work later formed the basis for Carolus Linnaeus of Sweden who named the genus Alpinia in his honor. Alpini's work, Plantes des Egyptiens, published in 1792, is an invaluable reference for researchers even today because his work is based upon direct observation. In addition to his work on Egyptian plants Alpini is credited with publishing the first account of the coffee plant in Europe, another plant used therapeutically in the Cayce system.[16] He was appointed professor of botany at Padua where he served until his death February 6, 1617.

Seville, Spain, is the home of another of the famous early contributors to herbal and botanical knowledge, Nicolas Monardes [1493?-1588]. Monardes received his medical degree in 1547 from the University of Alcalá[17] in Alcalá de Henares, Spain. He practiced medicine for over forty years before publishing his famous Joyful Newes out of the New Found Worlde in 1565. The work was translated into English by long time Seville resident and merchant John Frampton. Monardes wrote on plants imported from the "New Worlde" providing some of the earliest illustrations of plants used therapeutically in the Cayce system including tobacco, passion flower, sarsaparilla, Balsam of Tolu and Balsam of Peru. Monardes established a botanical garden in Seville where he cultivated and studied the effects of imported drug plants. Though his work was published in Latin and English as well as his native Spanish and is often cited, much of it is thought to have been borrowed from other published sources or simply based on hearsay.

---

15 1553-1617 Alpin, P. *La Medicine des Egyptiens I-II.* Cairo 1980. Alpin. P. *Plantes des Egyptiens* Cairo. 1980.
16 See Volume II.
17 The University of Alcala in Alcala de Henares was founded in 1504 by Franciscan Cardinal Ximenez de Cisneros, confessor to Queen Isabella. At this time Spain was a leader in medical science in Europe.

Two British Contributors

Two of the most popular and frequently cited British herbalists are John Gerarde and Nicholas Culpepper. These two are closer to us in time and because of the times in which they lived are deserving of closer examination.

During the time of Gerarde and Culpepper there were three categories of medicine in England: Physician, Surgeon and Barber. There were also three general categories [differentiated by the degree of training and formal education] in the practice of pharmacy: Apothecary, Herbalist, and Hedge Witch, or village practitioner. Herbalists and Hedge Witches acquired knowledge of their profession through association with another practitioner and maintained their practice based upon on their reputation, skill and success. Apothecaries were trained through long, formal, apprenticeships and had loosely defined legal relationships with physicians. The mortar and pestle used in signage in many modern drug stores and chemist shops remains a symbol of the apothecary.

Physicians of this time often combined medicine with metaphysics, diagnosed illnesses, prescribed medications, bled patients and set broken bones but would not dream of performing "Chiurgery" [from the Greek "hand-work"] as it was not within the scope of acceptable medical practice. Surgery, as it is practiced today, is an outgrowth of the profession of barber who was also a tooth puller and a blood-letter. The barbershop was often the closest thing to an emergency room available to the common people of the time. The red and white pole still used in advertising some barbershops today comes from the early practice of winding bloody bandages around a drying pole.

While the Barber Surgeons Craft Guild was organized in Edinburgh, Scotland as early as 1505, the acceptance of surgery by the medical profession was slow and fraught with many legal and social challenges. Considered only a simple manual craft it was not incorporated into the medical curriculum until 1803 and shortly thereafter the Royal College of Surgeons of Edinburgh, Scotland, one of the oldest surgical corporations in the world, was established. Both Gerarde and Culpepper lived on the cutting edge of this intense time of change.

John Gerarde [1545-1612] had been originally apprenticed to a barber-surgeon in London but he soon became the warden of the Barber-Surgeons Company. A proponent of the apothecary movement, he compiled a catalog of plants in 1596 and published his famous Herball in 1597. He was given charge and use of the gardens owned by William Cecil Burleigh [1520-1598] in the Strand and at Theobalds and also cultivated his own garden in Holborn [now within the city of London] where he grew his own medicinal plants and trees.

Some researchers and historians contend that Gerarde's work is not totally original and that he borrowed heavily from the work of others, among them Belgian botanist Rembert Dodoens. Some credence must be given to this. The Dodoens manuscript, Stirpium historiae pemptades sex sive libri XXX [1583], was being translated into English by one Robert Priest who died before the completion of his work. The publisher John Norton handed the unfinished manuscript over to Gerarde, who in addition to completing the translation, altered the arrangement to fit the system of French botanist Matthias de l'Obel[18] and added information of his own. Gerarde had somehow obtained a series of woodblocks originally used at

---

18   *L'Obel [1538–1616] also spelled Lobel, also called Matthaeus Lobelius* French physician and botanist whose *Stirpium adversaria nova* [1570; written in collaboration with Pierre Pena] was a milestone in modern botany.

Frankfurt, Germany, to illustrate Eicones plantarum written by Jacob Dietrich of Bergzabern,[19] [better known as Jacob Tabernaemontanus]. The illustrations were not original but had been borrowed from Bock, Fuchs, Dodoens and de l'Obel. Just how these exquisite woodblocks were acquired by Gerarde is not known, but they were used to illustrate his Herball. Unfortunately a few wrong descriptions were placed with some woodcuts and mythical plants were included such as a "barnacle tree." He introduced many helpful new plants in his book also but created some lingering confusion when a few plants such as the common potato were mistakenly identified. Fortunately a second revised edition edited by Thomas Johnson appeared in 1633 correcting many of the original mistakes. The woodcuts, in wide use as illustrations today, are still erroneously attributed to Gerarde.

Nicholas Culpepper [1616-1654] was a prolific author, but he is best known for his most famous The English Physician: or an astrological Discourse of the Vulgar Herbs of this Notion. Being a Compleat Method of Physick, whereby a man may preserve his Body in Health; or cure himself being sick for three pence charge, with such things only as grow in England, they being most fit for English Bodies. This work is better known today by its less weighty title: Culpepper's Herball, The Compleat Herball or more simply The Herbal.

Culpepper enjoyed two years of formal education at Cambridge but left to be married before finishing his course of study. Upon the untimely death of his wife, of whom little is known except that she was killed shortly after marriage by an unfortunate lightning strike, his guardian and maternal grandfather William Attersol arranged for Culpepper to be apprenticed to Daniel White, an apothecary in Temple Bar, a commercial district in London in this period. At this time [November of 1634] apprentices were required to fulfill a seven-year bachelor apprenticeship for a fee of fifty pounds. Daniel White soon went bankrupt and left for Ireland leaving Culpepper to find another master - without the balance of his fifty pound fee.

Culpepper next apprenticed himself to Francis Drake in Threadneedle Street where he was able to trade Latin lessons in exchange for his fee, room and board. Unfortunately Drake died, leaving Culpepper's apprenticeship again unfinished. Culpepper married a second time in 1639 automatically ending his apprenticeship two years short of journeymanship. His fifteen-year-old wife, Alice Field, brought a considerable fortune to the marriage and the couple bought a house and land for gardens in rural Spitalfields.

Culpepper worked from time to time, acting in the capacity of a journeyman, for Samuel Leadbeaters with whom he had been apprenticed in the Threadneedle Street apothecary; however, in June of 1644 the Society of Apothecaries forced Leadbeaters to stop using the unlicensed Culpepper. Unable to practice his chosen profession but fortunately blessed with sufficient funds to free him from the necessity of earning a living, he began an intensive period of study, research and prolific writing.

To understand Culpepper and the magnitude of his contribution it must be understood that at this time in British history physicians and apothecaries were at legal, philosophical, and political odds over who should prescribe and administer medicines. Culpepper was not without his opinion in the controversy. His criticism of the physicians, who were trying to bring every discipline under their legal jurisdiction, was based on the fact that nearly all their knowledge of pharmaceuticals was theoretical or highly specialized whereas the apothecary was very knowledgeable about the medicines he compounded and was in daily

---

19   Jacob Dietrich von Bergzabern [?1520-1590] was a pupil of Otto Brunfels and Jerome Bock

contact with the patient. In Culpepper's view this placed him in a better position to recommend, prepare and administer the appropriate remedies and more importantly to judge their efficacy. Culpepper also had very strong feelings about the practice of medicine in his day and had great contempt for the firmly entrenched "pay or perish" system of the medical profession. It is a fact that apothecaries were often the only source of health care for the poor in a time when only the very wealthy could afford to see a doctor. He felt strongly that apothecaries should be recognized as a separate and independent medical profession, not at the beck and call, nor under the legal jurisdiction of medical doctors. Because of his views Culpepper was very popular with the "man on the street" but he was often attacked in print by various warring factions within the so-called legitimate medical community.

Just as Leonhard Fuchs before him had done, Culpepper set about the Herculean task of translating the official Latin Pharmacopoeia into the vernacular. As word spread of the completion of the translation in 1648, he incurred the wrath of the medical establishment, but came under even greater public attack and censure when it was published a year later by London printer, Peter Cole. Cole was as active in the resistance to the established medical community as Culpepper and recent research suggests that Cole may have actually commissioned Culpepper to translate the Pharmacopoeia, or at the very least have underwritten the project. He certainly provided Culpepper with William Reeves to act as a secretary to take dictation, and Reeves remained with Culpepper as his secretary and assistant even as Culpepper's health declined.

With the publication of his <u>Herball</u> in 1652 Culpepper became so popular that he was effectively insulated from any further attacks from the medical community, and even though he was in poor health he was finally able to practice his profession without fear of further retaliation. He died on January 10, 1654 at the age of 38, two years after the publication of his <u>Herball</u>.

The official cause of Culpepper's death is recorded as tuberculosis and general debilitation, but questions about this are being raised today. He had served as a Roundhead at the First Battle of Newbury in September of 1643 where he was wounded in the chest. This wound had never properly healed and had plagued him throughout his life. Certainly the debilitating effects of this contributed to his early death but there is some question as to whether he may have suffered from tuberculosis or lung cancer. He was addicted to tobacco and is described as having "smoked continually."

Culpepper was a practical visionary. He is remembered as an astute and effective political activist and as someone who, with friends like Peter Cole, made very real and practical contributions to bring about social change. As an unlicensed apothecary/physician he practiced medicine among the poorest of the poor in the east-end of London and courageously fought throughout his life for the rights of everyone, regardless of their social or economic class, to affordable medical treatment.

DEVELOPMENT OF A UNIVERSAL BOTANICAL LANGUAGE

There have been uncounted numbers of individuals over the centuries who have made critical contributions to the development of a universal botanical language and all are worthy of study. It is expedient here to single out only three individuals whose comprehensive treatment of the overall subject matter is of such significance that they stand out amidst all others.

A system for identifying plants was developed in 1583 with the publication of <u>De Plantis</u> by an Italian botanist named Cesalpino. Andrea Cesalpino [1519-1603] studied both medicine and botany at the University of Pisa in Italy. He served as the Director of the Botanic Garden at the University of Bologna and became physician to Pope Clement VIII. In 1583 he published 16 books of which 15 volumes describe 1500 plants. His <u>De Plantis</u> and his work in the systematic mounting of plant specimens prepared a foundation for the continuation of this effort 25 years later with the birth of John Ray [1628-1705] in County Essex, England.

John Ray [sometimes seen as John Wray] was a Cambridge University Fellow and junior Dean and at an early age became an ordained priest in the Anglican Church. He was an expert in languages, mathematics and natural science. Among his many contributions is the proof that a living tree conducts water. He was so renowned for his discoveries that in 1667 he was inducted into one of the modern world's first scientific societies, the Royal Society of London. Ray's <u>Catalogue of Cambridge Plants</u> and his <u>Synopsis Methodica Avium et Piscium</u>, published after his death, are monumental systematic works on the classification of plants, birds, mammals, fish and insects. Ray's search for a natural system led him to classify plants by their shape or overall morphology. He was the first to divide flowering plants into monocots and dicots. Ray died at Black Notley at the age of seventy-six and is still referred to as the father of natural history in England.

The challenge of developing a universal botanical system was next taken up by Carolus Linnaeus [1707-1778] who was born in Sweden two years after the death of John Ray. Linnaeus entered the University of Lund in 1727 to study medicine. From his earliest childhood he had a passion for natural history and shared his father's love of plants. He transferred from Lund to the University in Uppsala largely because of its larger botanical holdings and it was at Uppsala that he first began to recognize the flaws and weaknesses in the rather chaotic and limited arrangement for botany. Unlike Ray, who had based his system on morphology, Linnaeus followed along the lines of Alpini, and began work on a system of classification based on the reproductive organs of flowers. He began work on his own method as early as 1730. In 1735 while in Holland studying medicine he completed work on <u>Systema naturae</u>, setting forth his new taxonomic arrangement for not only the plant kingdom but the animal and mineral kingdoms as well. He could not afford its publication so the costs were met through the generosity of his friend, teacher and admirer, Jan Fredrik Gronovius.[20] Later in 1736 Linnaeus published <u>Genera Plantarum.</u> Most scholars agree that this work must be considered the starting-point of modern systematic botany. His binomial Latin nomenclature is still a world wide standard and for the purposes of this study, allows the Cayce readings to speak with one voice amidst the many languages of the world.

---

20   Jan Fredrik Gronovius [1690-1762] Dutch botanist.

THE CAYCE MATERIA MEDICA

The materials of medicine culled from the thousands of transcripts produced by Cayce over the 40 odd years of his career yield a diverse and complex system of surpassing internal coherence.

Similarities between Cayce and the Egyptian, Babylonian, Greek, Ayurvedic and Chinese systems are significant, as their shared philosophical approach treats the patient as an integrated unit. Body, mind and spirit are all addressed in diagnosis and treatment. Focus on the simple alleviation of symptoms is minimal, and yet in Cayce there are three more distinct differences.

First, the origins of the information are not obscured by myth nor lost in the mists of time, as it is widely known as the largest body of revealed information in the world.

Second is the role of the muskoskeletal system which is inextricably interwoven throughout most all of the over 9000 physical transcripts. In the detailed descriptions of etiology and treatment almost the entire collection is predicated on the fundamental principles of osteopathic medicine.

The third is certainly of the greatest significance and unique to this researchers experience. The Cayce model does not just describe symptoms, diseases and treatments, but actually *gives the causes*. Causes which, when analyzed from one transcript to another, are frequently so similar as to reveal the most likely etiologies of a given disease. It is as if each individual is revealed through an internal photographic slide, the state and functioning of the anatomy and physiology frozen, as it were, for all time. Not only is the functioning of each physiological system described in exquisite detail but where relevant, the effect and influence of the mind and emotions are revealed as well. In a similar fashion, treatment recommendations, when analyzed from one transcript to another, yield treatment outlines which have the potential to present the Cayce information in a form appropriate for controlled clinical trial. A mathematical process of taking information given for individuals and translating it into a form appropriate for general use, resulted in the publication of medical Research Bulletins, which for a time were researched and published by the Edgar Cayce Foundation.

Extracting useable information for general application from this complex body of information is possible, because when viewed as a whole, it is comprised of what might be called, for lack of a better term, individual informational categories or data patterns.

These data patterns are not readily apparent by reading only a few transcripts but only by reading all transcripts on a particular subject, and recording all findings including the timing, duration and frequency factors. It is critical in this process to include every transcript, which sometimes requires analysis of hundreds of cases on a single subject. The advice given to this researcher by Gladys Davis Turner so many years ago retains its timeless relevance: *"If you are looking for answers from the Cayce material, don't just read one reading, read them ALL."*

It is an undeniable, albeit unfortunate truth, that a great number of cases were at death's door by the time information from this unorthodox source was sought and all too often no follow up information exists. One of the most poignant is that of a 32 year old medical doctor, a cancer specialist himself, diagnosed with leukemia and barely conscious at the time the information was given. Cayce advised one cubic centimeter Tincture of Iodine be combined with the patients' own blood and at the time of the next transfusion this was to be *"given back into the body."* The information clearly states the patients' <u>own blood</u>

[whole blood] is to be used and goes on to emphasize the critical need for extensive research, testing and the careful monitoring of each individual patients' response. Cayce goes on to state unequivocally that a positive result could be expected within weeks and remarkably that help and relief would be obtained *in fifty percent of all cases.* [2208-1 May 12 of 1940] Tragically the doctor was not able to undertake or direct his own treatment and he died five days later on May 17th.

There are far too many cases such as this, where potential help and hope for many different kinds of disease has lain unrecognized and unused by science for over sixty years. And yet, those few who sought help early enough such as a young music teacher from Hopkinsville, Kentucky diagnosed with scleroderma [transcript series 528] had successful recoveries. Her experience has saved many others from this dread disease, and fortunately, records such as hers yield valuable information about what to expect during the often long healing process.

Most illustrative of what is needed to bring to light the help and hope yet locked within the Cayce material is the example found in the landmark work of Dr. John O.A. Pagano. His experience with just one disease culminated in the publication of his book Healing Psoriasis: The Natural Alternative [21] wherein he details thirty years of success in working with patients suffering from psoriasis. Fortunately for the millions of psoriasis and eczema sufferers around the world, Dr. Pagano outlines both cause and treatment, detailing each step in the treatment and recovery process. All this information is made freely available in his book.

It is encouraging to learn that discoveries are being made which provide some scientific basis for some of the simple Cayce home remedies. A study at Miami University, Oxford, Ohio has yielded evidence for the efficacy of the white Irish potato eye poultice, recommended by Cayce as a home remedy to dissolve or prevent cataracts and to treat eye infections. Science has determined that bacteria have evolved proteins that bind to specific types of sugars present in epithelial cells in the body. This binding effect, sometimes described as "sticking" initiates a localized infection allowing the infection to spread to other tissues. Scientists found that the Irish potato contains agents which effectively inhibit this binding effect. Associate Professor Marjorie Cowan published the results of this study in 2000 in an abstract entitled *Inhibition of Bacterial Adhesion by a Potato Extract and Implications for Plant Antimicrobial Screening.* [22] The results of the Cowan study may inspire a few other researchers to take a closer look at what else the Cayce information has to offer.

Culled from the 9, 306 surviving copies of physical records are nearly 5,000 prescriptions for various eliminants, laxatives, and tonics. Only rarely is the mechanism of an individual plant described. In many cases taking tonics or formulas is precisely timed with osteopathic or chiropractic spinal adjustments and treatments, specific exercises and dietary changes. Most of these herbal formulas can be made at home.

21   John Wiley & Sons, Inc. http://eu.wiley.com/WileyCDA/
22   Abstract at the 2000 American Society for Microbiology Meeting. Gassert, M., .R. Terlecki and M.M.Cowan.
Inhbition of Bacterial Adhesion by a Potato Extract and Implications for Plant Antimicrobial Screening

SMART FORMULAS

Modern medicine does not acknowledge that there may be a distinct response by one or more physiological systems when acted upon by different kinds of eliminants or tonics, or even that there might be a need for such. Yet hundreds of Cayce formulas are described as "assisting in the elimination process" of *individual internal organs*. Further, specific compounds are said to *"reestablish harmony"* between individual organs, or to increase or decrease *"activity"* in their individual functioning. Dr. C. Norman Shealy, founder of Holos Institutes of Health, Inc. in Springfield, Missouri suggests that the concept of addressing the functioning of individual organs and their interaction is not a part of modern medicine. Dr. Shealy states: *"It is both a metaphysical concept and one that has been prominent in homeopathy and more natural medical fields."*

These Cayce "smart formulas," and their as yet scientifically unrecognized targets, remain an informational category finding or data pattern within the Cayce material that is as yet un-addressed by researchers.

The importance of eliminations and of being more aware of the potential effect of internal pollutants is graphically illustrated in the following excerpt, which indicates the mis-direction of bodily drosses or waste products manifests as various diseases. This is a concept held long ago by the Egyptians.

943-1 M
2. [Q] What is cause and cure for the psoriasis conditions on my body and scalp?
[A] This, as we find, has been given - as to what would cure and relieve the condition. With the present physical condition, of course, it is a great deal better that these manifest themselves in such a manner, than that they be kept in! As is known, psoriasis is - itself - an infectious condition that affects the emunctory and lymph circulation, and causes an improper coordination of the eliminating forces of the system, as in this body. Would this not be thrown off in the epidermis, or the lymph and capillary circulation, with this particular condition of this body, the intestinal tract would be full of pinholes; or, were it to go to the lungs, there would be tuberculosis; were it to go to the valves of the heart, it would be heart trouble - as would be called; were it to go to the liver, it would be cirrhosis of the liver; were it to go to the spleen, it would be a hardening of one end of it; were it to go to the brain, it would be softening of the brain; were it to go to the glands of the throat or thyroids, it would be that of goitre; or were it to settle in some other portion - were it to SETTLE - it would become a tumor of some character or nature.

Companion Plants

Just as the Cayce information is unique in its philosophical approach to diagnosis and treatment the way in which plants are used and formulas compounded is correspondingly unique. The Cayce method frequently calls for compound formulas calling for from three to as many as twelve or more "companion" ingredients. Indian turnip for example, is never prescribed by itself but is usually seen with wild ginseng. Dogwood bark is most often paired with prickly ash, sarsaparilla or yellow dock. Podophyllum, leptandrin [leptandra] and sanguinaria are almost always prescribed together. Why certain plants are always paired or combined is not explained and, unfortunately no one ever asked. This leaves yet another question to be answered by science. In a very few cases, an explanation of the mechanism of individual plants is given, but in the Cayce system it is not so much a question of what an individual plant does or is used for, but *what they become and do when combined.*

"In The Order Named"
And lastly, there is the unusual, possibly unique to Cayce directive, given in over 400 transcripts for the compounding of multiple ingredient formulas: *"In the order named!"*

In the compounding of some formulas certain common and well-known "carriers" are used - such as strained honey, simple syrup, wild black cherry, sage, distilled water, or grain alcohol. In the Cayce model these seem to act as a platform or foundation upon which all other ingredients are ever so carefully placed like living chemical building blocks, *each in their precisely ordered sequence.* This sequence or order, if recommended in the transcript, must be strictly followed for the formula to work. In a few cases researchers will find that a follow-up transcript states that the original instructions were NOT followed, reiterating that the formula should be made again, but this time to make it, *"in the order named."* Perhaps the chemical changes that occur as a result of the admonition *"in the order named"* are yet another unrecognized process worthy of scientific inquiry.

Don't Change It!
Finally, for those who may be interested in the commercial production of some of these tonics, eliminants, formulas and supplements, it is critical to note that preservatives are not to be used *unless called for in the original formula.* A transcript will often stipulate that a formula should be made fresh each time it is to be used, made only in enamel or glass, never aluminum, and stored in a certain way. The formula is to be used within a certain length of time followed by the injunction that the addition of preservatives will have a negative effect. It is well to remember the words of Dr. Harold J. Reilly,[23] physician, physiotherapist and friend of Edgar Cayce, who gave this author the following advice in regard to working with any kind of information in the Cayce readings: *"Until we know how this works, don't change it!"*

Some of the plants and methods in this study have fallen out of medical fashion but their efficacy will always be as timeless as Mother Nature herself. Some plants are considered by landowners and farmers as simply troublesome weeds. Many are pulled or sprayed with chemicals to rid lawns and fields of their undesirable presence. Some will thrive anywhere while others have stringent climate requirements. A few are illegal to grow in some countries and others are only found in remote or exotic places and cannot be grown by the home gardener. Many can only be gathered in the wild and a few, when handled or used incorrectly, are poisonous. A useful few, however, can be encouraged to grow along fence lines or simply allowed to live quietly behind the garage, ready for use should the need arise.

---

23   The Edgar Cayce Handbook For Health Through Drugless Therapy Harold J. Reilly, D.Ph.T.,D.S. and Ruth Hagy Brod. Macmillan Publishing Co., Inc. New York. 1975

A Final Word of Caution

Even though the use of natural or herbal remedies is as old as mankind and has become remarkably fashionable at present, it is well to remember that the words "herbal" or "natural" are not automatically passports to the harmless. Mixing different herbs or using one or more for too long a period of time can be very harmful, and the plants in this study are no exception. Natural or herbal products should be used judiciously, and the advice and counsel of qualified health care professionals should always be sought and heeded. While the question in transcript 1179-4 was not about an herbal formula the answer is certainly still true in all things:

"For there's no such thing that if an application can't help, it can't hurt! Because if it is helpful, mis-applied it must be harmful! – this is natural."

And finally, for those who would too readily self-diagnose and self-treat, notice should be taken of the advice given in the very last sentence of transcript 1173-8 for a 28 year old young man suffering from arthritis and dealing with the after effects of pleurisy. After receiving complete and detailed instructions for the treatments he *should* follow for his recovery, he asked if he should take "Pineapple Culture Bulgarious Bacillus." The response was that it would be all right to take it occasionally adding:

"But do not overdo it, see? as has been indicated, by continuing to be dosing with this or that and the other, without the understanding."

Let us then proceed thoughtfully, not by dosing with this or that, or to misapply or overdo, but to first gain understanding.

Jeanette M. Thomas

CAYCE PLANTS

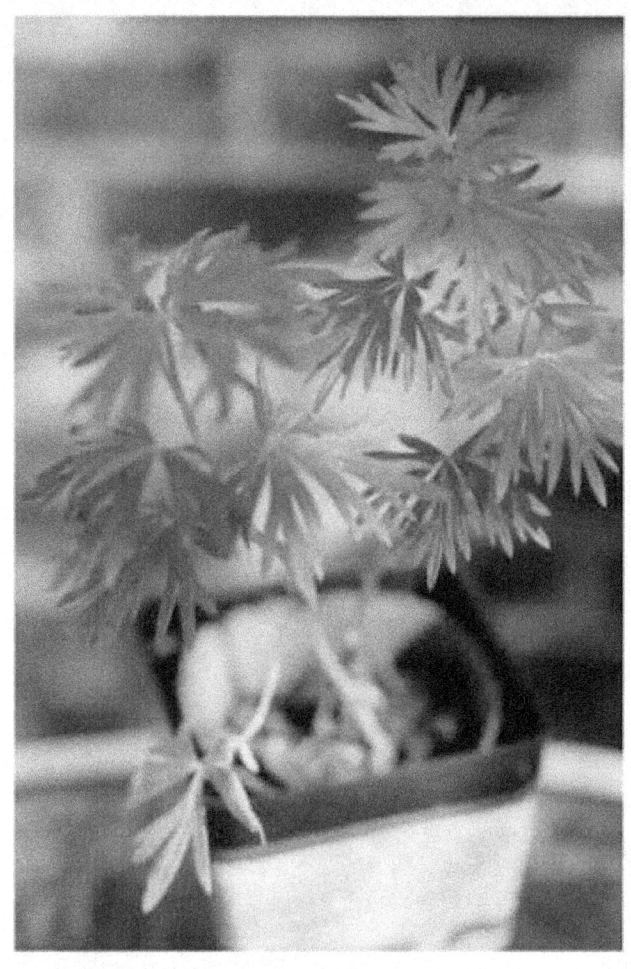
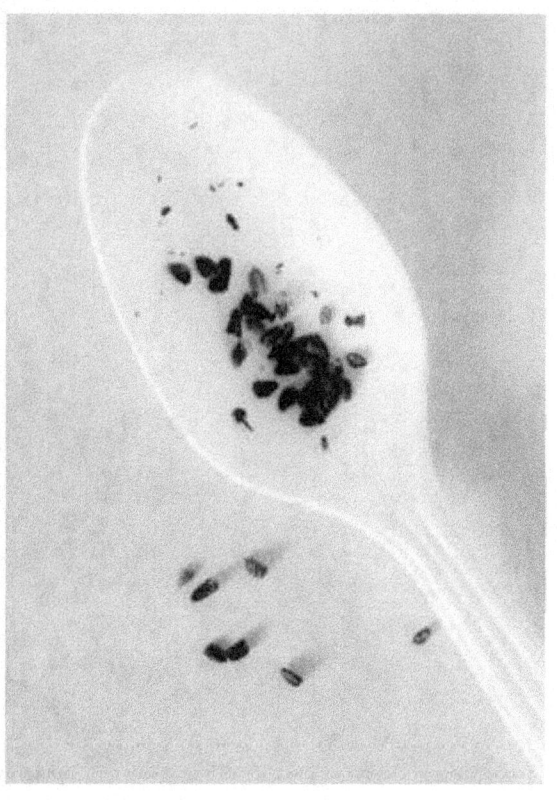
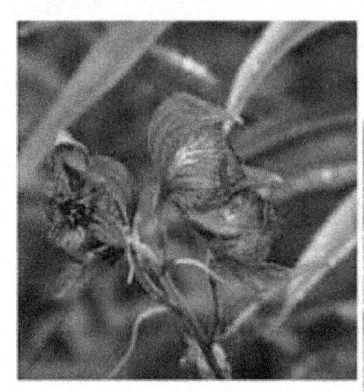
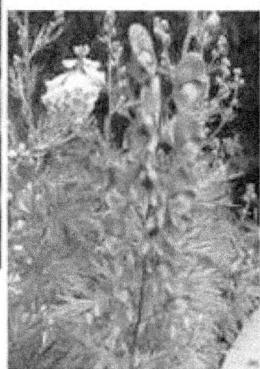
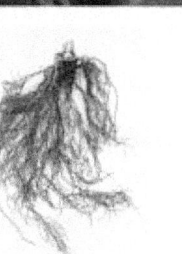
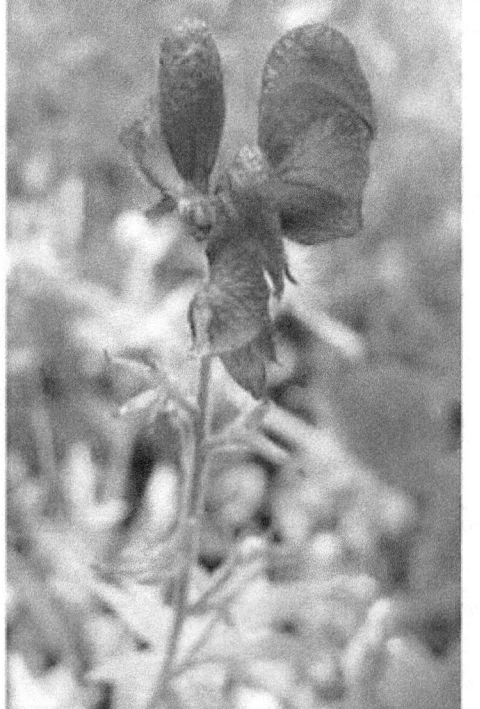

Aconite
Aconitum Napellus, Fam. Ranunculaceae

Common and Regional Names
Monkshood, Blue Rocket, Friar's Cap, Auld Wife's Huid, Wolfsbane

History and Common Usage
These beautiful blue, white or yellow relatives of the buttercup are found in the lower mountain slopes of the northern portion of the eastern hemisphere, from the Himalayas through Europe, to Great Britain and to the United States. More than 100 species belong to this family of plants.

Aconite has long held a place in folk medicine for use as a pain reliever and among some cultures it was considered an anti-inflammatory, but it is far more famous as a poison. Poisoning is an ancient art with records of poisons and poisoners found among the early Sumerians, Egyptians and Greeks. Pliny the Elder speaks of aconite in rather drastic terms:

"But who, I say, can sufficiently venerate the zeal and spirit of research displayed by the ancients? It is they who have shown us that aconite is the most prompt of all poisons in its effects..."[24]

Aconite is dangerous if ingested but the greatest danger is when there is an unknown or unsuspected sensitivity or allergy to handling the plant. It is important to recognize the symptoms of aconite poisoning because immediate medical help can be critical for survival. Because chest and epigastric pain are common symptoms of aconite poisoning it is often mistaken for a heart attack and goes untreated. It is critical to inform health care personnel of any potential exposure so that appropriate measures can be taken. Symptoms can begin with minor sensations of tingling and especially if any part of the plant has been swallowed this can escalate quite rapidly to numbness of the tongue followed by a sensation of warmth of the tongue and mouth sometimes accompanied by a sensation of ants crawling over the body. Labored breathing with chest pains and an irregular weak pulse occurs very quickly. A slow pulse, cold and clammy sensations, a feeling of "bloodlessness," giddiness and an inability to walk without staggering can also be present. The patient remains clear minded until the end.

Dr. Alfred Swaine Taylor [1806-1880] was Professor of Medical Jurisprudence at Guy's Hospital Medical School in London and is considered one of the early specialists in forensics and toxicology. He is rather famous for his statement: *"A poison in a small dose is a medicine, and a medicine in a large dose is a poison."* Properly used by knowledgeable health care professionals, aconite is a useful medicinal plant.

Both the American and British pharmacopeias of the Cayce era list aconite as an official drug plant. Never used on broken skin a combination of aconite and opium [or a tincture of aconite combined with a tincture of opium called laudanum] was prescribed to relieve the pain of neuralgia; lumbago and rheumatism. Painful areas of the body were painted with a tincture or liniment [sometimes an ointment was used] resulting in a numbing sensation. Aconite was sometimes combined with belladonna as a liniment. Tincture of aconite was also administered to slow the heart rate in the early stages of dangerous fevers and to diminish the pain of neuralgia, pleurisy and aneurysm. Physicians of the Cayce era also used aconite to treat or prevent cardiac failure.

Description

Aconite is a hardy, perennial plant that attains a height of 4 to 5 feet under favorable growing conditions. Cultivated in perennial shade gardens *Aconitum napellus* has blue to purple flowers consisting of five parts. The upper most petal turns downward shaped somewhat like a downward-opening hood giving rise to its common name, monkshood. The flowers have between two to five pistils. The follicles split open at the ends to release the seeds.

Growing Conditions and Propagation

Preferring moist soils and woodland areas aconite is frequently found growing with its poisonous cousin the larkspur. Some recorded cases of aconite poisoning have come from misidentification with the larkspur.

Aconite can be grown from seed, young plants can be purchased at a local nursery or through mail order catalogues, or from roots or root divisions from a neighbor's garden. It thrives in any ordinary garden soil and does best in moist shaded areas. Once established it self-propagates through "daughter roots" which develop from the crown of the parent root. Care should be taken to prevent young children and animals from chewing on any part of the plant. Even touching the leaves to the lips can produce numbness and tingling and in the case of toddlers could have quite serious consequences. If there are any cuts or open places on the hands gardeners should consider wearing gloves when working with aconite. In spite of the potential dangers of the plant it has been safely grown for hundreds of years and its beauty far outweighs any extra precautions required to have the lovely flowers in the garden.

Harvesting

For extract of aconite the leaves and flowers are gathered just as the flowers begin to bloom. In temperate zones this is usually in June.

The root should be harvested from two year old plants at the end of the growing season when the plant has died down, but before the buds have formed from which next years new growth develops. The strength of the alkaloid in the root varies from plant to plant, from season to season, and is considerably lessened if the "daughter roots" have been allowed to form. Roots that are roughly ¾ inches in diameter should be saved for drying.

The roots should be washed under cold running water and cleaned of all rootlets. They can be dried whole or sliced to speed the process. Spread them out on trays large enough so they are not touching one another in a warm shaded area for about ten days, turning them occasionally to speed evaporation. A gentle heat source can be used to speed the drying process. Drying is complete when the roots are brittle. They should snap when bent. The core of the root should be whitish in color and starchy, if not they should be discarded as they are not safe to use.

Use in the Edgar Cayce Readings

Aconite, as a companion plant, is mentioned over 80 times as a topical application for the relief of pain, but is never recommended internally. It is most often seen combined with laudanum, a tincture of opium, which as stated above is no longer available. There are 4 cases where iodine was combined with aconite. The mixture is painted on the skin of the painful area with a camel's hair brush to numb the nerves bringing relief from pain and in a few instances is said to bring about beneficial changes in circulation.

The following are typical examples of how aconite is used in the Cayce system:

4666-4 M 35 Nasal Catarrh
4. Make also a weak solution, or add half a teaspoonful Tincture of Iodine, half a teaspoonful aconite, half a teaspoonful Tincture laudanum, to two TABLESPOONSFUL of 85% [eighty-five percent] alcohol, and paint the antrums and back of the ear and along the left shoulder where the reaction comes from the stress on the muscular tissue in the system attempting to adjust the conditions through eliminations

2504-17 M 64 Ataxia
…However, there are conditions - as is seen, as is produced from the tendency for hindered circulation - that is, unless altered or changed, will not be for the better physical forces. These, as we find, have to do with that of the SYMPATHETIC, or of the circulation through the lymph TO the brain proper, and the effect as may be created - especially in the locomotary centers, in those of the lower extremities, in that of the brachial center. These are not at all times satisfactory.

2. We would, when there are the tendencies for the reaction, bathe those points - or centers - with an equal portion of tincture iodine and aconite, applying over same an oiled cloth in sweet oil; then applying mechanical or pad heat. This will produce a tendency for an equalization in these particular centers.

5736-1 M 37 Epilepsy
8. When specific conditions arise, as those in the lumbar or small of back, or those in the extremities of the body - from the base, or that portion of the system that is affected, not the limb itself but from the radial centers - we would apply first a solution that would be of aconite, with a very WEAK solution of iodine, and laudanum. Then apply Epsom salts packs, a solution made as heavy as may be carried. This we will find will bring relief very sure, and in a short period. Do not use these until these become necessary.

341-29 M 21 TEETH
…There is an indication in the mental forces of the overtaxed MENTAL body, and this is produced much by the STRAIN as is experienced through the PHYSICAL forces - especially in the nerves, as is SEEN with teeth. Many conditions have existed here that are retractions, yet there is seen - especially in the upper right molar - ONE that will need OPENING and TREATING the nerve exposed. Use in same iodine and aconite, equal parts, and we will correct the condition. This will be necessary for the relief of that portion of the system.

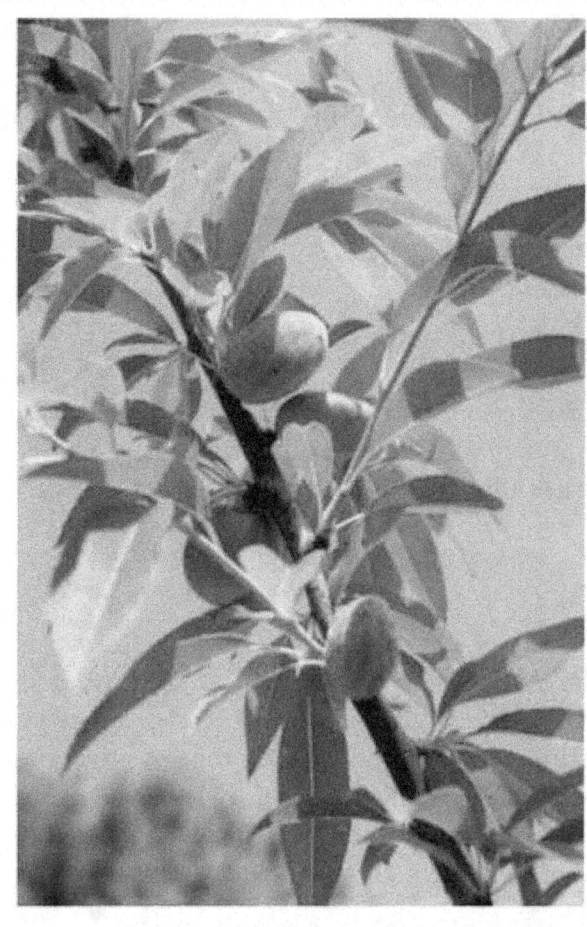

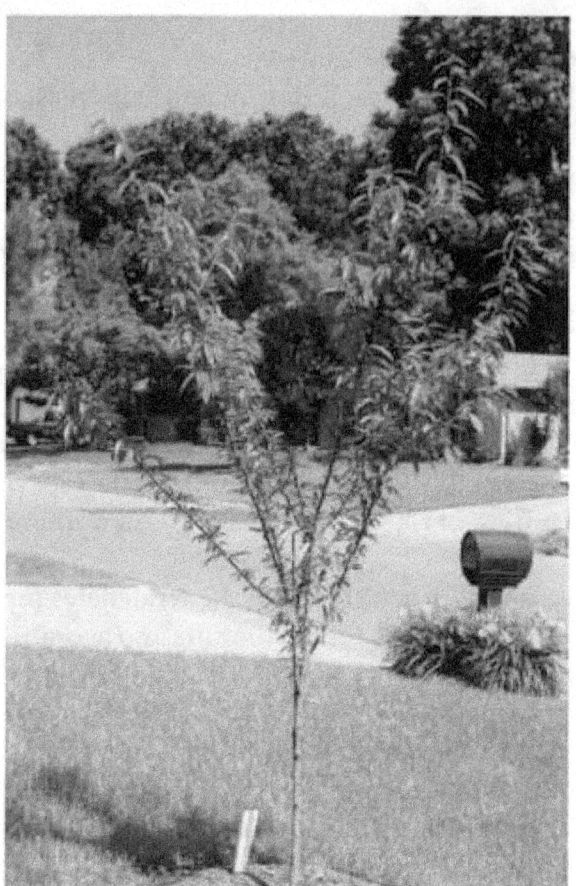

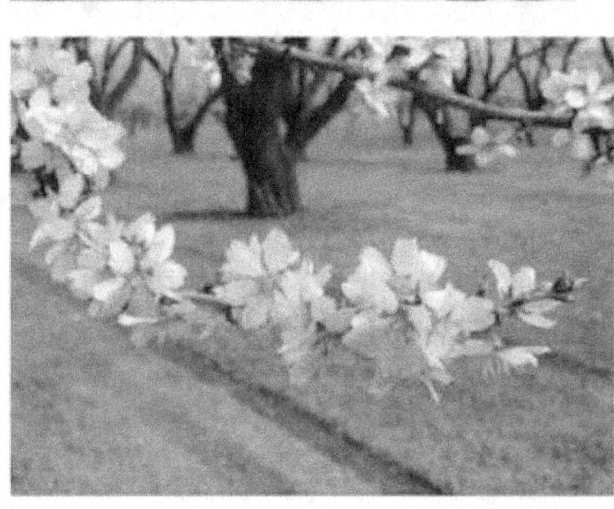

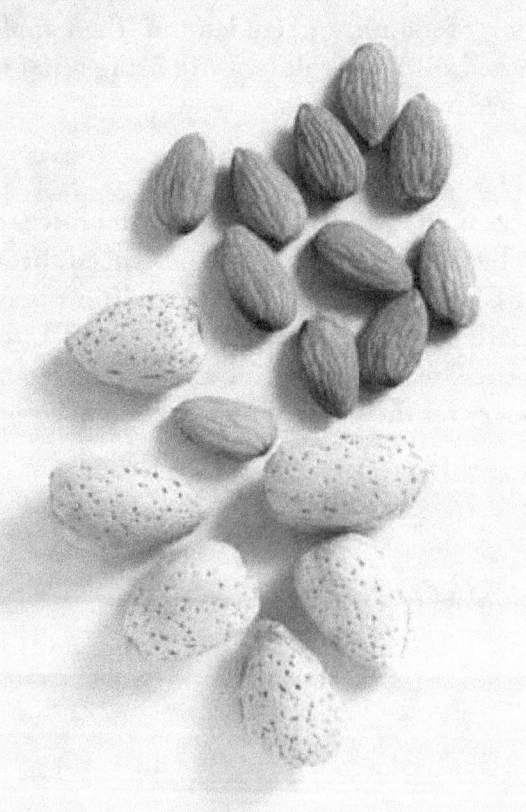

ALMONDS
Prunus dulcis, also *Prunus communis* and *Prunus amygdalus, Fam. Rosaceae*

Common and Regional Names
Jordan Almonds, Sweet Almonds, Greek nuts

History and Common Usage
The almond is believed to have originated in the hot, dry climate of the present day Middle East, along the shores of the Mediterranean and in what is today known as northern Africa, China and Central Asia.

In an area of Israel referred to as the Dead Sea rift recent evidence has been found of the wild almond[25] being eaten by early humans during the Early and Middle Pleistocene.[26] At the Acheulian site of Gesher Benot Ya'aqov pitted stones used to crack hard shell nuts have been found together with remains of both wood and nuts.

Evidence of the cultivation of almonds has been found dating to the time of the ancient Assyrians and Persians and the nut is mentioned in the King James version of the Judeo-Christian Bible[27] in Genesis 43.11.[28] *And their father Israel said unto them, If it must be so now, do this; take of the best fruits in the land in your vessels, and carry down the man a present, a little balm, and a little honey, spices, and myrrh, nuts, and almonds.* In 1351 B.C. they were placed in the tomb of the young Egyptian King Tutankhamun. The Book of Medicines makes extensive use of almonds in prescriptions for numerous conditions including lung complaints, liver disorders and nose bleeds. The Syrians distinguish, as does Pliny the Elder, between the bitter and the sweet. Pliny also refers to almonds as Greek Nuts. They have been used as food, their oil for lighting, cooking, perfumes and cosmetics for millennia. Almond milk was an early discovery and the nuts, ground into flour have long been used in making cakes and bread. The oil has been used medicinally to treat a variety of skin conditions and is an efficacious ingredient in many brands of toilet soap manufactured today.

The almond received the scientific name *Amygdalus communis* from Carolus Linnaeus in 1753. In 1801 August Johann Georg Carl Batsch[29] changed the name to *Prunus amygdalus.* Yet again in 1964 at the International Botanical Congress in Scotland it was renamed *Prunus dulcis* and its other names, such as *Prunus amygdalus* and *Prunus communis* were officially designated as synonyms.

Almonds were introduced into the United States in the 1800's in the area known today as Santa Barbara, California. A Catholic priest of the order of St. Francis, by the name of Father Junipero Serra,[30] is credited with introducing them from Spain when he came to the United States in 1769 to found the missions through which later evolved the state of California. Whole nuts were brought for use as food and seeds and at first were only grown on small plots for the early missions and individual families. It was not until the mid 1900's that commercial plantings were begun. Growers experimented in different parts of the country but once established in the favorable climate of the Sacramento and San Joaquin valleys the almond successfully took its place as a significant cash crop. California remains to this day

---

25 *A. communis* ssp. *microphylla*
26 Proceedings of the National Academy of Sciences of the United States of America. February 19, 2002.
27 Electronic Text Center, University of Virginia Library. King James Edition 1611
28 Generally thought to be dated to 1450-1410 BC
29 1761-1802 Director Botanical Garden Jena, Germany
30 Born Miguel Jose on the island of Majorca, Spain 11-24-1713. He died at the Mission of Carmel 8-28-1784.

the largest US grower representing 75% of the worlds market. Over 25 varieties are grown in California alone. The major cultivars are Texas [syn. Mission] Ne Plus Ultra, IXL, Peerless, Jordanolo, Eurkea and Drake. Nonpareil is the most popular variety representing 60% of the crop.

The best quality and the "right kind" of almonds are often identified by the name Jordan. The name Jordan Almonds has come to mean the very large nonpareil variety that can often be found in hard-shelled sugar coating in an array of pastel colors. Jordan Almonds are even available in silver and gold for special occasions.

There are two kinds of almonds. The sweet, which is the well-known edible almond of the world's market and the bitter, *Prunus Amygdalus, var. amara*, also called *Amygdalus Amara*. The bitter almond is native to Western Asia and North Africa and is widely cultivated in Spain, Turkey, Morocco, Tunisia and Egypt. The raw bitter almond is as poisonous as the kernel of its cousin the peach unless it has been treated by heating. Bitter almonds contain high amounts of cyanide in their seeds, bark and leaves, a poison that causes convulsions and death. The main chemical components of bitter almond oil are benzaldehyde and hydrocyanic acid from which prussic acid is extracted.

Because of their toxicity raw bitter almonds may not be marketed for unrestricted use in the United States. Imports cannot contain more than 5 percent of bitter almonds. Almond paste, and pastes made from other types of nuts, must contain less than 25 parts per million of hydrocyanic acid [HCN].[31]

In the United States at the time the Cayce information was being given purified bitter almond oil [treated by heating] was used as a medicinal delivery agent and was legal only for medicinal purposes. Yet purified bitter almond oil has long been used as a flavouring agent in various confections, especially in making marzipan. A synthetic flavouring is now in widespread use by the scientific name of benzaldehyde and is sold as an artificial essential "oil of almond." This is a derivative of the bitter almond and can be safely added to foods, massage oils, perfumes and soaps.

An interesting historical note is the use of bitter almond oil in the manufacture of Macassar Oil, which is a hair oil for men widely used in the 19th Century. It was originally made in Macassar, today called Sulawesi, a district of the Island of Celebes, a very odd shaped island located in the center of Indonesia in the Indian Ocean.

Macassar Oil was made with bitter almond oil, although sometimes the cheaper safflower oil was substituted, it was colored red with alkanet root, a plant commonly called dyer's root or Spanish bugloss and then scented with oil of cassia. The practice of protecting the backs of chairs or sofas with "antimacassars" came from the use of this hair oil. The antimacassar protected upholstered furniture from the staining propensities of this colorful and aromatic hair dressing, which kept the unruly locks of well-groomed Victorian gentlemen neatly in place.

The almond, because of the way it is recommended in the Cayce model, skirts along the edge of a bitter modern medical controversy. Almonds are a source of amygdalin, commonly known as Vitamin B[17]. Vitamin B[17] is also known as the controversial substance Laetrile,[32] which was banned by the American

---

31   Requirements of Laws and Regulations Enforced by the U.S. Food and Drug Administration [1977]

32   National Cancer Institute. Laetrile/Amygdalin [PDQ®.] 6/22/2004

Food and Drug Administration during a period of heated debate and legal dispute over its use in the treatment of cancer during the 1960's.

Amygdalin is most abundant in the poisonous seeds of the *Prunus rosacea* family which includes the bitter almond, apricots, blackthorn, cherries, nectarines, peaches and plums. It is present to a lesser degree in the sweet almond. It is also contained in grasses, lima beans, maize, sorghum, millet, cassava, linseed, apple seeds and many other foods that in general have been deleted from the menus of modern civilization. Amygdalin is found in any natural food containing *nitriloside* which has been used and studied extensively for well over 100 years. Nitriloside was first isolated in France in 1830 and was used as an anticancer agent in Russia in 1845. The use of Amygdalin in the treatment of human cancer dates back at least to the year 1843, although the ancient Chinese are reported to have used bitter almonds in the treatment of tumors some 3,000 years ago.

Natural B[17] is most abundant[33] in the kernel of the apricot, which is as poisonous as the bitter almond in almost any quantity. The exact action of Amygdalin in its effect on cancer cells is still only theoretical, and treatment of cancer with Vitamin B[17] is not within the scope of acceptable medical practice in the United States. Laetrile is now synthetically produced in the laboratory and those wishing to avail themselves of the drug cannot do so in the United States, nor can it be purchased through the mail. As recently as 2000 the FDA has taken legal action against those selling Laetrile across state lines.

At the time of this writing there are pending changes in USDA rulings in the United States which may, unfortunately, make the availability of raw almonds in the United States a thing of the past.[34] March 1 of 2008 was the deadline for changes requiring the pasteurization [heating] or chemical treatment of almonds before sale. This is due to the alleged dangers of salmonella, [there were 2 outbreaks, one in 2001 and one in 2004]. Those who wish to have natural, raw almonds available for health purposes should, climate permitting, plan on growing their own.

Description
The almond is a small tree attaining 25 to 30 feet in height at full maturity. The trees live and produce for nearly 50 years. The bitter almonds have white flowers and the sweet have pink, somewhat resembling the blossoms of its close cousin the peach. The bark of the almond tree is smooth and gray and its 3 to 4 inch leaves are medium to dark green, shiny and oval shaped. The almond makes a lovely landscape choice and can be grown for shade as well as nuts. In a favorable climate it will naturalize.

Growing Conditions and Propagation
Propagation of the almond today is mostly by budding and grafting. Often the sweet almond is grafted to the stock of the peach, and the trees are kept compact by pruning in order to make mechanical harvesting of the nuts easier. If whole raw or unprocessed nuts still in their hulls can be obtained, they can be planted in any ordinary garden soil at a depth of roughly 2 to 3 inches. Planting in the fall is best in most areas and germination will take place the following spring. Twice as many raw almonds should be planted to allow for uncertain germination response. Only the most vigorous seedlings should be allowed to grow. Young trees, certified disease free and suitable for the local climate can also be ordered from any reputable nursery and will do best if planted in January in most areas. Pioneer is a Heritage variety that does well in most home gardens.

---

33   Roughly 2% to 3%
34   http://www.almondboard.com/files/Rule.pdf

The almond likes deep, well-drained and loamy soils, in full sun, with a soil pH of 6-7. They require 180 to 240 days to produce a crop so mild winters are necessary and if bees are not available for pollination then two trees should be planted, spaced between 20 and 30 feet apart for cross pollination.

Because it blooms earlier than most fruit trees, the almond is prone to frost. In the British Isles the almond will grow and produce beautiful flowers but fruiting is very rare due to the cold climate and short growing season. They are quite drought resistant and can even survive short periods of standing water. They do not thrive in regions of high humidity where they are more susceptible to diseases. They begin to bear between 3 to 4 years of age and enter their period of maximum production after 6 or 7 years.

Harvesting
When the hulls of the nut begin to split, especially when splitting is noticeable in nuts growing inside the canopy of the tree, they are ready to harvest. A plastic tarp, sheets or blankets are laid on the ground and the branches are knocked with a light padded club or pole, being careful not to bruise the bark. Limbs can also be shaken by hand. The hulls will still be "green" or pliable and the shells containing the almonds are easily removed from the hulls by hand.

Sometimes, because of lack of moisture, poor soil, disease or insect infestations the hulls of some nuts are not easily removed. These are called "sticktights" and are a sign that growing conditions need attention. The nuts are safe to eat but crack and fragment easily.

The choice of the drying process is largely dependent upon local conditions. In dry climates the nuts can be left to dry on the ground and collected by hand or by raking. They can be put on mesh or trays and left in the sun and taken in at night. Where rain and humid conditions are present, small amounts can be satisfactorily dried in a very low oven. Once the nut breaks cleanly it is ready for storage, and if kept dry and cool can be stored for very long periods. Almonds keep best if they are stored in their shells in mesh bags and kept in a cool, dry place away from heat and light.

Nuts can also be canned in glass jars and stored away from the light in a cool place but once canned they are pasteurized and are no longer raw. Raw almond meal can be stored in an airtight container for a year; raw whole almonds for 2 years, and in the shell they will keep for 36 months. Raw shelled nuts can be stored in freezer bags from which as much air as possible has been exhausted and in the freezer will keep for years. Which ever method is chosen for storage, it is important to keep the nuts in airtight containers because they easily absorb odors.

The following guidelines from the Almond Growers Association of America are for raw nuts sealed in plastic bags and packaged in cardboard cartons:

Raw Natural Almonds
Stored in the shell	36 Months
Whole almonds	24 Months
Sliced	36 Months
Almond meal	12 Months

Use in the Edgar Cayce Readings
The almond is not a companion plant. As with the Ayurvedic and traditional Chinese medical systems, the Cayce model emphasizes diet as a critical treatment modality, often prescribing specific foods for

certain conditions or combinations of foods to be taken or avoided. Raw almonds are mentioned as a dietary item often to be eaten in combination with raw filberts as a source of easily assimilated calcium, and in a few cases certain individuals are said to benefit from this to a greater degree than by drinking milk. The almond is also described as combining phosphorus and iron in a more easily assimilated form than any other nut. It is also said to be an alkalizing food and better for the body than black walnuts or English walnuts which, in one case [543-9] are said to contain too much of the "fusel oils.[35]"

The 658 series is very interesting because information was sought by an enterprising 60 year old woman who wanted to develop her own line of cosmetic products including a skin care product based on almond cream. In the 1930's she asked a number of questions related to the development of skin care and hair care products. Cayce has this to say in 658-2 about her almond cream: *"…we will find how that it cleanses the pores, how that it makes for the removing of lines, how it makes for the addition of pliability, and get away from that roughness and also from that leathery expression or feeling that comes to so many as the years come."* Sadly there are no further records on her formula.

Perhaps of greater interest are the intriguing statements pointing to research potential on almonds and the subject of cancer. It should be emphasized that treatments for cancer in the Cayce system involve a number of modalities, including exposing the body to mercury quartz ultra-violet light combined with a product invented by Cayce called carbon ash,[36] a range of hydrotherapies, massage and spinal treatments. Also included are psychological and attitudinal suggestions, such as prayer, meditation and the use of affirmations, electrotherapies, occasionally surgery and radiation, and very critical dietary changes for the duration of the treatment period, including the addition of a few raw sweet almonds to the diet.

Another reference Cayce makes regarding almonds and cancer appears in case 659-1. He suggests that a form of vitamin in certain nuts, such as the almond is a helpful preventative of cancer. The word preventative suggests the efficacy of the vitamin in almonds may be primarily effective before the onset of the condition.

In a 1941 transcript [1206-13] Cayce tells a sixteen year old young lady that if she would eat two almonds a day, she would never have skin blemishes and would never "be tempted" towards cancer. Similar information appears in 1158-31 stating that those who would eat 2 or 3 almonds each day need never fear cancer. Then a 1943 transcript [3180-3] for a 20 year old woman urges her to avoid chocolate and coconut, but that nuts, especially an almond should be taken each day regularly, and she will be able to prevent accumulation of tumors or such conditions through the body. One other case [3515-1] given for a 56 year old woman who had breast cancer suggested surgery and then during the healing process that she eat an almond a day so that there would be no recurrence of this nature in her system.

In other transcripts Cayce volunteers the information that there are nineteen different kinds of cancer and speaks of the development of a serum he called niccolite.[37]

---

35   An oily, colorless liquid with a disagreeable odor and taste. It is a mixture of alcohols [largely amyl alcohols] and fatty acids, formed during the alcoholic fermentation of organic materials. After imperfect distillation of these fermentation products it becomes an impurity in the distilled liquor. Fusel oil is used as a solvent in the manufacture of certain lacquers and enamels [it dissolves nitrocellulose]. It has a detrimental effect on the human system.

36   The Heritage Store, P.O. Box 444 WWW, 314 Laskin Road, Virginia Beach, Virginia 23451. 757-428-0100, 1-800-862-2923. http://www.heritagestore.com

37   See 4444-1 through 2, 2514-4 re niccolite, 281-15 re niccolite, 4977-1 nineteen different kinds of cancer and blood injection, 1242 series about different kinds of cancer, 254-114 dealing with the spiritual rather than the mechanical and 659-1 on biotin research by Vincent du Vigneaud of Cornell and volunteered statements about almonds and cancer.

Statements volunteered by Cayce on the types of cancer and the almond raise questions such as [1] does the disease we know as cancer actually express itself in the forms as Cayce describes? [2] In what kinds of cancer are almonds effective, and [3] at what stage in the disease process could they be effective, that is, do they need to be taken BEFORE the development of the disease in the manner of a preventive.

This author has known of far too many individuals who, upon being diagnosed with cancer, immediately began to eat raw almonds and yet succumbed to the disease. Perhaps taking almonds AFTER the fact is like having a polio vaccination after paralysis has set in, or perhaps powerful unrecognized emotions can over-ride their effect. Only scientifically conducted clinical studies will provide answers.

The following are typical dietary suggestions including the recommendation that almond milk be a part of the diet:

1419-5 F Adult
7....The rolled oats make for too much acidity. The steel cut oats would be well. Then at another time use a combination of dates, figs and almonds; these would be cut or ground together; these may be warm or these may be cold; and they may be taken with a little milk - this combination would not be given so often, but it will be found to be most beneficial as an aid to better eliminations.

2028-1 F 5
13. Fruits and nuts may also be taken occasionally, but ONLY the almonds and filberts in the nuts - and more of the juices or the milk from crushing these, given with the foods for the body.

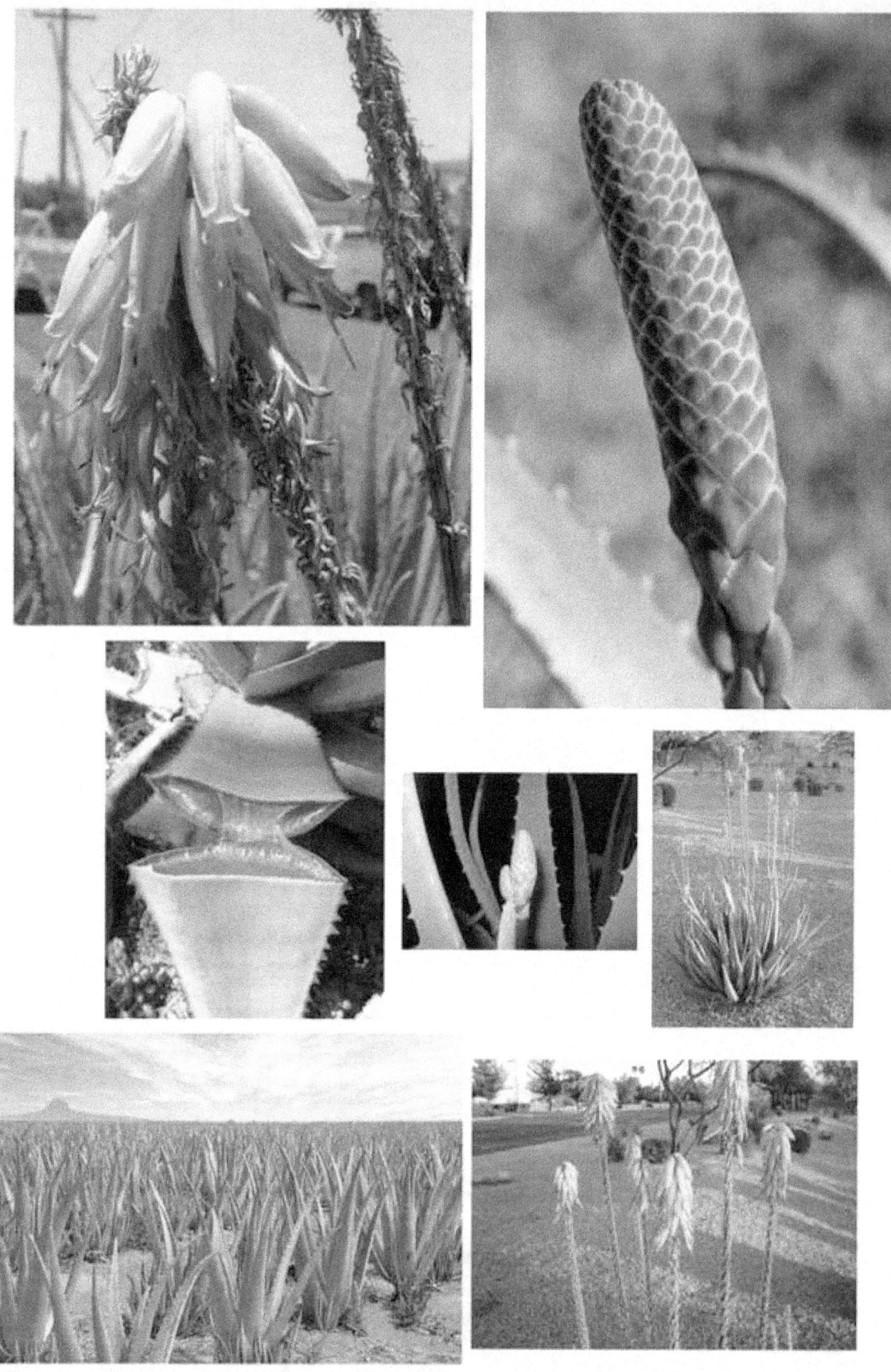

ALOE
Aloe vera, Fam. Liliaceae

Common and Regional Names

True Aloe, Curacao, Socotrine, Soccotrina or Zanzibar Aloe; Cape Aloe, Barbados Aloe, Medicine Plant, Burn Plant, First-aid Plant, Miracle Plant

History and Common Usage

Aloe can be said to be either blessed or burdened with many names. Among the commercially significant are: *Aloe Perryi* [Baker], commercially called socotrine; *Aloe ferox* [Miller], also called cape aloe [which also happens to be the tallest member of the family with stems 10 to 15 feet long], and *Aloe vera* [Linnè], also called curacao. There is even a poisonous member of the family named *Aloe venenosa*. Other members of the aloe family include *Aloe spicata* [Baker], indigenous to Africa and *Aloe chinensis* [Baker] probably an original native of Africa but introduced from China into the Dutch Colonies of Curacao in 1817. *Aloe africana* is a native of the Cape Colony, Africa and is considered by most scientists as a source of inferior aloes, "aloes" being the official name of the juice extracted from the plant for use in medicine. From this juice the active principles of the plant called aloins[38] are extracted. [The two most active principles are barbaloin and isobarbaloin.] It is important not to confuse *Aloe vera* with *Agave americana* another plant very similar in appearance and commonly called the American aloe. *Agave americana* belongs to a completely different family called *Amaryllidaceae*.

The historical trail is further obscured by there being too many names for the "true aloe" and the word aloe being used in the names of other plants and trees. Further confusion is caused by a number of faulty translations. The aloe, among many other helpful plants, certainly accompanied early man on his travels and has now been widely disseminated throughout the globe, its tradition having entered into every culture. In addition it has gained a foothold in every suitably warm climate, naturalizing and undergoing adaptive changes resulting in new names causing even more confusion in identification.

Historical sources past and present point to the area of the Indian Ocean; more specifically the Island of Socotra[39] in what is today the Republic of Yemen as the country of origin. [Socotra is also believed by most botanical historians to be also the place of origin of Frankincense trees.] Other scholars cite Arabia or North Africa as the region of origin. Both archaeological and extant written records provide ample evidence that the earliest use of the plant was in Egypt and its image decorates the walls of homes and temples to this day. It was also used by the Sumerians, Hindus, Mayans and the Chinese. The Persians record its use, as do the Greeks as cited by Dioscorides. It is grown today in Greece, Italy, India and the African continent. The plant is widely known throughout Asia and the Pacific and is found in the folklore of Japan, the Philippines and Hawaii. Aloe is a popular and common decoration throughout a great many cultures around the globe, used on walls, tombs, vases and other types of pottery.

There are some widespread and very popular anecdotal traditions about the *Aloe vera*, one being that it was used to anoint the body of Jesus. *Aloe vera* was not the plant mentioned in the Bible at all. It was actually *Lign-aloes*. *Lign-aloes* is another example of translation corruption between a plant and a tree in the use of the word aloe. *Lign-aloe* is a corruption of the Latin *lignum-aloe*, a wood, not a plant resin. Dioscorides refers to it as agallochon, a wood brought from Arabia or India, which was odoriferous with

---

38   Smith and Stenhouse first identified the active principal called Aloin in 1851

39   Sometimes seen as Soquotra or Sokotra

an astringent and bitter taste. This may also be *Aquilaria agallocha*, a native of East India and China, which supplies the so-called eaglewood or aloeswood, which contains both resin and oil. Most scholars believe that it was the aromatic resin of *Aquilaria agallocha*, also commonly called aloes that was recorded in the Bible as being used to anoint the body of Jesus in preparation for burial.

Another legend of the aloe is that the Macedonian general, Alexander the Great,[40] took possession of the Island of Socotra after his campaign in India in order to control the cultivation, supply and distribution of this valuable healing plant. This remains an unsubstantiated anecdote, albeit a charming one.

There are approximately 325 species of aloe distributed throughout Africa, Arabia and Madagascar, all marvelously adapted over eons to their individual climate. Aloes, the died and purified juice, is found in pill form in early British and American pharmacopoeias, never prescribed alone but always combined with other herbs such as cascara sagrada, or myrrh or with asafoetida, and even soap and water in the treatment of constipation. Aloes has been known and used as a laxative or purgative since the most ancient of times and the gel, or sap of the plant has been known for its healing properties throughout recorded human history.

Description
Aloe vera is a fleshy, lance-leaved perennial, which grows directly from the ground, without a stem or stalk. It attains heights of 12 inches to several feet, depending upon the variety grown. Some species grow to be 3 feet tall, others upwards of 60 feet in the wild. *Aloe vera* is found between 3 to 5 feet tall under ideal conditions but readily adapts its size to existing environments. It is characterized by a rosette of large, upright, succulent leaves, sharply pointed at the tips with firm triangular-shaped teeth spaced at regular intervals at the tips of the leaves where the edges are slightly scalloped along the margins. The leaves vary in color from gray to clear light or bright green and are sometimes found striped or mottled in coloration. Often younger leaves will display pale spots and older leaves will be a gray or bright green without any patterning.

When aloe reaches an age of between 3 to 5 years of age the plant begins to bloom. The greenish-red or light green, cone-shaped buds begin to grow from the base, usually from the center of the rosette, on long smooth stems. The buds are characterized by tightly overlapping scales in which the flowers are formed. The flowers are tubular in shape, usually yellow, sometimes pink, orange or red in color [depending upon the degree of hybridization]. They are usually densely clustered at the tops of the stem or stalk and when cultivated in stands make a handsome and colorful display. The flowers usually appear from June through August, depending upon the climate zone. Small angular, tannish seeds are borne within the flowering capsules.

Growing Conditions and Propagation
Fertilized by insects and the wind, *Aloe vera* propagates naturally through casting of seeds, and the enlargement of its rosette base through offshoots, increasing the circumference of the base of the plant year by year. Aloe is easily propagated by cutting a side leaf with a root base, and simply planting the shoot into prepared soil or in a pot to a depth of 1 inch to 1 ½ inches. Some gardeners recommend treating the wound on the mother plant with powdered sulphur with a light dusting on the shoot before planting as a preventive against soft rot. The newly planted division will then grow to form a new rosette by developing additional leaves. This type of propagation can be done at any time during the season from a plant in the garden or from one grown in a pot.

---

40   356-323 B.C

Aloe vera is a frost-tender succulent which thrives in lowland, subtropical areas. Aloe will tolerate almost any soil but has a preference for sandy areas. It likes full sun however; in some very hot climates the plant requires some shade at midday when the sun is directly overhead. In the United States, the warmer states of Florida, California, Nevada, New Mexico and Texas provide a climate suitable to naturalization of the plant and in many of these areas it is illegal to pick or transplant from the wild. There are some climates where the plants can be successfully grown outside year around but must be covered at night as protection against frost. The older and larger the plants become in these areas the more successfully they resist damage from cold nighttime temperatures. In areas where temperatures fall below 50°F for any length of time aloe must be grown in pots and as a house plant.

Aloe vera can be grown from seeds and do best in soil that is predominantly sandy. Whether sown outdoors or in pots the seeds should be only lightly covered and kept moist. Too much water and soft rot will contaminate the seedlings so a fungicide is recommended as a precaution. *Aloe vera* seed takes about 3 weeks to germinate and if planted in pots or containers the tiny seedlings will be ready to make the transition to outdoors in about 12 to 18 months.

Harvesting
Aloe is harvested for its gel, buds and juice. The gel is used in skin care and skin care products, the treatment of burns, wounds and infections and the dried juice is used in powdered form [usually in pills] as a laxative or purgative.

There is no known method for preserving or storing the gel [although there are a few commercial products on the market making claims for 90% or more pure aloe] so keeping a live plant in a pot for immediate use in the home remains the best solution. Always select leaves from the outside of the plant and cut them at the level of the soil, never in the middle of the stalk which only wounds and weakens the plant. They can be peeled and the gel rubbed immediately upon the affected skin. Leaves not used right away can be wrapped in plastic cling film and stored in the refrigerator between uses.

The juice of the aloe can be obtained in the same manner as the ancients. How much juice is obtained depends upon how much of the plant will be sacrificed. In commercial operations the entire plant is cut for "bleeding" and entire fields are harvested. Water the plant well the night before harvest. Cut as many leaves from the outside of the rosette as desired and place them on a slight incline to allow the juice to drain into a container. A stainless steel stockpot works well with a clean board leaned against the edge to hold the leaves in position. The cut edge of the stalk should be as close to the bottom of the board as possible so that the liquid can drain directly into the pot. The leaves will drain for a month or more and during this time the juice in the pan begins to evaporate naturally.

When no more of the yellowish exudate is forthcoming discard the leaves and bring the juice to a low boil. Simmer and watch carefully until the juice begins to thicken and then pour it into a glass container [an 8 X 8 glass cake dish works well] to continue evaporation until it hardens. Once it has hardened it is ready to be pulverized into powder. The powder is then stored and kept from light and moisture.

While boiling reduces the severity of the action it still can cause considerable "griping pains" and it brings about a congestion of blood in the pelvic region which can be extremely dangerous. It should never be taken during menstruation or pregnancy and never under any circumstance given to children.

It is worth emphasizing that this powdered extract is a slow acting but extremely powerful laxative which is never taken alone but always in combination with cascara sagrada, asafoetida, myrrh, or belladonna to lessen the intensity of its reaction. In 2002 the United States the Food and Drug Administration banned the use of aloe and cascara sagrada as ingredients in over-the-counter laxatives.

Use in the Edgar Cayce Readings
Aloe, or aloes, is mentioned only 19 times. The bud is used alone and aloes is used as a companion plant. Aloes is recommended in combination with agar in an over-the-counter product called Alophen. Oil of aloe is used in one case, combined with butterfat, tobacco and "oil of the buckeye kernel" as an ointment for the relief of hemorrhoids.

A rather unusual recommendation for aloe is in a steam sitz treatment; and in the 4 cases, only the bud of the aloe is used. This most unusual use of the aloe bud may indeed be unique to Cayce, as use of the bud in this way has not been found in any materia medica known to this researcher to date. A steam sitz bath was recommended in case 5671-6 for a 34-year-old woman suffering from vaginal pruritis. In the first treatment powdered aloes was substituted instead of the bud as had been stipulated. In a second check reading the opening statement in paragraph 1 states: *"Now, in some respects we find conditions not so good; produced mostly by the improper application of the steam baths - for, instead of the aloes being in the form as in CONFORMITY to the properties as given - that PULVERIZED, or anhydrized, is too STRONG, and irritation has been the result."*

The advice continues in paragraph 3: *"and do not add the aloe unless it is obtained in its ORIGINAL state – for the GUM of same is that as is necessary for the addition to the properties, so that the tendency is to penetrate more into the organs themselves, as the ACTIVITIES of same produce relaxation and contraction."*

Aloe buds can be used fresh or dried. For drying the buds are harvested early in the morning, when they are fully developed, but before they show signs of opening. Cut from the stem they are then partially dried in the sun, or a gentle, artificial heat source, until they feel "rubbery." They are then sealed in plastic freezer bags or sterile glass jars. They should not be frozen.

It is interesting to note that while traditional herbal lore uses the gel of the plant for relief and treatment of sunburn the gel is not recommended by Cayce for either skin care or sunburn. In cases of sunburn the information turns instead to pure apple vinegar, soda water, Glyco-Thymoline or even witch hazel as an additive in a steam cabinet.

One enigmatic reference is found in a life reading for an 18-year-old young woman as to aloe or myrrh as being *"influences innate to the entity for weal or woe."*

1714-1 F 18 Life Reading
13. In the one before this we find in that land known as in the French period, or during those of the Louis's - the 15th, and during that period when Richelieu ruled with the greater strength. The entity one to whom Richelieu oft went as one seeking counsel from the incenses burned during that period. The entity then in the name of Katrina, and the entity gained and lost through this experience; gaining in the UNDERSTANDING of the influences of incense, or of odors, or of such as are cleansed by fire, and lost in the APPLICATION of same as respecting the influence over men. In the present, much of that as is to be met in a karmic influence is the PROPER application of these same INFLUENCES, as may be used for the DEVELOPMENT of peoples, individuals, men, women, understand, excel; for especially are SOME of those of the aloe, or of the myrrh, those

influences innate to the entity for weal or woe.

The following excerpts are examples of the use of aloe in the Cayce system:

222-1 F 34 VENEREAL DISEASES:GONORRHEA
16. Also use those douches in the vagina at least once each three days, or every third day, Creolin, and use in sitz baths those of Myrrh and of Aloes and small quantity. That is, one aloe with twenty [20] drops of tincture of myrrh in BOILING water, and sit over same, so the steam may enter the exposed regions of the vagina and uterus. This will take longer but surer, for the blood stream is in poor condition for the operative method. [Cancer: Incipient? Gonorrhea?]

2711-2 M 58 HEMORRHOIDS
16. LOCALLY, apply those properties as would be found in a combination of THIS character; using this as an ointment following the stools, or WHEN there is irritation. RESTING, keeping feet up, will also aid these conditions - as well as aid the general HEALTH of body, with the taking of the medicinal properties and the manipulations [which should be had at least ONCE each day]. This salve [Tim], or ointment, would be made in THIS manner:

17. To 1 ounce of OIL of butterfat, add 1 dram of very fine POWDERED tobacco, 2 grains or 2 minims of oil of aloe, and 2 minims of oil of the buckeye kernel. Stir well together and use as an ointment.

4333-1 F Adult DEMENTIA PRAECOX [Author's note:Schizophrenia]
9. Keep the body where it will not harm self or others, yet do not have the body remain alone too often or long.

10. And osteopathically reduce the lesion in the lumbar and sacral region. It would require at least forty [40] such general adjustments for the effective reaction from such adjustments may only be meted or seen active in those periods of menstruation; when these properties are used as the property to react with the forces in the system:

11. Each day while such periods last, there should be prepared as this, in an earthen or crock container, at least sufficient in size that the body may sit over same with ease: Place one [1] gallon of boiling water in crock, and add twenty [20] drops of Tincture of Myrrh, with forty [40] drops Fluid Extract of Tolu, with one [1] Aloe; and expose the parts to the steam arising from same, and prepare the vagina in such a manner that these fumes may enter the vagina proper, see?

12. In the periods between there will be the constant correction; and keep the mind directed towards spiritual application of the better things, and within the three to four [3 to 4] moons, there will be found the RETURNING of the full equilibrium in this body, [4333].

5663-1 F 36 Sterility
9. At least two to five days before the periods of menstruation, for two to three moons, we would use a steam sitz bath. The STEAM; not sitting in the water or bath - but prepare as in THIS manner:

10. Two gallons of BOILING water poured into a container, see? To this water [plain water] add a pinch of alum, one aloe bud, fifteen minims of tincture of myrrh, and tolu gum [pure tolu gum] the size of a pea - English pea.

11. When this has been prepared, then sit OVER such - so that the puba and the vagina is exposed to the STEAM from same, for five to eight minutes.

12. Do this three to give times - that is, from two to five days before [once each day] - before the regular periods. ONCE after the cleansing, or after period - see?

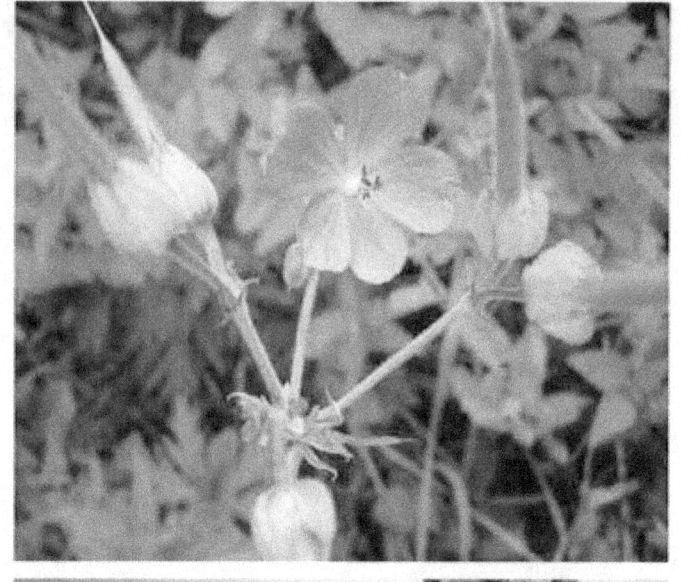
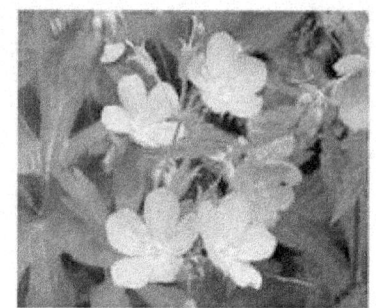
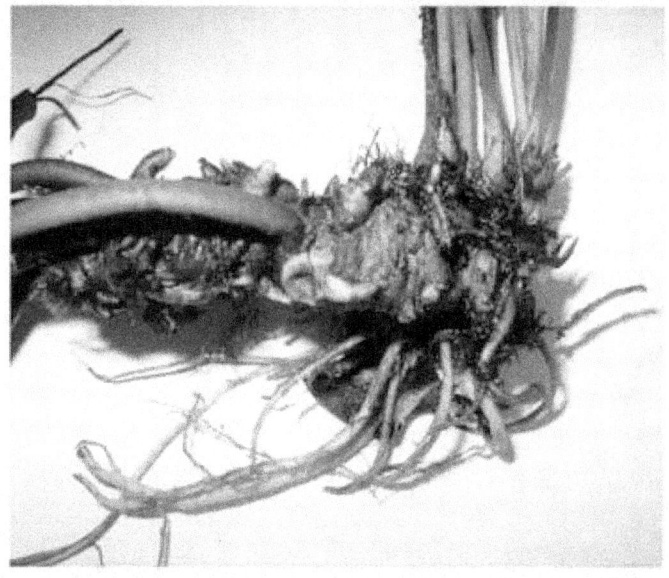
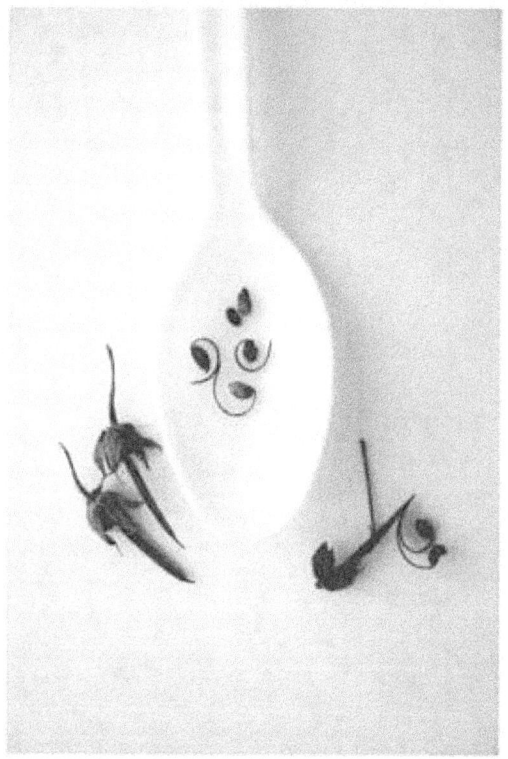
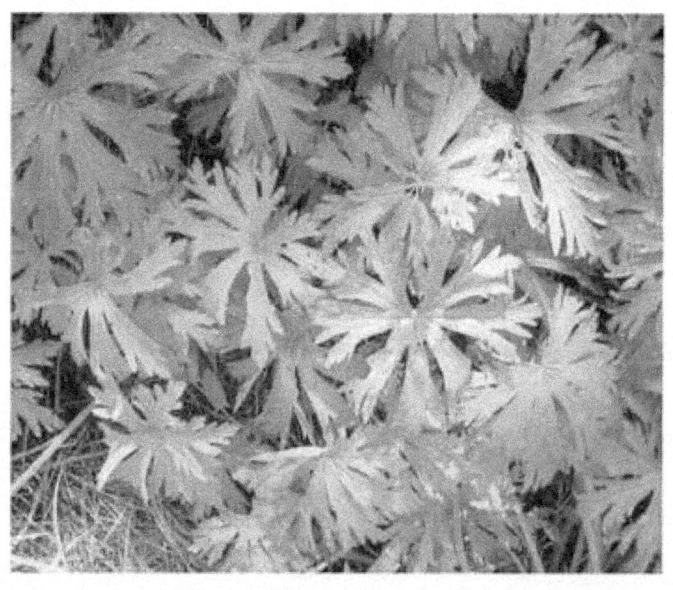
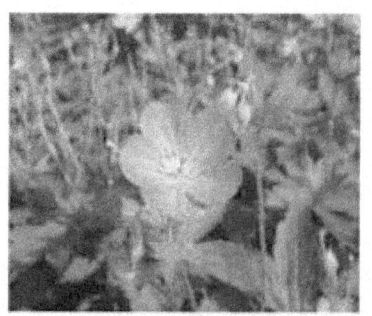

Alum Root
Geranium maculatum, Fam. Geraniaceae

Common and Regional Names
Cranesbill, Spotted Cranesbill, Wild Cranesbill, Storksbill, Alum Bloom, Wild Geranium

History and Common Usage
Alum root is found in moist woods and along the edge of hedges and thickets in low grounds from Newfoundland to Manitoba and south to Georgia and Missouri and is also widely distributed in Europe and Scandinavia. In the United States the plant is most abundant in Indiana, North Carolina and Virginia. This plant differs from the other native species of geranium in that it has a perennial rootstock and its flowers are much larger than others members of the geranium family.

Alum root is cited in a number of historical sources as having been used by the Native Americans who first introduced it to the early settlers. The Native Americans used the plant internally in the treatment of diarrhea and what is today called irritable bowel syndrome, in cases of cholera, kidney complaints, ulcers and dysentery. They used it externally as a dressing on purulent wounds, in the relief of hemorrhoids, and for throat infections and inflammations of the mouth.

A tea to aid digestion can be prepared by boiling 1 or 2 teaspoons [5 to 10 grams] of the root in 2 cups of water for fifteen minutes. Up to 3 cups a day may be drunk, however, some sources suggest that if taken to excess it will cause an upset stomach rather than cure one.

American and British pharmacopeias from 1900 to 1940 list alum root as an official drug plant and describe it as "one of the best indigenous astringents." It was prescribed in the treatment of infants and given to those with delicate stomachs in cases of diarrhea, chronic dysentery and in various hemorrhages.

Description
Alum root grows from 12 to 18 inches up to 4 feet high. The leaves are deeply parted, usually in sections of 5, each division of the leaf being again toothed and cleft or irregularly notched. The plant will blossom and produce seeds at the same time throughout the growing season. The flowers range in color from pale pink deepening through rose and blue to a light bluish-purple. They have five petals and depending upon the climate will begin appearing in April to June.

The root is usually found in sections 2 to 4 inches long characterized by multiple stems and rootlets from which it produces new plants. The root is reddish-brown on the outside and white on the inside turning to a darkish purple inside after drying. There is no odor to the root. It has an astringent but not unpleasant taste.

The flower develops into what is called a five-celled regma[41] which looks like the beak of a bird giving rise to one of its popular names "cranesbill." Each cell contains one small black seed.

---

41   Regma – a kind of dry fruit, consisting of three or more cells, each which at length breaks open at the inner angle.

Growing Conditions and Propagation

Alum root is a perennial preferring the edges of swamps, woodlands, thickets and meadows thriving in moist areas characterized by rich loam. It propagates both by seed and from the root system which continuously sends up young plants giving rise to ever larger colonies of the plant.

Seeds are planted by pressing them into prepared soil in the fall or early spring in shady areas which are moist or can be watered frequently. Roots should be planted 2 to 3 inches deep, and plants can be transplanted at any time during the growing season.

Harvesting

Both the leaves and root of the plant are used in traditional herbal systems. The root is best gathered while the plant is flowering. They should be washed with a soft brush under cool running water and the many stems and rootlets should be removed. They can be used fresh or sliced into smaller pieces for drying, although most roots are not large enough to make this necessary. The leaves should be collected and dried at first bloom, just before seeds begin to develop when their active principles [tannic and gallic acids] are at their highest levels.

Use in the Edgar Cayce Readings

Alum root is used alone and as a companion plant. Only the root is used in the Cayce system and its use reflects both herbal and official medical recommendations. It appears in 9 transcripts where assimilations were disrupted, kidneys affected, and where ulcers, colitis and diarrhea are all described. There are 3 females in this group, listed as 1 adult and one 50 and 51 years old respectively. The 6 males ranged in age from 59 to 6 months of age. [Case 348 had 4 of the 9 transcripts]

Of the group, 7 individuals were told to use alum root as an ingredient in fusions and tonics in combination with other herbal materials such as Indian turnip and wild ginseng.

In 2 cases a piece of the root was recommended to be carried *"in the pocket"* to have on hand to be chewed occasionally throughout the day to treat the kidneys or to address problems of diarrhea. In the remaining 7 alum root is one ingredient in compound formulas taken as a part of a total treatment regiment for colitis, duodenal ulcers and kidney conditions. The following 5 excerpts are typical ways alum root is used in the Cayce system:

5631-1 M Diarrhea
7. Then begin with small doses of THIS as a compound: to 6 ounces of distilled water, add:

> **Alum root..........1 ounce,**
> **Indian Turnip.....20 grains,**
> **Ginseng [wild].....1 dram.**

Reduce by slow simmering to 1/2 the quantity. Strain while warm and add 2 ounces of grain alcohol with 1 ounce of simple syrup. The dose would be a few drops in the beginning, every hour, until there is relief through the alimentary canal, and a tendency for the stopping of the diarrhea.

348-23 M 53 Diarrhea
8. Begin with a small piece of Alum Root [dried] to be put in the mouth and chewed - a little piece of this the size of an English pea - put in the mouth about half to three-quarters of an hour after

each meal, and gradually chewed - and the juice swallowed. This will gradually correct the condition through the digestive system

Perhaps one of the most interesting recommendations for alum root was not given in a physical reading but in a life reading warning of a "summer complaint."

4714-1 M 6 mos. Diarrhea
5. One that is destined to suffer with that condition in early childhood known as the summer complaints, or that of the looseness to the intestinal tract, to detraction of the physical body, unless warned against same. With this, use those properties as would be found in herbs of alum root, camphor and such natures - alcohol mixed with same.

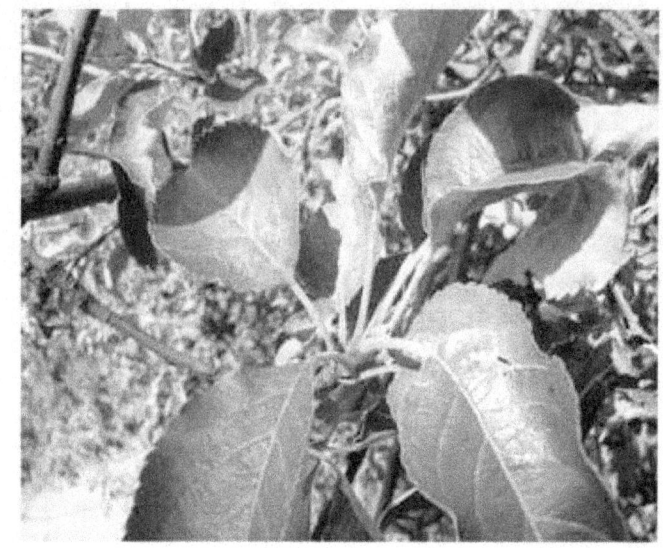
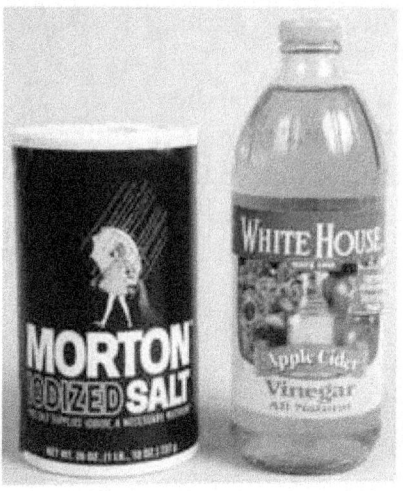
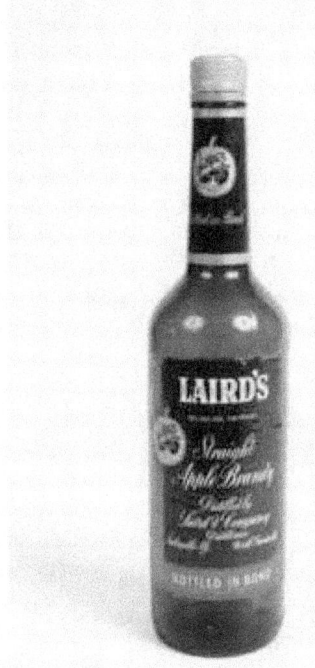
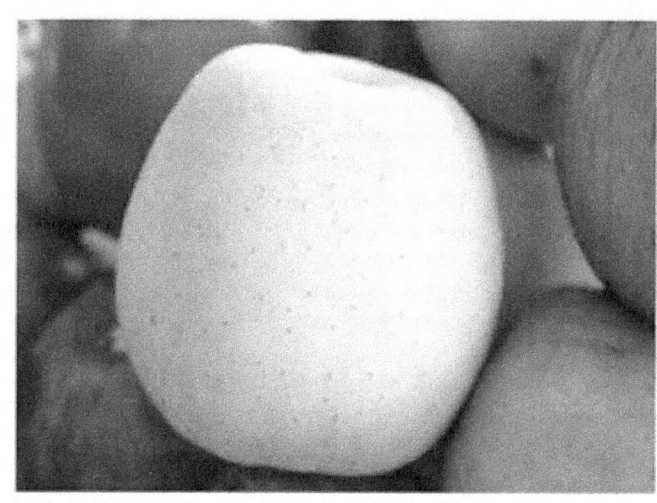
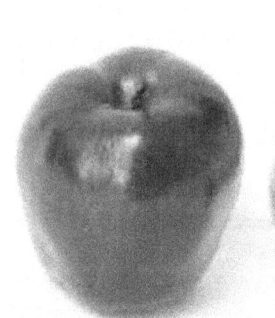
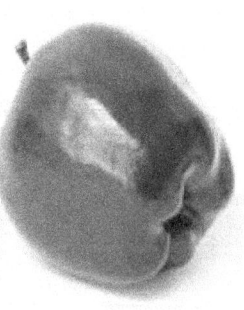
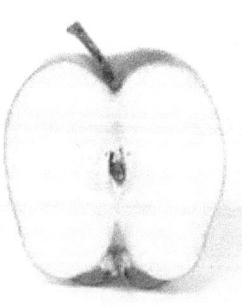
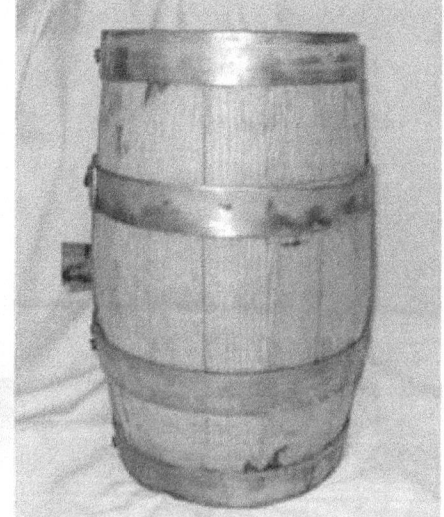

APPLES-APPLE BRANDY-APPLE CIDER VINEGAR

Malus pumila, Fam. Rosaceae

Also seen as *Malus domestica, Malus sylvestris, Malus communis,* and *Pyrus malus*

Common and Regional Names

None

History and Common Usage

The history of the apple parallels the known history of man and it grows in every temperate region in the world. Most scientists believe it originated in the general region of what is present day Russia and Asia. Recent research has traced Mala domestica to the Kazakstan region between present day China and Russia where scientists have identified a 300 year old tree still producing fruit.42 Archeological sites throughout Europe yield evidence that apples were sliced and preserved for winter use by drying by Mesolithic peoples, a practice still in use today.

Pomology, the branch of agricultural science that deals with fruits and nuts, is known to have begun development in China 6,000 years ago. These ancient records of crossbreeding, budding and grafting procedures and techniques used for apples, peaches, apricots, plums, pears and other kinds of fruits have made possible the great variety of fruit enjoyed today.

Scientists estimate there are now at least 10,000 different kinds of apples, all developed from the 25 to 30 original wild varieties. The original wild apple, referred to as a crab apple [Malus sylvestris] developed distinct characteristics in evolutionary response to the climate and other conditions in which it grew. This resulted in some being better in the warm seasons, others after the onset of winter frost while some could only be used after being frozen on the tree. A few were sweet and fragrant, others were sour in the extreme. Pliny the Elder says of the sour variety: "There are some small wild apples also, remarkable for their fine flavour and the peculiar pungency of their smell. Some, again, are so remarkably sour, that they are held in disesteem; indeed their acidity is so extreme, that it will even take the edge from off a knife."43

Apples were known to the Egyptians but the climate was not suitable to their cultivation even though Ramses II is recorded as having the trees planted in his Delta garden. Some scholars debate whether it was the apple or the apricot being referred to in Egyptian records, however the Sumerians clearly differentiated between apricots and apples leaving records of one or two prescriptions calling for apples and apple juice recorded in their Book of Medicines.

The apple itself does not command a large presence in folk medicine but there are references to it in every language and in every culture. There are apple sayings, metaphors and similes for almost every occasion: "The apple of my eye," "the apple doesn't fall far from the tree," he or she is "a bad apple," - "one bad apple spoils the barrel" and "comparing apples and oranges" are all a part of every language.

One of the most enduring American legends is that of Johnny Appleseed. John Chapman was born in Leominster, Massachusetts in 1774 and was definitely a man born with a mission. At about 18 years of age he began traveling to establish apple orchards throughout what is today Ohio, Indiana and Illinois. Never married, he was a devout advocate of the Church of the New Jerusalem based upon the revealed information of Emanuel Swedenborg, and was characterized by a life long concern for animals making him one of the earliest animal rights activists and conservationists in the United States.

42 FOREIGN TRAVEL REPORT, Plant Collection Expedition to Kazakstan, August 24 - September 19, 1996 http://
43www.usda.gov/wps/portal/usdahome BOOK XV. THE NATURAL HISTORY OF THE FRUIT-TREES

John did not believe in grafting. He preferred only Heritage or wild apples - trusting the results to Mother Nature. He established apples as a cash crop in the United States, becoming a legend in his own lifetime. John died in 1847, however the exact date and place of his internment are still in dispute. Some sources state he died March 18th others March 22nd. Some believe his grave is marked by a rock near the site of his original cabin, others say he is buried in Archer Cemetery. Both sites are in Fort Wayne, Indiana.

Well tended apple trees can live and produce up to 100 or more years. The oldest apple tree of record in the United States was planted by Peter Stuyvesant, director-general of the New Amsterdam colony in 1647. The tree thrived on the southern tip of Manhattan Island until it was destroyed 219 years later by a derailed train. The oldest apple tree of record in England is a Bramley's Seedling, sown in 1810, making it over 200 years old.

Apple juice is a refreshing favorite and pressing apples after the fall harvest for juice and cider is the stuff of festivals in many countries. At some point in history it was observed that apple juice or fresh cider fermented producing the alcoholic beverage known today as hard cider. This was soon followed by apple vinegar and the development of apple wine and apple brandy. The word vinegar comes from the Old French 'vin aigre,' - literally sour wine - and because of its flavoring and preservative qualities vinegar has entered into the kitchens of every culture.

Vinegar can be made from almost anything that has sufficient sugar to produce fermentation. There are quick vinegars and slow process types, some premium vinegars are not ready for use until they have aged at least 3 to5 years. It has been used in folk remedy traditions for centuries due to its ability to halt the activity of bacteria, both on human skin and in food. Vinegar appears in both the British and United States Dispensatories during the time the Cayce information was being given but is listed as an unofficial preparation.

Description
An apple tree can reach 40 feet in height with a crown of 20 to 25 feet in diameter. The bark is scaly and grayish brown in color. Trunk diameter is age dependant and many older trees can be 3 to 4 feet in diameter. They begin to produce fruit between their 5th and 7th year.

Apple leaves, 2 to 5 inches long, are medium to dark green, oval with slight serrations along the edges, occurring in an alternating fashion along the twigs and branches. Flower buds appear in April to June, depending on the growing zone and weather. They are pink turning to white as they open and mature. Apple blossoms are sweetly and unforgettably fragrant.

Since choosing a fruit tree is a long term decision the size of the mature tree and the use of the fruit should be carefully considered. There are full size or standard trees, semi-dwarf [12 to 16 feet] and dwarf varieties [5 to 8 feet tall].

Over time individual strains have been developed to meet individual needs and tastes. There are now varieties that are considered better for eating raw, or for baking. There are those favored for applesauce and apple butter, and others preferred for pies. Some are the variety of choice for making juice and cider. Some ripen as early as June, such as the Yellow and White Transparent, and some as late as October, such as the Arkansas Black Russet. Some ripen incrementally and are best eaten fresh through their season while others are good keepers and will store in a cold place until spring. [Apples should not be stored near carrots as the ethylene in the apples will adversely affect the taste of the carrots.] Apples freeze at 29° F and are best stored at 32-34° F. Each variety has different dormancy and chill requirements to be considered if the tree is to remain healthy and productive into old age.

The home gardener should assess the space available for a mature tree and determine preferences for sauce, pies or fresh fruit before visiting a reputable local nursery or consulting a local extension office.

Growing Conditions and Propagation

Apples grown from seed will be nothing like the parent tree. They are the superstars of evolution, successfully adapting to every climate, but not always producing edible fruit. Grafting is the only sure means of having a true-to-parent variety.

There are varieties that are self-pollinating, assisted by wind and insects, and some that are partially self-fertile. Self-fertile varieties will set fruit without another tree, but will yield a better crop if they are cross-pollinated. Varieties requiring a pollinator will do very nicely with a crabapple near by, that blooms at the same time.

Apples require full sun, especially in the early morning to dry the dew from their leaves which helps prevent disease. They do best in sandy loam to sandy clay loam and good drainage is important. Soil pH should be near 6.5.

Apples are subject to a number of diseases and pests. There are times to spray and times not to spray. Regular pruning, management and prevention of apple blight, fire blight, canker, sawfly, leaf weevil, spider mite, mildew and a host of other such challenges is a field of special study. Good housekeeping in the orchard is a necessity if trees are to reach full maturity and produce abundantly.

Harvesting

As strange as it may seem it can be difficult to determine when an apple is ripe, especially if the appearance and flavor of tree ripened fruit is unknown. There are no absolute guidelines to determine ripeness. Some turn red before they ripen, but will be hard and taste woody or starchy. They will not "cook down" to a soft stage during baking and lack the full flavour of a ripened apple. This is often the case with apples in American supermarkets and unripe apples are difficult to digest.
The number of days from bloom is a good general indicator. The Jonathan variety, for example, is usually ready in approximately 135 days; Red and Golden Delicious require roughly 145 days. If the seeds are a rich brown color the time is right especially if a slice of the fruit, held up to the light has turned from light green to white. The ultimate indicators of ripeness, of course, are aroma and taste.

Use in the Edgar Cayce Readings

The apple, mentioned in over 300 transcripts, is not a companion plant in the Cayce system; however, brandy and vinegar derived from the apple is used extensively and usually combined with other products.

Cayce recommends the use of apple cider vinegar in cases of sunburn and there is even an unusual, albeit temporary, tanning lotion to be made using apple cider vinegar:

276-7 F 16
32. [Q] What is the best formula that will make my skin brown from the sun?
[A] Sun tan for some is good. But for those that have a certain amount of pigment in the skin, as indicated in this body, to make for variations as to the effect of weather or sun upon exposed portions of the body...to get a sun tan would not be well for this body; for it would burn tissue before it would tan. That which would be more effective...would be the use of vinegar and olive oil [not vinegar made from acetic acid, or synthetic vinegar, but the use of that made from the apples] combined with coffee made from resteaming or re-vaporing used coffee grounds. The tannin in each of these, and the acids

combined, would become very effective. But it will wear off, of course, in a very short time even - if used.

Questions were asked about apples in matters of general diet, and the answers provide valuable guidelines as to how, for some people, apples should be prepared and eaten. They are also recommended in an important mono-diet for therapeutic purposes. The fact that the apple diet results in weight loss is an often highly desirable byproduct.

Not all apples receive the Cayce stamp of approval, and the following explanation is offered as to why. There is further emphasis that only tree ripened fruit should be eaten:

4834-1 F Adult
4. The body shouldn't take things that produce acid. We have things that are not acid themselves, but change into acid when taken into the mouth. Normally there are glands in the throat which produce lactic fluid or pepsin, this body is not producing sufficient lactic fluid, so that whatever is taken is carried into acid. There are properties that are not acid themselves but are turned into acids when taken into the mouth, and properties that are acids that are not acids when taken into the mouth. Pear, which is acid, forms into iron and loses its acid, certain apples are acid, others are not. This body should take apples that have ripened on the tree.

Among the apples NOT favorably recommended are a few referred to as the "fall or woody stock" such as the Ben Davis and Winesap. They are not as desirable as the Jonathan, Arkansas Black or Black Arkansas, Oregon Red, Red and Golden Delicious, Arkansas Russet and Grimes Golden, which are recommended by name.

The word jenneting occurred in many transcripts such as in the case of a young man who wanted to be a pilot but was diagnosed as being color blind. Cayce described the malfunction and the young man was trying to correct the problem with Cayce's help. The 20 year old received the following:

24. NO raw apples; or if raw apples are taken, take them and NOTHING else - three days of raw apples only, and then olive oil, and we will cleanse ALL toxic forces from any system! Raw apples are not well unless they are of the jenneting variety. [GD's note: Dictionary of obsolete words gives re. jenneting: "A jenneting pear - an early pear resembling the jenneting apple." NOTE: Jenneting: A variety of early apple, so named for being ripe about St. John's Day, June 24th.] Apples cooked, apples roasted, are good. No bananas, unless you are in the territory where they are grown and ripened there. Do not use large quantities of potatoes, though the peelings of same may be taken at all times - they are strengthening, carrying those influences and forces that are active with the glands of the system. But beware of those things indicated; as for the rest, keep a well-balanced diet. [820-2]

Research by Gladys Davis in the 1960's concluded that the definition of the word jenneting meant *"A jenneting pear - an early pear resembling the jenneting apple...a variety of early apple, so named for being ripe about St. John's Day, June 24th."*

This calls into question the meaning of the word jenneting as it is understood to date because analysis of the strains of apples recommended by Cayce all ripen, not in the spring, but in the fall.

The varieties of apples favorably recommended by name by Cayce are:

Variety	Harvest date	Cold storage time
Jonathan	early September	January
Black Arkansas[44]	early October	December to April
Oregon Red	early October	October to May
Sheepnose[45]	early October	October to December
Delicious - Red	early September - Oct	October to May
Delicious - Gold[46]	early September - Oct.	October to December
Arkansas Russet	early September - Oct	October to May
Grimes Golden	early September - Oct	October to May

These apples also happen to be among a group called antique apples or heritage varieties. They ripen late in the season and keep well in storage. Some strains actually benefit from storage as in the case of the Black Arkansas or Arkansas Black. It is a very hard apple which softens during storage. The commonalities in all varieties of apple named by Cayce are:

[1] They ripen in the fall
[2] They are considered storage apples or "good keepers"
[3] They are all from a common strain characterized by a conical shape and "bumps on their noses" which is the most distinguishing characteristic of the modern and easily obtained Red or Golden Delicious, of which there are over 40 varieties today.

Dietary Recommendations
In a dietary context apples are mentioned in over 200 cases. Of the 200 dietary recommendations 148 individuals were told NOT to eat raw apples but to have them only cooked, baked or roasted and taken with cream. In this group Cayce said apples reacted within the system to increase acidity and were not well digested. Of the 200 there were 37 individuals who were told not to eat apples at all, either cooked or raw. Of the 15 or so who could tolerate them raw were to have them occasionally and eat only the "Jonathan" variety.

General Dietary Recommendations
3180-3 F 4 ...An almond a day is much more in accord with keeping the doctor away, especially certain types of doctors, than apples. For the apple was the fall, not almond - for the almond blossomed when everything else died. Remember this is life!

951-1 F 18 ARTHRITIS
8. ...Beware of apples and bananas among the fruits.

2923-1 F 60 ARTHRITIS:NEURITIS
14. ...Not raw apples, but cooked apples may be included....

837-1 M 45 ANEMIA:BRONCHITIS
17. ...Beware of raw apples unless used as a cleanser.

---

44   Also called Black Twig
45   Also called Black Gilliflower
46   Starkspur, a chance seedling of the Grimes Golden.

Apple Diet

The apple diet is perhaps the most widely known of the Cayce mono-diets. It is recommended in 24 cases and in 14 of the 24 the amount of time to remain on the diet is given as three days. The diet begins with a raw apple breakfast on the first day and continues to the last meal of the day on the evening of the third day. A normal diet is resumed on the morning of the fourth day. During this time only fresh, raw apples are to be eaten.

One exception to this was found in case 1621-1 for a 50 year old gentleman who was told to eat nothing but vegetables for four or five days at a time and only in the evenings was he to eat raw apples.

There is no mention of peeling them although if waxed fruit is the only kind available peeling is certainly advised. It is suggested that one should *eat all the apples you can!" [288-42]* one case recommends *"eat them, all you can, at least 5 or 6 apples each day, scrape them well, chew them up." [1409-9]*

Apple dieters are also to drink a lot of water but may not take other foods or juices. Coffee or tea may be taken but must be taken black, that is, without cream or sugar:

780-12 F 55
4. We would use first the apple diet to purify the system; that is, for three days eat nothing but apples of the Jonathan variety if possible. This includes the Delicious, which is a variety of the Jonathan. The Jonathan is usually grown farther north than the Delicious, but these are of the same variety, but eat some. You may drink coffee if you desire, but do not put milk or cream in it, especially while you are taking the apples.

5. At the end of the third day, the next morning take about two tablespoonsful of Olive Oil.

A cereal drink such as Pero or Postum is found recommended once, but again when on the apple diet should be taken without cream, milk, honey, sugar or artificial sweeteners.

The diet is nearly always concluded on the evening of the third day by taking olive oil. The amount of oil varies from case to case. Transcript 543-26 has this to say about Olive Oil: *"...it is a food for the intestinal system by absorption as much as by activity upon the organs of the assimilating forces..."* The amount of olive oil is always recommended "to the point of tolerance," however, suggestions range from one tablespoon to half a cup.

Case 820-2 contains a general statement as to the efficacy of the cleansing apple diet, *"NO raw apples; or if raw apples are taken, take them and NOTHING else - three days of raw apples only, and then olive oil, and we will cleanse ALL toxic forces from any system!"* The apple diet purifies the system, reducing toxicity levels. One case [1409-9 F 66] states *"this will get rid of the tendencies for neuritic conditions in the joints of the body."*

Transcript 567-7 suggested the apple diet as a test for intestinal worms and stated further *"...And this would remove fecal matter that hasn't been removed for some time!"* In 1850-3 it states that the apple diet *"is to cleanse the activities of the liver, the kidneys, and the whole system..."*

In the majority of cases a colonic irrigation or enema is not called for in connection with the apple diet. Only 1 case [1621-1] out of the 24 recommends that after the apple diet has begun the individual should have a thorough cleansing of the colon through a colonic irrigation. The information goes on to say that even this need not be done if the diet is repeated, suggesting that the colonic irrigation could wait until the next month when the special diet was to be followed again.

Apple brandy is used extensively both internally combined with other ingredients and as an inhalant. The following demonstrates ways apple brandy is used in the Cayce system:

Apple Brandy Tonics and Expectorants
304-47 M 83 Eliminations
8. We find that a helpful tonic, of course, at times for the heavy breathing, would be Rock Candy and Rye. This, of course, not too much, but for the strengthening and for the activities. Or, more preferably still, use the Rock Candy or the Honey in Pure Apple Brandy. The proportions would be two ounces of the Strained Honey, heated, before it is put in a pint of the Pure Apple Brandy. This would be shaken well, and the dose would be not more than a teaspoonful - two, three, four times a day. This will allay the cough and helpful for the digestion and the activities of the whole system.

427-6 M 23 Cough
9. Also it would be well to have prepared a compound in this manner:
10. To 1/2 pint of apple brandy, add:

> **Rock Candy.........................1 ounce,**
> **Glycerine..........................5 minims,**
> **Oil of Pine Needles................3 minims.**

Shake this before the dose is taken, and two or three times each day take a teaspoonful. And during the night, if there is trouble from coughing or from sweats, take a teaspoonful.

Egg Nog with Apple Brandy
1014-1 M 41 COLD:CONGESTION:DEBILITATION:GENERAL
32. Use milk rather in the meal that would be BETWEEN the morning and noon meals; that is, in a glass of milk there would be added the YOLK of an egg with apple brandy. Have the egg "cooked," as it were, with apple brandy; then ADD the milk. This should be at least a glassful, in the middle of the morning between the two meals.

Apple Cider Vinegar and Salt in Physiotherapy Applications
Apple cider vinegar is recommended combined with salt and applied to the body in the form of hot packs and is sometimes gently massaged into injured joints providing pain relief and to speed the healing of injured tendons and muscles. This application helps eliminate the stiffness and weakness that is the usual result of such injuries. There are approximately 59 cases where pain from fractures, sprains and other injuries, including muscle spasms have been reported as successfully treated.

Often severe headaches caused by muscle spasms of the neck and shoulders can be relieved by the simple application of vinegar and salt. Apple cider vinegar is poured over a cup or two of salt (iodized or plain) and heated in a stainless steel pan on the stove to the point of tolerance. [Never use an aluminum container] While seated in a warm bathtub for easy clean up, handfuls of hot wet salt are applied to the neck and shoulders and allowed to remain for 15 minutes or until relief is obtained. A hot shower will rinse away the salt but the odor of the vinegar will linger.

Apple Vinegar and Salt for Fractures and Sprains

The following is a common condition which often plagues professional athletes. It is easily corrected with salt and apple vinegar and a little persistence:

849-34 M 31
13. [Q] Should anything be done to help the cartilage that slips out of place in the right knee?
[A] Yes - this should be massaged, too, but preferably massage this with salt and pure apple vinegar - a saturated solution. Gently massaging this, it will absorb sufficient so that in a little while this will remain without any slipping.

In the case below a young man was suffering from a wrenched back, with the 5th rib injured. He had been suffering from pain and restricted movement for 5 or 6 months:

1710-2 M 23
4. Through the other shoulder we find ligaments and tendons have been strained; and these tend to make for conditions that are as severe almost as a break...

5. As we find in the present, over those areas where there is the disturbance with any exercise of any perceptible nature of the arm and shoulder, we would apply each evening for at least three or four evenings a saturated solution, or even heavier, of salt and apple vinegar. This would be applied almost as a pad, and then an electric pad placed over same for a period of an hour or more.

6. These Packs we would use each evening for at least three or four evenings, before we would have the corrections made; so that these will relax and tend to make it easier for the adjustments osteopathically to be better made through the dorsal areas, - from at least the 8th or 9th dorsal to the 3rd and 4th cervical. This would be gently done, but should not require more than three to four or five adjustments.

In the following a 60 year old lady had fallen and broken a wrist. She was concerned about regaining the full use of her hand:

501-2 F 60 INJURIES:Fractures
15. [Q] Will body be able to use right hand and wrist as formerly?
[A] As we find, it will...When this is loosened, then we would begin with the massage of the arm and shoulder, hand and wrist, with those first of the olive oil and the tincture of myrrh, heating the oil and adding the myrrh. Then in the next day or two use those of the pure apple vinegar with SALT - common salt - dissolved in same. Massage this into the joints, especially. That it produces burning, and when the attempt to move it produces the feeling as if it was grinding BETWEEN the bone itself, keep on using it! for it will not irritate more than that as is necessary. Use this about two or three times each week, the other on the opposite days, - see?

These 2 excerpts speak to the use of apple vinegar and salt in cases where fluid has collected due to broken bones, and the second deals with helping to deal with sprains:

903-35 F 41 FRACTURE
5. Thus, for the elbow, the massage with Pure Apple Vinegar and salt - the salt saturated with the vinegar. This will enable the fluids accumulated about the end of the bone here that is broken, or bent

in, to be dissolved so that it can come back to its normal position. For it is more the cartilaginous force than a set or calcified condition in the body.

3336-1 F 77 SPRAIN
11. In the area of the knee, where ligaments have been torn, use about twice each week this combination: Moisten table salt [preferably iodized salt] with pure apple vinegar; not having too liquid, but that it may be gently massaged into the knee cap, the end of the ligaments. While this will hurt a few times at first, if this is kept up each day for quite a while we will get better results here.

Apple Brandy and the Charred Oak Keg Therapy
Apple brandy is used in an inhalation therapy in 104 cases utilizing a small charred oak keg in cases indexed as pneumonia, bronchitis and tuberculosis. A charred oak keg[47] is a small barrel made from oak that has been burnt on the inside so as to char the interior. This charring produces both color and flavor in the whiskeys, Sherries and brandies that are aged in kegs. It is important to specify charring when purchasing a keg as they are sold either toasted or charred. Charring is required for this therapy. A keg that will hold a gallon [128 ounces] or a gallon and a half [192 ounces] of brandy is the most practical size.

In a near terminal case where lung tissue was so weakened by tuberculosis that the keg could not be inhaled the following method of using apple brandy is recommended:

1045-3 F 37
7. Also we find that the inhaling of the fumes from apple brandy would be most beneficial. For THIS particular condition in the immediate, it would be best that such fumes be from putting at least a tablespoonful of pure apple brandy in a quantity (say two tablespoonful) of very hot water (as in a croup cup) and allow the fumes or the vapor to be inhaled. In this manner (with the water in same) it will supply to the mucous membranes, to the lungs, to the throat, a moisture that would be most helpful for the body.

Hildick is the American brand recommended by Cayce and in 1944 Hildick and Laird were both produced by the Laird Company. The Laird family has been producing apple brandy and apple jack in the United States from the time of George Washington.[48] Hildick is no longer manufactured but Laird still produces an excellent straight apple brandy, which is unfortunately only available by special order in some states in the United States. Mr. Cayce used Laird for his personal use and recommended Laird in his correspondence.

The Cayce information uses the word "pure" which simply means that the brandy is not to be a blend or mixed with other spirits or adulterated with grain alcohol. Apple jack is NOT to be used although a re-distilled apple jack is acceptable. Laird has been producing apple brandy in the United States since 1780 and their 7 year old and 12 year old brandies are excellent choices for this therapy. In Europe Calvados is recommended.

---

47   Casks may be purchased in the United States from Brew U.S.A. : http://www.brew-usa.com/Oak_Barrels_Spigots-Oak_Keg_2_Gallon_Charred.html. Kegs can also be purchased from http://www.heritagestore.com/ located at 314 Laskin Road, Virginia Beach, Virginia 23451 757-428-0500.
48   http://www.lairdandcompany.com/products_applebrandy.htm
Laird & Company, One Laird Road, Scobeyville, N.J. 07724. Phone: [732] 542-0312 Fax: [732] 542-2244
1-877-GETLAIRD

The following excerpts are typical ways in which apple brandy is used as an inhalation therapy:

1564-2 M 44 TUBERCULOSIS

But prepare the keg in this manner: In at least a gallon or gallon and a half oak keg, charred inside, put half to a gallon of the Pure Apple Brandy [half a gallon to the gallon keg, you see; or that proportion]. Bore a hole in the top; not in the bung side but in one end, you see, that may be kept corked tightly. Then bore a small hole [which would be kept tightly corked] next to same, in which would be put a tube or metal from which there may be inhaled or drawn the gas from the Apple Brandy in the vacuum, you see. This may be inhaled once to twice daily, and we will find a great exhilaration from same; and after a few days we will see greater improvements in the activity of the properties for the keeping of a balance in the circulatory forces.

1172-1 M 16 TUBERCULOSIS:CURED

10. Prepare the apple brandy in a keg; gallon keg charred inside, or gallon and a half or two gallon keg. Anyway, put at least half a gallon of apple BRANDY in same; not others, but pure apple brandy that has been distilled, see? Keep this where it will keep warm; keep it corked tight; and prepare with a tube that may be kept corked, from which there may be inhaled the fumes - as the cigarette would be - into the throat and lungs; even at times swallowing same; not the brandy but the FUMES of same, see? These tend to cauterize as well as to make for recuperative powers.

In May of 1943 Mr. Cayce received a letter from a 19 year old young man hospitalized in the State Sanatorium in South Mountain, Pennsylvania:

3085-1 M 19 …Somewhat over three years ago I first entered a sanatorium for tuberculosis, and except for a brief five months of last year spent at home, it has been my habitation up until the present day. I'm nineteen years of age [being admitted first at age of sixteen] and in the consequence of the disease have experienced three break downs. My general physical condition is still fairly good however; that is, all properties excepting my lungs….

Treatment information was obtained in July of 1943. Cayce responded by saying the condition was serious but to carry out the regimen at home. It began with inhaling the fumes of a charred oak keg with Hildicks Apple Brandy 3 or 4 times a day, taking Acigest and Calcios,[49] he was directed to stay out of the night air but to enjoy the sun with his shirt off, and a diet was given that emphasized yellow vegetables. The regimen, so clearly outlined in this case, is typical for Cayce on tuberculosis and the directions were followed to the letter. Six months later in January of 1944, when a check reading was obtained, the information confirmed what the young man and his family already knew:

3085-2 M 19 TUBERCULOSIS

3. …The body is much improved. There is no active bacilli in the lung at present. To be sure, this is as yet latent and will require that the body take precautions as to keeping a well balanced diet, so that there are not again the effects of the digestion becoming upset, or the liver and the kidneys.

Mr. 3085, now in his 80's, continues in good health at the time of this writing, and still credits Edgar Cayce with saving him from pneumothorax surgery soon to be followed by what was in the 1940's, a certain and slow sentence of death.

---

49   Acigest is an over-the-counter supplement and Calcios is a calcium supplement that can be ordered from The Heritage Store.

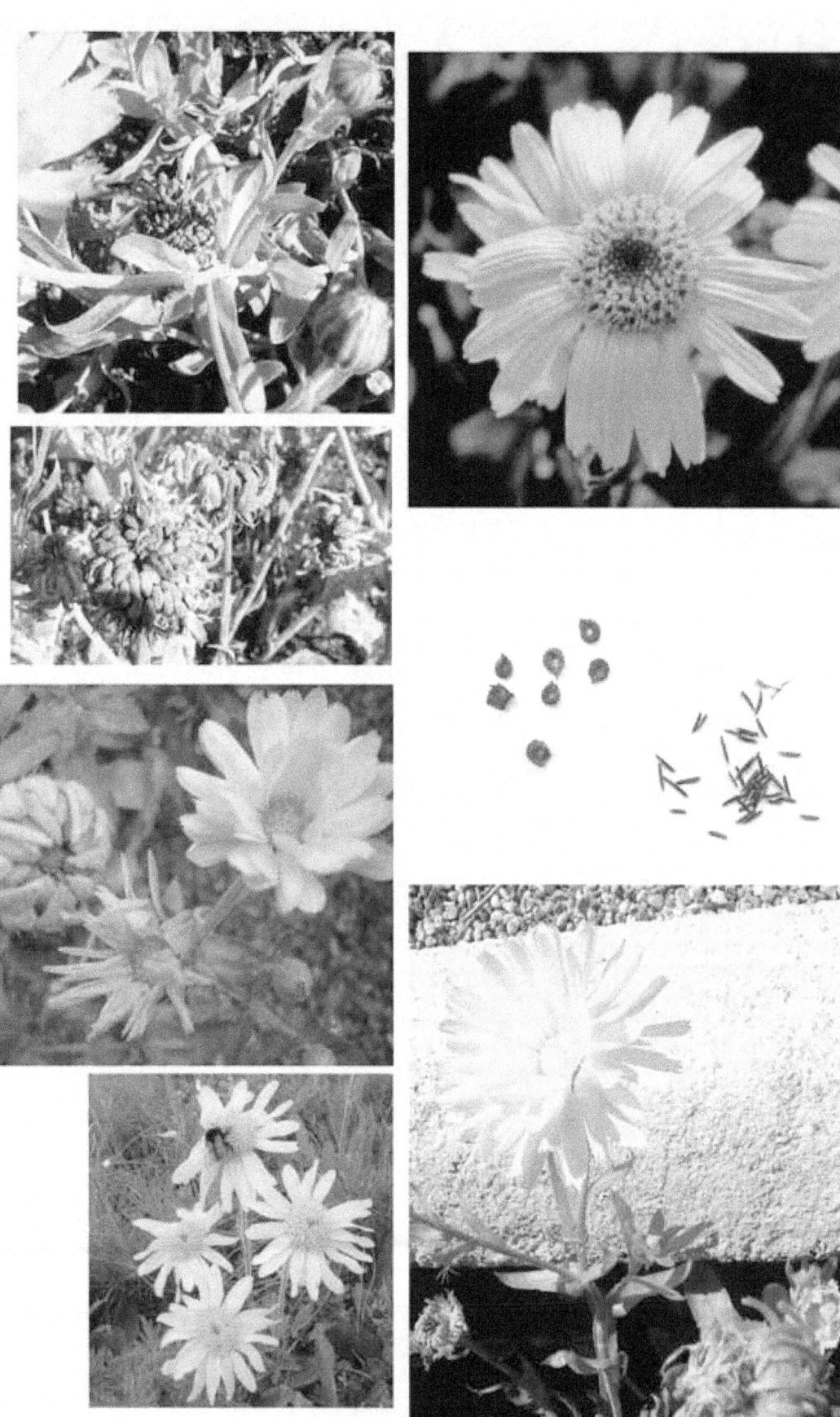

ARNICA
Arnica Montana, Fam. Compositae

Common and Regional Names
Mountain Tobacco, Leopard's Bane, Wolf's Bane, Sneezewort

History and Common Usage
The *A. montana* is both a North American and European native and the official species cited in the US Dispensatory and British Pharmacopeias during the time the Cayce information was being given. Other American natives are: *A. fulgens, A. sororia* and *A. cordifolia. A. cordifolia* is commonly used in over-the-counter preparations in the United States today and *A Montana* is in more common use in Europe. The flowers were official in many pharmacopeias from the 1700's on but the use of the root had fallen out of medical fashion by the 1940's. Arnica is widely distributed today growing wild throughout the mountainous regions of the United States and western and central Europe. The plant takes its name from the Greek word arnakis, meaning lamb's coat, because of its soft, felt-like leaves.

There are no records of exactly when or where arnica first entered into human use as a medicinal plant but it certainly would have been known in Neolithic times and both the root and the flowers have been used in North American and European folk medicine traditions for millennia. It is especially well known and used as a home remedy plant throughout Russia and Siberia.

Despite its widespread anecdotal tradition arnica can be a dangerous plant when used inappropriately. Some folk remedy traditions call for tincture of the root to be taken by mouth, but it is extremely dangerous to take internally. It is an active irritant and produces violent, toxic gastro-enteritis, which, in inexperienced hands, can cause fatal poisoning. It is also important to note that repeated or long-term topical applications of arnica will cause severe inflammation. Some people will have a severe reaction not unlike a bad case of poison ivy. If a reaction like this has occurred any further use will result in an extremely severe and treatment-resistant case of contact dermatitis, even years later. Arnica should never be applied on broken skin or used by people with very thin or sensitive skin. One good test of sensitivity, giving rise to its common name sneezewort, is if the fresh flowers cause sneezing when handled or their scent inhaled the plant should be avoided.

The Native Americans made an arnica based salve for sprains and sore muscles by heating 1 oz of lard with 1 oz of the fresh flowers. They also made a simple tincture for use as a liniment by steeping 2 teaspoons (heaping) of the fresh or dried flowers in a pint of boiling water until cool and bathing the sore area. Weary travelers would sometimes bath their sore feet in this arnica flower footbath. This fresh tincture, made without grain alcohol, does not store and must be made fresh each time.

A tincture which can be stored is made by pouring a pint of 70% grain alcohol (diluted with distilled water) over 2 ounces of freshly picked flowers. Sealed in a clear sterile glass jar it can be left to infuse in a warm place or put out in the sun each day. At the end of 7 days strain the liquid, pour it into a sterile container with an airtight seal and store it out of the light. To use as a lotion combine first with equal portions of distilled witch hazel.

Arnica is safely and readily available for internal use in commercially available homeopathic dosages. It appears in the POCKET MANUAL OF HOMOEOPATHIC MATERIA MEDICA AND REPERTORY[50] by W. Boericke, M.D. as the treatment of choice for injuries, falls, blows and contusions. It is recommended as a remedy in cases of emotional shock, where anxiety, panic and fear are experienced. Arnica based preparations are used today by cosmetic surgeons to reduce pain and swelling for their surgical patients. It is also available from many manufacturers in the form of a salve for use on sore muscles or rubbed on the temples to ease the pain of headaches. Often these salves contain arnica, bee's wax, coca butter and other emollients and aromatics.

Description

Arnica is a low growing, herbaceous perennial. Its bright yellow, (sometimes orange-yellow) flowers resemble the daisy in shape. The flowers are borne from a single, medium-green stem, which grows from 1 to 2 feet in height. The leaves are large, medium to dark green, oval shaped and richly veined. They grow in a rosette fashion at the base of the stem. The stem often bears two leaves independently of the basal rosette and branches out in two or three short stalks, each bearing a single flower.

The root is brown, white on the inside, and covered with a somewhat thickish bark. Short, brittle, somewhat wiry rootlets grow from the bottom. The fresh root smells somewhat aromatic and has an acrid and bitter taste.

Growing Conditions and Propagation

Arnica is a long-lived perennial. It is pollinated by insects and wind and propagates naturally through seeding. It requires a winter dormant season and will not do well where summers are extremely warm. It is naturalized in mountainous regions and high meadows where winters are long and severe.

Seeds are sown directly into prepared soil in the late fall or early spring at a depth no greater than 1/8th of an inch and only lightly covered with loam, peat or planting medium to facilitate germination. In the first year of growth the plant will appear as a rosette, only sending up a stalk and coming to flower at the beginning of the second season of growth. The stem or stalk of arnica is sometimes quite "leggy" and plants have a tendency to lean. Plants can also be easily taken by transplanting from the wild. In some areas small plants can be found along city sidewalks and these endangered orphans appreciate a good home. Once established in the garden new plants can easily be grown through dividing and replanting roots. When conditions are favorable one plant will soon give rise to a small colony.

Arnica prefers full sun, thrives in rich soils, and appreciates the same care as any other cultivated flower in the garden. In the late fall a mulch of leaves and grass will help protect the plant through its first winter. Sufficient water, fertilizer and protection from invasion by insects will ensure its future.

Harvesting

The whole plant can be used in healing but the flowers and root are considered by most sources to contain the more active principles. The flowers can be collected at any time during their June through August blooming season but are always best if picked on the first full day of bloom. The whole flower head can be used but the individual receptacles should be checked for insects and larvae. Receptacles with signs of insect damage should be discarded. The fussy home gardener or Wildcrafter can collect just the petals, discarding the rest. The flowers are spread on screens or spread on cloth to dry. Some sources recommend drying in the open sunlight and others indicate that drying in a warm, dark place produces a superior product. The dried flower parts are best stored in sealed containers and kept out of heat and light.

The root is dug in the fall after the plant has died back and the leaves have turned brown. It is cleaned under cool, running water and the small, wiry rootlets are removed. Larger roots are sliced transversely for faster drying in a warm, dark place until they have reached the brittle stage. They should snap when bent. The dried root should be stored in a sealed container so that it will not take up moisture, and kept out of the light.

Use in the Edgar Cayce Readings
Arnica is a companion plant in the Cayce system, but does not command a significant presence as it is only mentioned in 4 cases. In 2 cases a massage using equal portions of olive oil and arnica was recommended as an application for bruises. In a third case 1 ounce of arnica was combined with other ingredients to make up a compound massage oil. In the fourth the use of arnica was equated to "any good massage" to remove the strain from bruises caused by a fall.

Following are the ways arnica is used the Cayce system.

288-51 F 36
19. (Q) Any special treatment for bruises [on arm] resulting from fall last Sunday?
(A) Use Arnica on same, or any good massage that will remove the strain.

318-3 M 2 Months
4. To bring about the better condition, then, would be through that manipulation of the portions of body in that way of the neuropath or osteopath, and by massaging into this portion of the system those of equal parts of olive oil and arnica, and keep this bandaged until the condition has the chance to heal and strengthen; of course, removing bandage when these manipulations and emplacements are made, which should be done at least every other day, see? and at each time this is done, massage in the system, gently, those properties as given, for the strengthening of the walls.

391-2 M 21
18. For the limbs, we would MASSAGE same thoroughly - as we SHOULD take a GENERAL massage 2 or 3 times a week, other than that as taken in the regular work-out; but in MASSAGING the feet use THIS - as put together to massage into the feet, the soles of the feet, and the ankles:

19. To 1/2 pint of Russian White Oil, add:

> Witch-hazel...................1 ounce,
> Rub alcohol...................2 ounces,
> Arnica........................1 ounce,
> Tincture of Myrrh...........1/2 ounce.

Shake this together and massage just sufficient as to what the body, or the pores of the skin, absorbs.

1129-1 F 32
10. Also we find it would be MOST helpful to have a rub along the whole of the spine and along the limbs with equal portions (or half and half) of Olive Oil and Arnica. Of course, this should not

be massaged over the whole of the area bruised, but where segments or the cerebrospinal and the locomotory forces coordinate in their activity. Heat the oil a little to pour these together and to stir. Then, shake them together and massage gently.

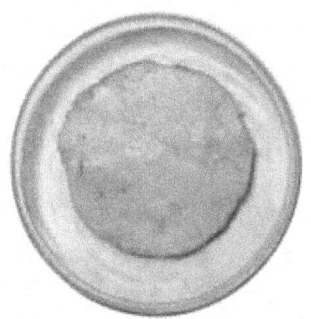

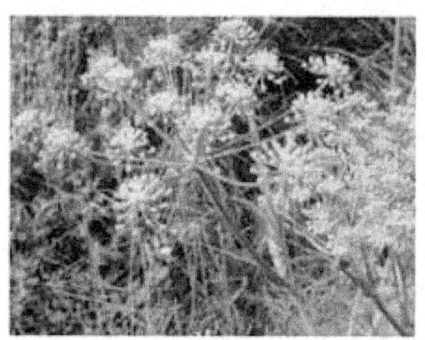

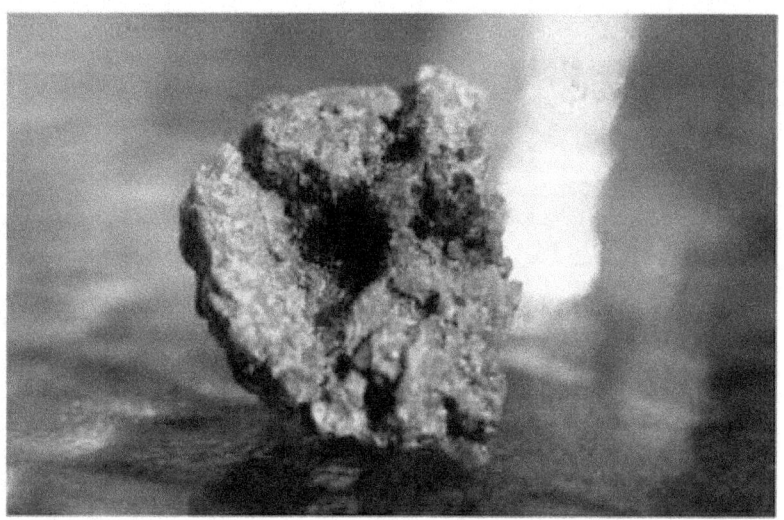

ASAPHOETIDA

Ferula Asafoetida and *Ferula foetida. Fam. Umbelliferae*

Common and Regional Names
Devil's Dung, Food of the Gods, Hing, Kandaharre Hing

History and Common Usage
Ferula asafoetida is native to the high mountain ranges of Afghanistan and to ancient eastern Persia. It is also either indigenous to India or it was imported there in such ancient times as to be beyond the time of memory.

Asaphoetida takes its name from the Persian *aza*, or *asa*, for "mastic" or "resin." Asa is a Latinized form of Farsi, and the Latin *foetidus* means "stinking." And asaphoetida does indeed smell. The odor of the fresh resin has been described as not unlike the smell of rotting fish or akin to rotting garlic.

The Latin name *ferula* means "carrier" or "vehicle." A related species (*F vulgaris*) is native to the Mediterranean and is mentioned in Greek mythology as the plant that helped Prometheus to carry stolen fire from the sun to the earth. It has been suggested that stone-age nomad tribes may have actually used the hollow stems of the plant to transplant fire from camp to camp. Another explanation could be that the stench of the resin carries.

While it was probably in use in native medical traditions from the time of antiquity, and is cited in some records as early as the 12th century, it did not come to the attention of so-called western medicine until 1844 when Alexander Lehmann, a German scientist, discovered and described the plant.

Asaphoetida has long been used as a spice or condiment but is not much appreciated by western palates. It is found in a South Indian (Tamil) spice mixture called *sambar podi*, and is said to be popular with some Brahmins in India who refuse to eat garlic. It is an important ingredient in early Persian cuisine and traces of its use can be found during Roman times. During the Middle Ages in Europe it was used as a flavoring agent in cooking mutton. As a spice asafoetida comes in powdered form and pure resin. Powdered asafoetida loses its aroma after a few years but the resin holds its own year after year. The pure resin has a very strong odor and must be used and stored with care. It is necessary to fry the resin in hot oil for a few moments to dissolve it in the hot fat. This disperses the flavor throughout the food and the high temperature improves the flavor.

Asaphoetida, again fried at a high temperature before continuing the preparation of a dish, will provide an interesting alternative to onion and garlic. A piece of resin the size of an English pea is considered a very large amount and would only be used to flavor a very large pot of food. For those who prefer more delicate flavors a tiny piece of resin can be stored in a jar with pine nuts, a practice developed by the ancient Romans. When the pine nuts have absorbed the aroma and flavor of the resin the nuts can be used to flavor dishes.

The medical use of asafoetida is lost in antiquity and its efficacy as a stimulant, antispasmodic, emmenagogue and a vermifuge have long been known and widely accepted among many indigenous cultures. It relieves gastric irritation and is used among some native cultures in combination with raw morphine and quinine in the treatment of sick headaches. It has been used in the treatment of nervous disorders such as depression and agitation or irritation. It has also been used as a remedy for bronchial cough but its greatest benefit remains as a remedy for disorders of the alimentary tract and as a laxative. Asafoetida is officially listed in modern pharmacopeias as a carminative and a placebo.

Description
Asafoetida is a very large perennial often growing up to 6 or 7 feet in height. It is a coarse plant with a very large, fleshy root from which the resin is obtained. The main trunk or stem of the mature plant is about 6 inches around at the base. The branches or stems are radical, that is they grow from the root base and are quite large, often extending 6 to 10 feet in length, bearing flowers of a pale yellow or greenish yellow color. The fruit containing the seeds is a flat, thin oval, reddish brown in color and with a strong and unpleasant odor.

The fleshy and bristling root of the plant is several inches in diameter with a coarse and hairy aspect. It is similar in shape to a parsnip but the bark is wrinkled and somewhat blackish in color. The internal structure of the root is fleshy and white.

The Tibetan asaphoetida called *Narthex Asafetida* is closely related to the *Ferula*. Some of the asaphoetida used commercially today comes from this variety.

Growing Conditions and Propagation
Asaphoetida is self-fertile having both male and female flowers and it is pollinated by insects and wind and propagates by seeds. It prefers a desert habitat and is indigenous to the high and dry mountainous regions of present day Afghanistan and eastern Iran with extremes of temperature and poor soil. It is not hardy in sustained temperatures colder than -10° F. The plant is monocarpic, that is, it only flowers once [usually in July] and then the plant goes to seed and dies.

Seeds are preferably sown in a protected environment in the autumn. In the following spring the young plants should be placed in prepared soil in a permanent location. Asafoetida needs full sun. If grown in areas where temperatures do not fall below their life zone tolerance the plants should be mulched for their first winter outdoors. Out of its native habitat gardeners can expect that an asafoetida will grow for at least 5 years before it flowers and dies.

Harvesting
The plant is ready to yield gum-resin when the leaves have begun to decay at the end of the growing season. The root-leaves are then twisted off close to the root and the soil is cleared from the crown of the taproot. The large root crown is then covered [burlap is a good choice] and protected from sunlight throughout the period of harvest.

The resin of the plant is harvested by successive cuttings made to the upper part of the large root, which has to be protected from sunlight during the entire process to prevent lose of the resin through evaporation. Thirty to forty days after the leaves are removed a thin slice of the crown is removed causing the milky juice to bleed from the root and the root is carefully re-covered. The milky juice hardens naturally and can be scraped off and preserved in a clean container but one left open to the air. This allows for further hardening through evaporation. Another cut is made and the hardened sap of the plant is again scraped away from the root and saved. This process continues until the root will yield no more juice.

Next the resin must be purified. This is done by heating the accumulated "tears" of resin in a glass or stainless steel pan over low heat and when liquefied the resin is poured through a cloth similar to a jelly bag to remove impurities such as bits of bark from the root or grains of sand. Squeeze the bag to save as much of the liquid as possible.

The residue is then cooled and formed into small balls of a size desired for use in flavoring foods. These "tears" or small amounts of the pure resin will keep for many years if stored in a cool place in sealed containers.

The hardened resin can be quickly pulverized in a home blender or food processor into a manageable powder, but only if it is kept very cold during this process. Once the powder has been obtained it too should be stored in airtight containers and stored in a cool place.

Use in the Edgar Cayce Readings

Asaphoetida is used as a companion plant but the Cayce system departs somewhat from traditional and modern medical use. It is recommended 7 times as an extremely effective remedy against flu, cold and congestion when small amounts are taken in combination with common aspirin.

In 2 cases the amounts of aspirin and asaphoetida are not given. In 5 cases the amount of asaphoetida is to be 5 grains and the amount of aspirin is given as 5 grains.

In the remaining individuals the amount of aspirin recommended varied. In 2 cases asaphoetida and aspirin was to be swallowed with a "gill[51] or two" of HOT spirits frumenti[52]

The following analysis of the ratio of aspirin to asaphoetida shows the variations in dosages in the 7 cases:

Reading	Aspirin	Asaphoetida	HOT spirits frumenti	Alopen
286-2	5 grains	3 grains		
288-21	2 aspirins	5 grain pill	1 jigger	1 pill
341-25	amounts not given			
900-381	10 grains	5 grains in pellets		2 gills
1010-8	10 grains	5 grains		
1073-2	10 to 15 grains	5 grains	a gill or 2	
3518-1	2 aspirins	5 grains		1 pill

This is a typical recommendation for Asaphoetida and aspirin:

1010-8 F 64 FLU
3. Then we would take ten grains of Aspirin with five grains of Asaphoetida - the properties that will make for an allaying of the temperatures that arise from the influence of too great an activity of the leucocytes splitting up, or the mucous membranes becoming irritated or inflamed by the cold or congestions.

4. These, as we find, taken once in the evening, again in the morning, should make for a relief.

---

51   A gill – 4 fluid ounces.
52   Rye whiskey

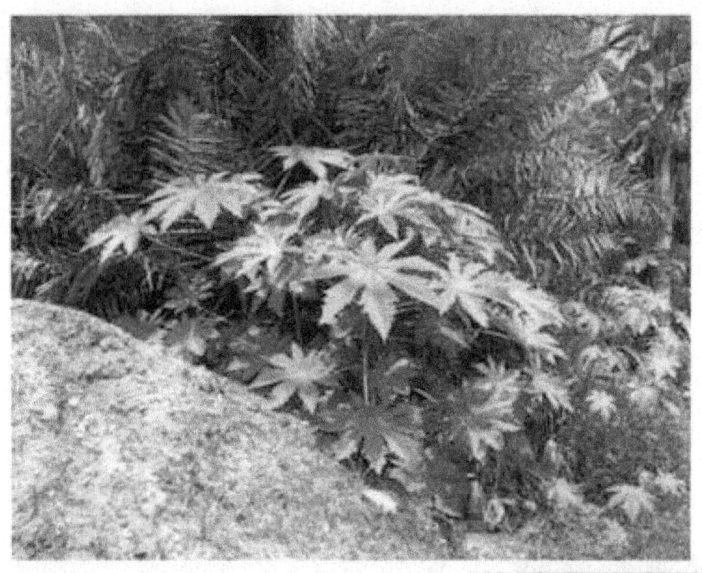

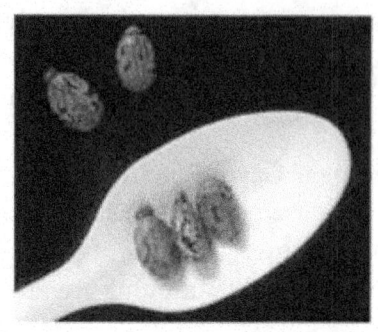

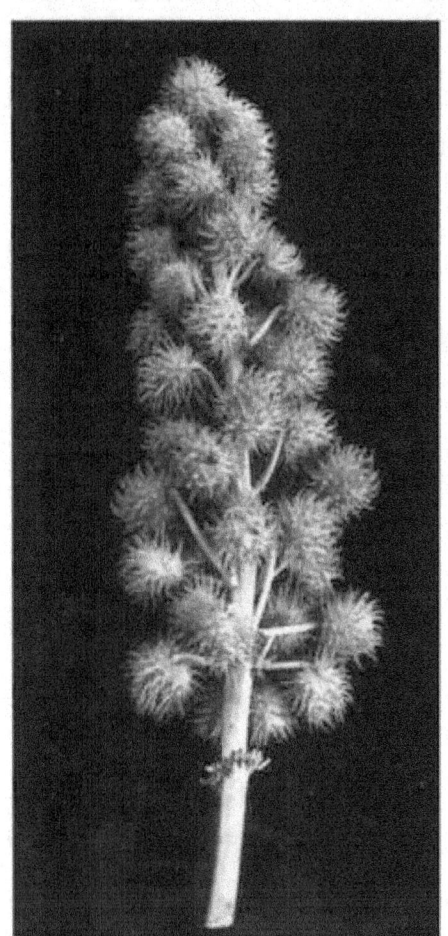

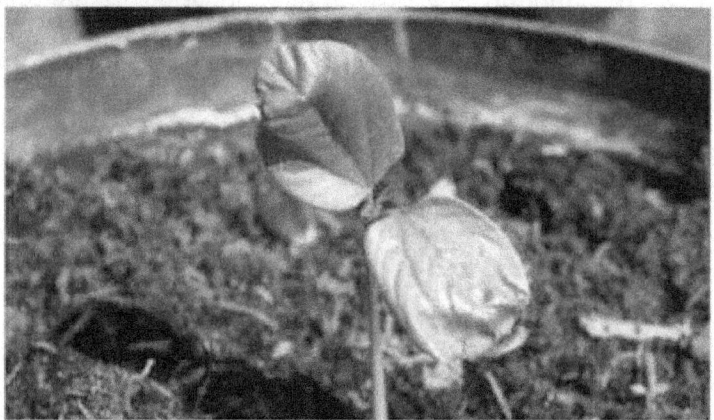

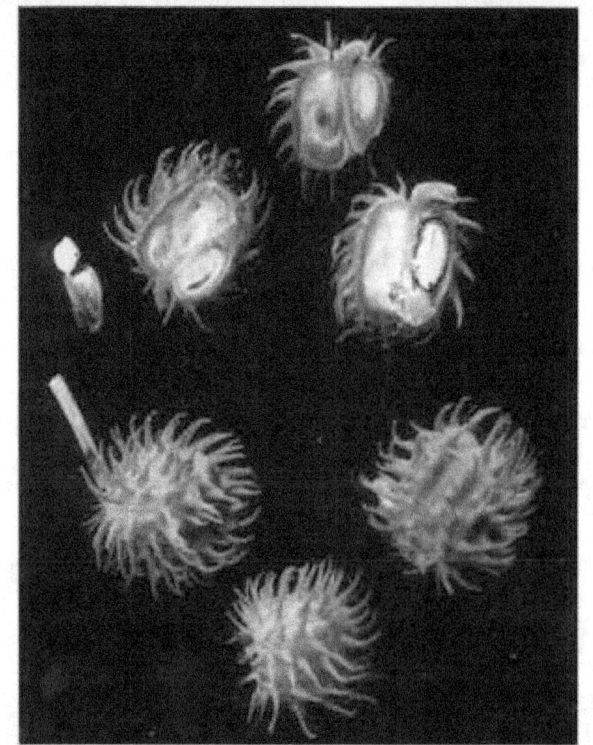

CASTOR
Ricinus communis, Fam. Euphorbiaceae

Common and Regional Names
Mole Beans, Castor Bean, Mamona, Ricino, Mamoeira, Mexico Seed, Jonah's Gourd, Oil Plant, Wonder Tree, Palma Christi

History and Common Usage
The history of *Ricinus communis* is as old as the human use of plants. Knowledge of castor is recorded in the Ebers Papyrus: *"To know what is made with the ricinus-plant according to that which was found in old writings as something useful to men."* Castor is also mentioned in the very earliest surviving records from the Greeks and Romans being mentioned by Pliny the Elder as a "drastic purgative." The present scientific name of the plant, *Ricinus*, means tick in Latin, and was so named by the Romans for its resemblance in shape to an engorged dog tick. The seeds are brownish-tan in color and mottled in distinctive patterns. No two seeds have the same pattern.

The Greek historian Herodotus knew of *Ricinus communis* referring to it in his writings as Kiki.[53] Five hundred years before the birth of Christ, he records that the oil was used in "earlier times" by the Egyptians as he found the seeds in their "ancient tombs" during his travels there. In his Account of Egypt Herodotus describes the use of the castor plant as follows:

"And for anointing those of the Egyptians who dwell in the fens use oil from the castor-berry, which oil the Egyptians call kiki, and thus they do:--they sow along the banks of the rivers and pools these plants, which in a wild form grow of themselves in the land of the Hellenes; these are sown in Egypt and produce berries in great quantity but of an evil smell; and when they have gathered these some cut them up and press the oil from them, others again roast them first and then boil them down and collect that which runs away from them. The oil is fat and not less suitable for burning than olive-oil, but it gives forth a disagreeable smell."

The Syrians do not seem to have used the plant as it is not listed in The Book of Medicines. It remained in use as a purgative in the practice of Graeco-Roman medicine until Arabian physician Mesue[54] [Jahiah Ebben Masawaih] began to promote the use of senna. More palatable than castor oil, senna is also much milder in action and therefore more comfortable to use. Senna is also recommended by Cayce in over 200 cases.

Ricinus communis is thought to have originated in what are today the geographical regions of Asia and Africa. Present day India is certainly one of the places of origination and the plant is known there by several ancient Sanskrit names, the oldest being Eranda, which has now passed into several other Indian languages.

The name castor, sometimes erroneously seen as "caster," entered the official London Pharmacopoeia in 1788. A British physician by the name of Peter Canvane,[55] a member of the Royal College of Physicians in London, England, is credited with resurrecting its medical use after investigating the use of the oil. He properly identified the plant and discovered the Spanish referred to it by the common name Palma Christi or "Palm of Christ," a name by which it is still known by today. Since the 1780's it has been

---

53   Coptic language for the word Egypt as well as the castor plant
54   777-857 A.D.
55   Peter Canvane. 1720-1786

retained as a purgative in many pharmacopoeias around the world. Castor oil has also been used as a lubricant, a lamp fuel, as a source of "Red Turkey" dye in the textile industry and as a dressing for leather. In folk remedy traditions dating from the time of antiquity to the present, a *small* dose of castor oil can be used to induce labor.

Today *Ricinus communis* is grown commercially for a dizzying array of uses ranging from organic manure, to its derivatives being used in food additives, textile chemicals, disinfectants, paper, plastics and rubber, perfumeries, polyurethane, pharmaceuticals, [glycerine being one of the best known derivatives] paints and other coatings, inks and adhesives, lubricants. Castrol is a well known brand name for use in jet engines and racing cars, cosmetics [lipstick or shampoo may contain over one third castor oil] and in electronics and telecommunications.

Castor is commercially grown in India and Brazil, the West Indies, Africa, Asia and the United States. The 100 year old H.J. Baker & Brothers is the largest American manufacturer in the industry. Over 18,000 acres are presently under cultivation in the United States in Arizona, Oklahoma and California.

In ancient times the oil was extracted by the simple method of heaping seeds in bowls set in the hot sun and collecting the exuded oil. In parts of India today the oil is extracted by boiling the seeds in water and skimming off the oil. The oil – thick and viscous with a strong odor - is then strained and bleached in the sun before storage. Oil is commercially produced today by heating the beans in large ovens after which the warm beans are broken up by grinding, flaking, or rolling and the oil extracted by means of a continuous screw press exerting pressure as high as 30,000 pounds per square inch. Smaller extraction operations produce what is called cold pressed oil through cold expression [water cooled extrusion] but further clarification and purification of the oil must still be done by heating the oil to 140°F for 20 minutes before it is safe to use.

The leaves, stalks and roots of all varieties are mildly poisonous if eaten but the poison is concentrated in the shells of the seeds. Called ricin, or ricinoleic acid, it was first described in 1889. Another toxin is present in the seeds called *ricinus communis agglutinin* or RCA for short. RCA is only toxic if injected into the bloodstream where it causes disintegration of red blood cells. Poisoning by ingestion of the castor bean is due to ricin which penetrates the intestinal wall resulting in life threatening dehydration accompanied by painful bloody diarrhea within hours.

The oil itself is not harmful provided no cross-contamination occurred during production. Because it is water-soluble ricin does not partition into the oil during the extraction process and ricin is rendered harmless by heating to 140°F for 20 minutes. This makes heating the oil a very critical step in the extraction process.

Research today suggests that ricin can be targeted to specific cells, such as cancer cells to kill the cells. RTA-immunotoxins [a 267-amino acid globular protein found in ricin] have been successfully used to destroy T lymphocytes in bone marrow transplants.[56] This area of research shows promise for the future.

---

56   Woo BH, Lee JT, Lee KC. Stability and cytotoxicity of Fab-ricin A immunotoxins prepared with water soluble long chain heterobifunctional crosslinking agents.
College of Pharmacy, SungKyunKwan University, Suwon, Korea. 1994 Dec;17
SB Kornfeld, JE Leonard, MD Mullen and R Taetle Department of Medicine, University of California, San Diego. Assessment of ligand effects in intracellular trafficking of ricin A chain using anti-ricin hybridomas Cancer Research, Vol 51, Issue 6 1689-1693, Copyright © 1991 by American Association for Cancer Research

The 21st edition of the United States Dispensatory lists castor as an official drug plant citing its use as a purgative and an emollient. It also indicates that research, now 80 odd years old, revealed ricin produced an antitoxin exactly analogous to those produced by the body against bacteria when injected in small amounts. This information may someday shed further light on the mystery of the healing properties of the oil recommended so often in the Cayce system, yet still does not address the remarkable efficacy of the oil when applied to the *outside* of the body in the form of abdominal packs.

Description

Ricinus communis is the only species in its genus. It is not a true bean but a member of the spurge family. There are several varieties of *Ricinus*, some boasting reddish or purple leaves, and there are two pigmented garden varieties suitable for northern climates called *R. Bronze King* and *R. Africanus*. The original ricinus varieties have been improved upon through selective breeding to produce dwarf hybrids capable of producing a ton of beans per acre for commercial growers. These plants yield 50% of their weight in oil. Hale and Lynn are two such cultivars.

This shrub-like plant has greenish stems that grow in ringed sections similar to bamboo. The stem color varies from green to tan as the plant ages. In the tropics the plants can resemble a tree sometimes found 30 feet in height. They are usually found between 10 and 12 feet tall with large umbrella-like alternating leaves with between 5 and 9 sharply pointed and serrated finger-like lobes. The leaves can grow as large as 30 inches across and make dramatic additions to large floral arrangements. The flowers are small and very exotic in appearance. They are born on stems within the interior of the plant emerging from the stalk and stems closest to the stalk. They are produced in narrow, upright clusters, first as greenish buds that later develop into short fringe or string-like petals in a variety of brilliant colors of red, pink and yellow depending upon the variety grown.

The seeds from which the oil is obtained are produced in greenish blue, soft spiny round pods. Each three lobed pod contains three seeds. The mature beans or seeds are dark brown to black or even brownish reddish in color with irregular white or tan spots and if the shell remains intact are usually not harmful even if swallowed. Once the seed coat or shell is cracked or chewed and ingested signs of poisoning can manifest up to 18 to 24 hours later. The symptoms of castor bean poisoning are abdominal pain, vomiting and diarrhea followed by severe dehydration, a decrease in urine and a decrease in blood pressure. If death has not occurred in three to five days the victim usually recovers. Children must be treated immediately as dehydration can become life threatening in a matter of hours.

Horses are extremely susceptible to the ricin toxin. Immediate medical intervention is critical to their survival if even the smallest amount of seeds, seed cake or meal have been ingested. Horses cannot vomit so immediate lavage of the stomach represents their only hope of recovery. Castor should not be allowed to grow near pasturelands used by any grazing animals. Young children are also especially at risk. Plants that are grown where unsupervised children are present should at least be docked and not allowed to flower and come to seed.

Castor seeds are also known in the United States as "mole beans." The seeds are left in mole tunnels as edible bait. An interesting historical endnote on the subject of poison is the suspected use of ricin in 1978 to assassinate Georgi Markov,[57] a Bulgarian journalist who spoke out against the Bulgarian government. He was stabbed with the point of an umbrella while waiting at a bus stop near Waterloo

---

57   1929-1978. Writer and political dissident. http://www.rferl.org/specials/markov/

Station in London. A perforated metallic pellet imbedded in his leg had presumably contained the ricin toxin. Since the poison was administered by injection it suggests that the poison was *ricinus communis agglutinin* or RCA.

Growing Conditions and Propagation

Castor is pollinated by insects and wind. Where winters are not too severe it proliferates from an underground root system producing whole colonies of plants. These colonies spread year after year preferring to grow along stream beds and rivers. The stalks are usually found from ½ inch to 6 inches in diameter. When naturalized in tropical zones it is considered a long-lived perennial taking on the aspect of a tree rather than a shrub or plant and the trunk or stalk can be 8 to even 12 inches in diameter. In warmer Mediterranean countries such as Algeria, Egypt, Greece and the Riviera it attains an average height of 10 to 15 feet but in more northern climes it shrinks to 4 to 5 feet. *Ricinus communis* is classified as an annual in the temperate zones. Seeds have been documented to ripen as far north as Christiana in Norway.

The plant is very ornamental and fast growing. It prefers a well-drained soil, preferably a moisture retentive clay and does best in full sun. It will flower and bear seeds simultaneously in its first year. *Ricinus* propagates through natural seed casting and through its roots. Seeds can be sown outside in their permanent location when there is no danger of frost. They can be covered with an inch or two of soil or simply scattered on the surface of the ground.

In colder climates the seeds are started indoors in pots filled with two thirds loam and one-third leaf mold and kept where the temperature will remain above the minimum of 60°F required for germination. This can take up to three or four weeks. Once the seedlings are established they should be planted in their permanent location provided all danger of frost is past.

Ricinus communis makes a good screening plant. If grown as an annual where cold temperatures are below its tolerance, the plant can still reach 6 to 8 feet in height during the summer. High wind will easily damage its tender leaves and break the stalks of young plants. It makes a beautiful showing in sunny, moderately sheltered corners. If the plants are successful and naturalize, it bears repeating that great care must be taken to prevent accidental exposure or ingestion of seeds by humans and animals.

Harvesting

The fruiting structure of the plant can grow to 24 inches in length. As the blue-green, soft, spiny, three lobed pods mature seams can be seen resembling a thin white line. This line, seam or suture spreads to actually split the spiny sections [called carpels] apart as they mature and dry, revealing a tan inner capsule or shell. At maturity the shell cracks open quite suddenly expelling the seed. This sudden action of seed casting is called dehiscence and it is quite audible. In order to collect as many seeds as possible the entire stem is cut from the plant when the white lines are clearly noticeable and spread or hung to dry.

During the drying process seeds can be expelled as far as thirty feet. The heavy stems are spread on tarpaulins or sheets to facilitate collection and need to be protected from rain. They can also be hung vertically on lines or poles, shielded on all sides by tarpaulins or sheets. When drying is finished, the seeds which are not expelled naturally are extracted by hand hulling. The capsules are rubbed between gloved hands, winnowed or shaken on coarse screens to remove extraneous materials, or picked over by hand. It is important to keep the seeds that are gathered by hand hulling separate because expelled seeds have a higher rate of germination than those harvested by hulling. The naturally expelled seeds are stored in brown paper bags in a dry place and will retain roughly 70% viability for up to 2 years.

In cases of extreme emergency beans can be crushed and mashed with a hammer on cheesecloth and the material applied directly to the body in the form of a primitive pack or poultice. To avoid accidental poisoning from ingesting the raw ricin the hammer should be washed, well rinsed and stored where it will not be accidently used to crack edible nuts. Even if heated to the required 140 degrees for a full 20 minutes, oil extracted at home should never be used internally.

Considering the labor-intensive nature of extraction, not to mention the danger of accidental poisoning should insufficient heat be applied to render the ricin harmless, it is safer and cheaper to avail oneself of oil purchased through commercial sources.

Use in the Cayce Readings
Castor is not a companion plant in the Cayce model. Considered the flagship of all Cayce plants castor is mentioned in over 500 transcripts. The testimonies for its efficacy are legion. It is often used as a massage oil, especially recommended for sprains and joint injuries, rarely recommended internally, and is most frequently to be applied over the abdominal area in the form of a pack.

Flannel, preferably well used flannel, is the material of choice for the pack, and provided it is properly stored, it can be used and re-used time after time proving a most economical home health remedy. Generalized directions call for using the pack one hour a day for three days in succession as follows:

2645-1 F 60 Eliminations
14. First, begin with the application of Castor Oil Packs over the liver area, for at least an hour each day for three days. Use at least three thicknesses of flannel, preferably old flannel - not new. This would be saturated in Castor Oil and applied over the liver area. Let this extend well over the liver AND the caecum area on the right side. Apply as warm as can be well stood, and then apply the electric pad - after covering same so as to prevent soiling of linens or the clothing, and allow this to remain on at low heat for the full period.

15. Rest for three days, then have the Oil Packs again for three days, one hour each day.

While 3 days in succession is generally recommended there are acute situations which call for the packs to be used 5 days in succession:

2153-1 F
7. In the beginning, then - we would apply hot Castor Oil Packs directly to the body, over the lower portion of the liver, the lacteal duct center, and extending to the caecum area. Use at least three thicknesses of flannel that is soaked or saturated in Castor Oil. Apply this as warm as may be handled comfortably, though not too hot. Then cover it with cloths, and an electric pad put over same. Let this remain on for at least an hour each day for five days.

The pack is stored in a covered plastic or glass container which is pre-heated if desired in a low oven or on a heating pad. The type of flannel is not specified. The information only states from time to time that "old flannel" is desirable. Over the years of working with various types of material and hundreds of patients, Dr. Harold J. Reilly came to recommend wool flannel as it was cheap and readily available, and because cotton flannel becomes almost too heavy for comfort when completely saturated. While it works very well, wool is actually mentioned only once in the over 550 cases where castor oil packs are mentioned:

650-1 F 22 ADHESIONS:PELVIC CELLULITIS
9. ... begin with the Castor Oil packs over the LIVER area and the ducts of the assimilating system [that is, the whole right side from the upper rib area to the hip]. [Use three to four thicknesses of flannel or wool material, dipped in hot Castor Oil.] Keep these packs hot, applying them for two to three hours each day.

In the following old flannel is recommended:

2645-1 F 60 Eliminations
14. First, begin with the application of Castor Oil Packs over the liver area, for at least an hour each day for three days. Use at least three thicknesses of flannel, preferably old flannel - not new. This would be saturated in Castor Oil and applied over the liver area. Let this extend well over the liver AND the caecum area on the right side. Apply as warm as can be well stood, and then apply the electric pad - after covering same so as to prevent soiling of linens or the clothing, and allow this to remain on at low heat for the full period.

The exact physiological mechanism of the pack is so far unclear; however abdominal packs are used in a wide range of disorders. It is used in the treatment of conditions ranging from arthritis, cirrhosis of the liver, scleroderma, gall stones, to improving the immune system, or as a simple aid to improving assimilations and eliminations.

Clarification by Cayce of the action of the pack within the body appears in only a few transcripts. For example in 1055-1 for a 50 year old man suffering from stomach lacerations and adhesions the information states: *"The effect of the Castor Oil Poultice or the Castor Oil Pack is to loosen the adhesion..."* In transcript 19-4, a case of a 52 year old man with severe intestinal difficulties including a prolapsed colon the information advises castor oil is used to: *"... arouse the liver to activity; that is, across the liver area extending over the duodenum and the upper portion of the bowel; with those of castor oil packs as hot as the body can well stand them..."* In case 1151-31 the information states: *"The Castor Oil Pack is to act upon the nerve forces and the energy activities through the liver itself."*

Certainly one of the most hopeful applications of castor oil is in the treatment of scleroderma, a disease at present thought to be an incurable auto-immune disorder. Cayce states that scleroderma is caused by a tubercle germ:

2514-1 F 22 SCLERODERMA
8. We find that this arises from those conditions that are a part of the combination of disturbances - producing a tubercle in the superficial forces in the lymph and the emunctory portions of the body in the skin itself.

Other cases suggest the same cause for this rare and dreaded disorder:

528-3 F 28 SCLERODERMA:CURED

3. …very subtle nature and unless there can be some activities produced in which there is assistance to the vitality of the body, in resisting the inroads of a tubercle in the nature in which it is involving not only those areas through the respiratory system but even the structural portions of the body, from which the blood supply attains or gains its division of a supply of element from which the red blood cells are builded, we find that the condition will rapidly continue to make inroads.

Mrs. 528 recovered and provided the following testimony years later:

528-16 F 30 SCLERODERMA:CURED

R17. 3/61 HLC taped an interview with Mrs. [528] via telephone in …, KY She said: "I became ill about eight months before I obtained the first rdg. for the condition [528-3] on 1/14/37. I was examined at the Haggert Clinic in Nashville, Tenn. At first I had symptoms something like flu or malaria. That is what they first thought I had. There was a generalized aching all over the body, and a low grade temperature. By the time I had the rdg. I was hard - all the flesh from the hips to the knees was just as hard as it could be. I was not suffering pain, except just the aching. All the upper part of my body was swollen, and when I smiled my face was so swollen that I couldn't see out of my eyes. I had a pone [hardness] all down my back, and my arms were swollen. I was swollen all over my body except from my knees to my feet, and from my hips to my thighs the flesh was HARD. My condition was getting progressively worse at the time I obtained the reading. The main treatment, as I remember, was Castor Oil Packs. I had to lie in these packs for three hours at a time, three times a day; in for three hours and out for two hours, and there was some medication but I have forgotten what it was. A little later the Wet Cell Appliance was recommended, and I did use it. Later on the olive oil rubs were advised.

"In a week's time after beginning the treatments the swelling began to leave my face, and it just gradually left. By the summer of 1937 the swelling was just in my thighs a little bit. In September of 1937 I went back to work, as an organist at the Methodist Church.

"Yes, I completely recovered. In 1942 I got married and am still married but have no children. I am still active as an organist and have had no return of the trouble."

3108-1 F 67 SCLERODERMA:CURED

8. Then the effect this has upon the general nervous system, not only from the sources of the disturbance – an infection in the epidermis that causes this consuming, and thus is a form of tubercle of the skin force itself. Yet in the type of circulation produced it brings the acids in conjunction with the activity of air upon those portions of the limbs, and along portions of the buttocks and back, and gives a great deal of pain as well as discoloration, and changes that gradually come about in the texture as well as of the skin itself.

The treatment for scleroderma consists of a number of therapies including the wet-cell appliance, dietary changes, use of the charred oak keg as an inhalation therapy [See commentary on apples], massage with various oils and the most important and unusual of all – wrapping the affected areas of the body in warm castor oil packs and leaving them on for long periods of time.

Internal Use

Internal use of the oil as a laxative is limited to 5 cases. Statistically the Cayce system seems to favor the abdominal pack over using the oil internally as a purgative. One of the 5 cases provides this humorous answer to a 49 year old gentleman suffering from a severe case of lumbago:

348-18 M 49
11. [Q] In the present would it be better for the body to remain in bed or without moving about?
[A] It'll move when you give it the Castor Oil, and that'll be soon enough!

On the rare occasions calling for castor oil to be taken by mouth, it is considerately recommended to combine it with something like root beer to make it more palatable.

Crushed Beans

As mentioned above packs of crushed beans can be used, if oil is not available:

2514-6 F 23 Scleroderma
13. [Q] In case Castor Oil cannot be obtained in the future, could anything be used as a substitute?
[A] Mole beans may be rolled and used as packs - or the Castor bean. But it will not be so this cannot be obtained, for such conditions.

Even the castor bean meal is recommended in one case:

5449-3 F Adult Cholecystitis
We would apply castor oil packs, or castor bean meal will be more effective in this particular condition but will be more RADICAL in its action. Castor oil packs, though, over the liver area - these kept up for a period sufficient to produce a reaction; that is, don't put on one pack and then not put on any more for a week or so - for that would mean very little. It would be like trying to stop a millpond by putting up a little log or a little mud in same. Keep these up continuously for four, five, six, seven hours - as fast as one is cool place on another, until there is a REACTION.

Recommended as a massage oil castor is used for a great variety of physical conditions; it is however, very messy. It can be cleansed from the skin by sponging the area with a solution made from one heaping teaspoonful of common bicarbonate of soda to a gallon of warm water.

The following case is that of a woman recovering from mastoid surgery, the after effects of which affected the flow of nervous energy resulting in the formation of small moles and other skin problems. Among other treatments she was advised to have a weekly massage:

5300-1 F 65 ICTHYOSIS
5. Some aid may be indicated if there will be used a Castor Oil massage; messy, very messy, but massage all that can be massaged into the body, at least once a week, especially around the middle portion, around the diaphragm area, over the abdomen, parts of the feet, along the back, all that the body can absorb.

Castor Oil is recommended in cases of painful bunions and combined with baking soda to help remove warts:

303-13 F

8. (Q) What is the best way to remove warts?
(A) This one on the right knee is gradually leaving. Put equal portions of Castor Oil and Soda on the finger tip, massage this, it'll make it sore but it'll take it away also.

1688-9 F 31

16. (Q) Is there anything that can be done to make a bunion less painful?
(A) Massage same with Castor Oil, and occasionally - though not every night, about twice a week - mix baking soda with same. This will make it very tender, but - with the other massage - will remove the causes of it.

759-10 M 5

6. (Q) What will eliminate the warts from the hand and body?
(A) Massage them with Castor Oil.

7. (Q) How often?
(A) Every evening.

8. (Q) When should we see results from this treatment for the warts?
(A) In two to three weeks.

While testimonies to the efficacy of castor oil are legion, its reputation has frequently resulted in some creativity in its use, sometimes in ways not found in the Cayce system. Only a few testimonies are included here, and only those published on the current CD of the Cayce transcripts are cited as a reminder of the efficacy of this ancient remedy.

12/1/72
"About 3 months ago I had a large mole on my neck right at the collar. The shirt collar kept irritating it. I read about using Castor Oil, so I swabbed some on and put a band-aid on it. In about a week it started to shrink and I kept up the swabbing. Then by the end of the second week it was very dry with a thin strand holding on. A few days later it fell off and since hasn't come back."

R. J. Marciniak,
2651 W. Belden Ave.,
Chicago, Ill. 60647

6/29/75
"I have just finished reading an article from the July, A.R.E. Journal entitled, 'Laying On of Hands.'

"The story was very significant for me because I had an experience similar to that woman. I too had discovered a lump in my breast and was told to see a surgeon as soon as possible. My doctor told me he thought it was a cyst and not a tumor but in any event should be removed.

"I had read where Castor Oil Packs on external cysts, warts and moles were beneficial but I hadn't read where it was recommended for the breast. Well I applied the packs faithfully for about a week. I even fell asleep once with a pack on! Almost immediately the size of the lump decreased. During this time I meditated daily. I say this only because I often miss a day or two and I know meditation has a healing effect on the body.

"During the next month I continued the packs but only once every two days.

"It is now two months later since finding the lump and it has disappeared. I returned to my doctor and after examining me found everything normal. He asked if I saw the surgeon and I replied, "no"... Whatever - the lump is gone and I feel the Castor Oil had a lot to do with it."

Mrs. Richard T. Brand,
Yonkers, New York

R7. 1/75 Mrs. Vincent Martina, Rt. 1, Box 1, Wayland, N.Y. 14572 wrote: "Two years ago someone told me to apply castor oil to several large warts on my son's feet and spreading to his hands, which I had been trying to ignore as I had heard the cost involved with a dermatologist [something like $12 a wart for X-ray.]

"We put it on each wart daily and covered with bandaids. And within a few days out popped all the small ones and in a day or two more all the large ones, all leaving a neat little crater, which filled in no time.

"Have been broadcasting this all over ever since."

6/26/79
To Whom It May Concern:

I have had trouble with splitting, breaking fingernails for several years...always a source of embarrassment.

It would be difficult to estimate the amount of time and money that I have spent over the years to correct the problem.

... I began to massage a drop of Castor Oil into each nail and cuticle area daily, about a month ago. THE RESULTS HAVE BEEN SOMETHING ELSE!

If this is not a part of your file, perhaps someone would like to experiment with the idea and test it. I'm sure there would be many who would be grateful for such an easy, inexpensive cure for splitting nails.

A. Mitchell
C.N.S., INC.
Box 8331
Coral Springs, FL. 33065

2/4/2002
To Whom It May Concern:
I am writing this short testimony to speak to the effectiveness of the use of Castor Oil Packs in my own life.

In 1951 I had abdominal surgery and many years later, about 1974, I developed severe pains in my lower abdomen in the area of the surgery. I went to several doctors, including a homeopath. I had many tests and after a great deal of diagnostic work no one was able to tell me what was causing such pain.

In about 1980 or 1981 I was introduced to the Edgar Cayce readings and learned of the abdominal Castor Oil

Packs. I followed the readings, using the packs for 5 days in succession for 1 or more hours at a time. I then rested from the treatment for 2 days. I continued this process for 2 months. That was 21 years ago, and I have not experienced that disabling pain since.

You are free to use my name and I will be happy to tell anyone about my experience.
Sincerely yours,
Mildred N. Latimer
Virginia Beach, Virginia

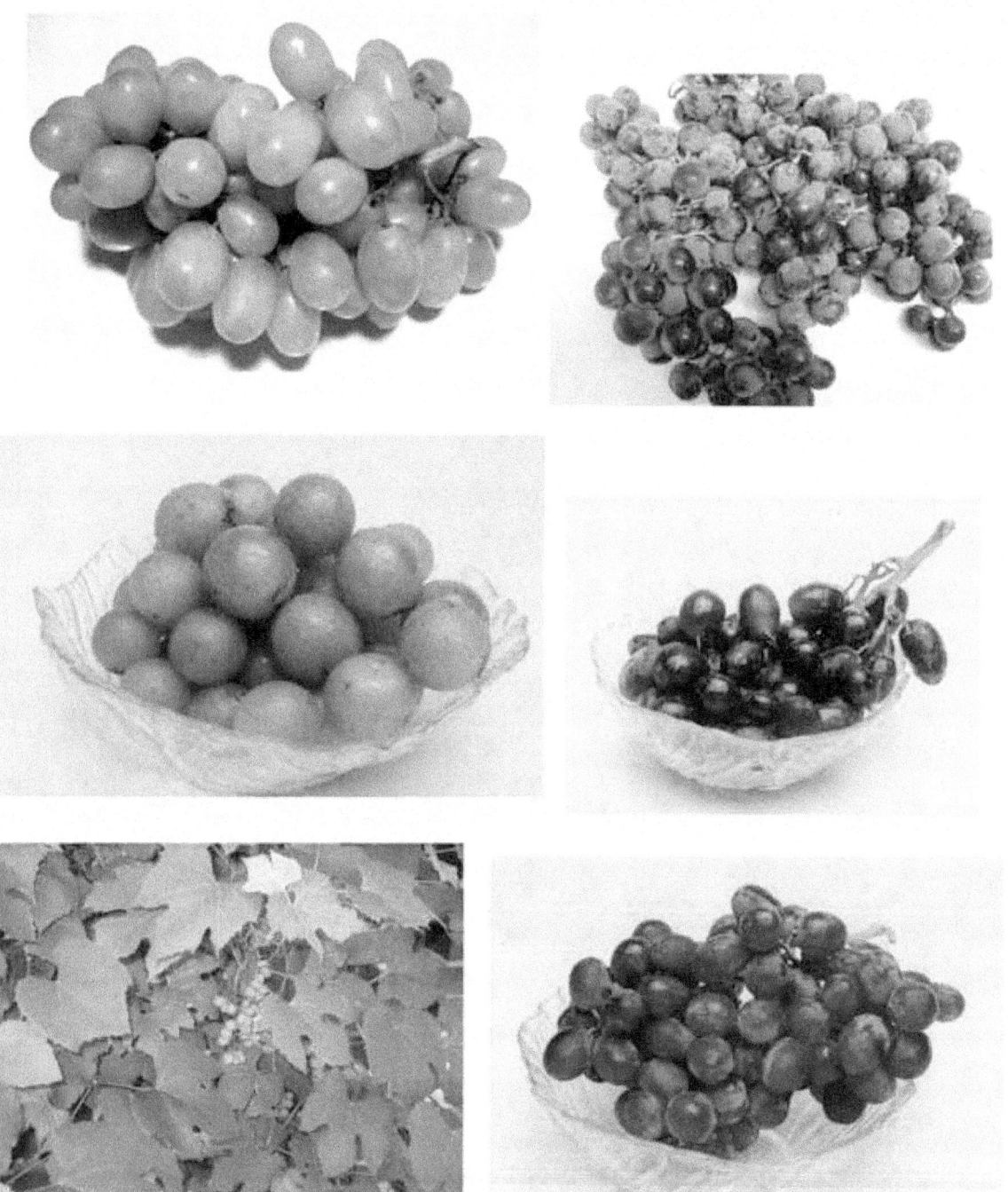

GRAPES

Vitis vinifera, Fam. Vitaceae

Common and Regional Names
None

History and Common Usage

The ancestor of the modern grape dates to some 23.3 to 5.2 million years ago making it a companion of the great mastodon. Fossilized remains of grape seeds, vines and leaves have been found in Northern Hemisphere deposits dating from the Miocene and Tertiary epochs. Thought to have originated in the area of the Black Sea grape take its place along side the fig as the two earliest cultivated plants on earth. They have been used as food and as a source of both fresh and fermented beverages for eons.

The practice of fermenting grape juice began very early. Excavations from the Neolithic[58] period yield proof of winemaking at the Hajji Firuz Tepe site in the northern Zabros Mountains of modern day Iran. Dating from 5400 to 5000 B.C., intact jars unearthed at the dig contained traces of grape wine and beer. Clearly winemaking practices were already in widespread use during this early time.

Grapes have long been used in Chinese medicine, and the black grape is one of the special foods prescribed today for post-partum women to help regain strength and vitality after the demands of childbirth.[59] Grape leaves are edible and Middle Eastern cooks have long made extensive use of them in a great variety of recipes for stuffed grape leaves called dolmades. These tidy packages of leaf filled with rice and pine nuts, chick peas or various meats and spices are both elegant and tasty.

The ancient Egyptians left records describing the grape and its many uses in medicine as well as their age old wine production methods, subsequently passing their techniques and practices along to the Mesopotamian and Greek civilizations. Bowls of raisins have been found in Egyptian tombs and the grape vine and fruit decorate the walls of houses and many every day objects of Egyptian culture. The Book of Medicines lists over 20 prescriptions used by Syriac physicians calling for grapes and fresh grape juice, describing the use of wild and red grapes and raisins added to wine to treat constipation. Noah is described in the Judeo-Christian Bible as planting a vineyard on Mount Ararat after the great flood.[60] Pliny the Elder left records describing 91 varieties of grapes and catalogued 50 kinds of wine. The grape is thought to have entered what is today known as France at least around 600 BC with the Phoenicians, and the Romans carried vines with them in their later expansion into the Rhine Valley in what is today Germany and later to England.

In view of the nearly 8000 varieties known today, it is interesting to note that one species - *V. vinifera* – was the only species cultivated by man until the time of the early settlement of the east coast of America. Early settlers brought their European vines with them to establish vineyards, but their vines were soon destroyed. A disease called phylloxera, caused by the plant louse *Dactylospheara vitifolia* was, at this time, only present in the eastern region of the Americas. This event forced the early settlers to seek out wild indigenous American varieties to replace their stock.

---

58   8500-4000 B.C.

59   Post-Partum Care with Traditional Chinese Medicine. Dr. Andy Orr. Colby College, Waterville, Maine. February 25, 2007.

60   See Cayce transcript 311-3 and 364-6.

Among the 50 or so wild American species was the handy and hardy *V. labrusca* [a so-called "slip skin" grape] with a pronounced aromatic or "foxy" flavor. Developed by Ephraim Wales Bull,[61] a Concord native, *V. labrusca* later became known as the Concord grape because it was first extensively cultivated in Concord, Massachusetts. The Concord easily tolerates humid summers and bitter winters and produces flavorful juice, jams, jellies and a delicious wine and is favored in the Cayce system. Another American native is the Catawba classified as *V. labrusca* and the commonly called "muscadine," classified as *V. rotundifolia*. The muscadine shares the genus *Vitis* but is actually classified in a subgenus called *Muscadinia*. Both are very successful in the extreme hot and humid conditions of the American south where they are widely cultivated, their wines being regional favorites. They have not enjoyed the extensive commercial cultivation and development of the Concord.

Beginning around 1860 samples of wild American vines were transported back to Europe, unwittingly and unfortunately carrying with them the plant louse. It took a little less than 20 years to wipe out the age-old vineyards of France and Germany. European growers were forced to reach out to America for rootstock that had, over eons, developed some resistance to the pest. Hybridizing the surviving *V. vinifera* with American species represented the first systematic attempts to produce disease resistant vines in modern times.

Over eons specific varieties have been developed to meet individual tastes and needs. Strains that proved better for wine making were carefully and passionately cultivated. Special table grapes were grown for use as fresh fruit and even dessert grape varieties prized for their special sweetness were cultivated. Individual strains that dry and store well for the production of raisins were carefully nurtured, and later seedless grapes, developed first for canning, came along to answer the varied needs of the market place.

Wine making has become a worldwide culture and a global industry. There are presently 5 classes of wine: appetizer, red and white; table, dessert and sparkling. There are 17 or so types differentiated even further by the varieties of the grapes themselves that form either a single dominant - or their "generics and proprietaries" which are named by color or region. Perhaps no other plant enjoys such a varied, ancient and rich tradition in growing and cultivation as does the grape. There are schools of wine tasting and classes in wine making. The science of pruning, the study of climate and soil requirements, the exact amount of rain, not too much and not too little, are all now a part of the complex science of the world wide art of wine making and wine drinking.

The "fruit of the vine" drunk by the ancients was not anything like the wines of today. Lack of sanitation and refrigeration combined with uncontrolled fermentation left the enjoyment of the early wines to those who had acquired "the taste." Spoilage was a great problem and Greek wines were frequently dark, and flavored with honey, white barley and even grated goat's milk cheese.[62] Roman improvements in wine making and storage were maintained through medieval times by the Catholic Church through its great network of European monasteries. France and Germany, with their Benedictine and Cistercian abbeys, grew vines and developed important refinements in the wine making process. The technique of distilling wine in order to combat spoilage during long sea voyages can be traced to the Phoenicians some 3,000 years ago. The people of what is today southern Spain continue using the same methods producing excellent sherry and many fine brandies.

---

61   Bull is buried in the Sleepy Hollow Cemetery, Concord, Middlesex County, Massachusetts. A plaque reads: Ephraim Wales Bull, The Originator of the Concord Grape, Born in Bostin March 4, 1806, Died in Concord September 26, 1835, He Sowed Others Reaped.
62   National Grape Cooperative, Inc. IN THE VINEYARD – House of the Grape. January, 2002.

Freshly made grape juice has been enjoyed since the time of the ancients but it did not become a popular and widely available beverage until the discovery that heating foods and beverages destroyed harmful bacteria. This process, called pasteurization, is named after the French chemist Louis Pasteur who developed the process in 1876. Pasturization, combined with the work of Dr. Thomas Bramwell Welch in 1869, a dentist of Vineland, New Jersey, gave the world the first commercially bottled grape juice. Welch's grape juice was at first made only for use at the local church communion service but the Welch family later went on to produce not only juice from the local Concord variety but jams and jellies as well, and the business has grown to world wide prominence in the last 130 odd years. The company headquarters is still located in Concord, Massachusetts.

Grape wine and brandy have been used as anesthetics on early battlefields to dull the pain of the tortuous practice of surgery in the field. The grape appears official only in the form of grape brandy in the 21st US Dispensatory during the time the Cayce information was being given. It was described as a disinfectant and as both a stimulant and a depressant whenever alcohol was called for to dilate the vessels of the heart. Grape sugar in the form of dextrose also appears in the same dispensatory and was at one time injected into the blood stream to increase the strength of heart contractions and to better manage some cases of diabetes.

Description

The grape is a vine characterized by deeply lobed, medium green leaves, smooth and somewhat shiny on the top and slightly fuzzy underneath. The leaves are shed in the fall leaving behind vines that can be cut and woven into baskets, wreaths and other decorative items. The vines cling to taller plants and other structures by means of thin, pale green tendrils. The young shoots are also pale green, pliable and amenable to being trained to grow on trellises or other structures. As the vines age they take on a thick, woody appearance and the older, thicker parts are covered with a grayish shaggy bark. Commercial growers keep the plants trimmed to a convenient height for harvesting and support them on wire or wooden structures where each year the new shoots will produce fruit. Grape vines can grow to 60 feet in length.

Tiny buds open into equally tiny whitish flowers from which the fruit appears. Most varieties will produce fruit in the familiar pyramidal shape, born from the youngest canes or shoots hanging down in lovely, fragrant profusion. Grape varieties produce fruit ranging from nearly white to pale green, red, pink, purple, and blue-black and with a flavor to suit every palate. There are, for example, over 17 varieties of white grapes from which to choose in making white wines and 21 for making red wine. The home gardener should determine the type of grape desired and then consult a reputable nursery to determine which varieties will succeed in the local area.

Growing Conditions and Propagation

Grapes thrive in temperate zones and will tolerate freezing winters, yet they require full sun and warm summers to produce their best fruit. Wild grape vines are either male or female; they are fertilized by insects and reproduce by seeds. Most of the grapes available today are hybrids and can only be propagated by cuttings. All grapes need some kind of structure for support and ease of harvesting the heavy clusters of fruit. Most will tolerate ordinary soil, and unless the climate is extremely dry, established plants do not need to be watered. In some areas hungry birds will pick each grape as it reaches the ripe stage so covering the vines with netting may be necessary.

Grape vines that are properly tended are extremely long lived. The Greek village of Pagkratio boasts what may be the oldest living grapevine in the world. It is named the Pasanias Grapevine [also Pafsanias] after the famous traveler who was the first to mention it in his memoirs in the 2nd century AD.[63]

The oldest known cultivated grapevine was planted more than 400 years ago in the Lent district of Slovenia. This vine is named Stara trta and in spite of its age still produces approximately 35 litres of red wine each year.

Harvesting

Entire clusters of grapes are cut from the vines when they are ripe, ripeness being determined by color and fragrance. The grapes are picked from the stems and processed according to the desired use. Seedless grapes can be dried whole as raisins. Any grape can be juiced, crushed and processed for juice or wine or made into jellies and jams. The seeds should not be eaten.

Use in the Edgar Cayce Readings

Grapes are not classified as one of the companion plants nor used in internal prescriptions but they are used therapeutically. They are mentioned in over 340 individual transcripts. Fresh grapes are recommended in mono-diets in cases of colitis, toxemia and where eliminations need to be increased. It is clear that grapes have some as yet unrecognized anti-inflammatory properties as the cases in which they are recommended all describe some form of internal abdominal inflammation.

Grapes are used topically as an abdominal poultice to address inflammation of the intestines, bladder or kidneys in cases ranging from ptomaine and food poisoning to typhoid fever, colitis and peritonitis.

For therapeutic purposes any grape will do but seeded grapes seem to be favored if they can be obtained. Cayce states the seed of the Concord contains more of these effective anti-inflammatory properties than other varieties.

Alcoholic beverages are certainly not prohibited in the Cayce system although certain kinds of alcohol are more highly recommended than others. Beverages made with hops, hard liquor, or malted alcoholic beverages are generally warned against especially if taken in excess. This clearly comes from the standpoint of an adverse chemical action within the body and the resulting impairment of various internal physiological systems is described in detail. Red wine, however, is frequently recommended taken in combination with whole grain bread often called "black bread."

2548-1 M 36 VENERAL DISEASE:AFTER EFFECTS

36. [Q] Is beer or natural wine harmful to me?
[A] **Beer or ANY of the brewed or distilled liquors are harmful. For, they only add to the lymph disturbance - by exciting to activity throughout the mucous membranes of the whole body.**

We would refrain even from carbonated drinks. Ice cream and ices may be taken, but not carbonated waters. These also excite lymph activity, and with the burr in some of the tissues of the body is irritating.

---

63   Greek geographer and historian who traveled and wrote extensively in the 2nd century AD. He lived between 76 AD and 161 AD but his birth and death dates are not known. He is most famous for his DESCRIPTION OF GREECE.

The effect of too much alcohol on the liver is described in the following:

877-13 M 45 Dermatitis
29. [Q] The effect of alcohol, should it be strong or not?
[A] Alcohol in moderation is well for MOST bodies. But not too great a quantity taken as to cause a slow congestion in the liver area. But alcohols taken, evenings - very well.

As stated above wine is frequently recommended therapeutically by Cayce, red wine being preferred over white and champagne which is often given in small quantities in cases of severe debilitation. The difference between the action of champagne and red wine is described as follows:

325-68 F 63 CANCER:BREAST
5. [Q] What kind of wine is best?
[A] As indicated. One is strengthening, the other is a stimulation. The light wines or the champagnes or the like are for stimulation, while the red wines are strengthening - but these should be taken in VERY small quantities.

Often a small amount of red wine, usually 2 ounces or so, is recommended to be taken in the late afternoons, at least an hour before the evening meal, with a slice of rye or pumpernickel bread. This combination is often described as being *"HELPFUL to the body if taken ONLY with bread; for this produces an activity that is body, blood and nerve building, but wine taken in excess - of course - is harmful; wine taken with bread alone is body, blood and nerve and brain building. [821-]* The best types of wine to drink are described further as follows: *That which is well fermented, or grape juices or the like; these are the better, not too much of the sour nor too sweet a wine. Tokay, Port, Sauterne. [821-1]*

The time of day for this unusual pick-me-up is three or four o'clock in the afternoon. This recommendation is fairly consistent from case to case and often suggests that this combination is good for the digestion:

1530-2 F 50
22. We find that red wine in the afternoon – three or four o'clock – would be well, if it is taken as FOOD; NOT as a drink. Take about an ounce to an ounce and a half or two ounces of red wine or sherry wine – with brown or black bread, preferably. This will tone the digestive forces and make for better abilities for assimilation of foods.

Upon the repeal of Prohibition[64] in the United States one enterprising gentleman sought business advice in setting up a liquor manufacturing and distribution company. He received this bit of volunteered information about the best wine formulas in the United States at the time:

417-7 Male 39 [October 11, 1933]
25. [Q] Has he got the proper formulas for making wine?
[A] Best formulas in this country are those that may be obtained from the Pleasant Valley people, for these are natives of Switzerland, France and Germany! And this is the valley where so many grapes are grown, where their sauterne and dry wine is the very best Madeira or Rhine either![65]

---

64   [6] 1920 to 1933
65   [7] Authors Note: This is the Pleasant Valley Wine Company, also known as The Great Western Winery. It was established in 1860 in Hammondsport, New York.

In case 437-7 a 48 year old gentleman was suffering from Erythrokeratolysis hiemalis commonly called "winter itch." It is an extremely rare form of ichthyosis. The disorder is characterized by periodic attacks of red [erythematous] plaques that are distributed equally on the body. A layer of skin can actually be peeled from these plaques and the condition is uncomfortable in the extreme. This gentleman had been helped earlier in 1933 but failed to follow through with the recommended diet saying to Mr. Cayce in a letter: *"Life is really not much fun when you have to eat like that."* The condition returned with a vengeance in 1936 and he again turned to Mr. Cayce for help. In the process he was given some valuable information on why red wine has therapeutic value:

437-7 M 48
8. But do not have those combinations where there are too great quantities of any alcoholic-producing foods. Not referring to alcohol itself so much, for as we find RED WINE would be excellent if taken as a meal with black or sour bread, in the evenings or late afternoon. But refrain from combinations of starches, as white bread, potatoes, spaghetti, macaroni, or those things where there are great excesses of starch WITH sugars. These produce a fermentation that is an aggravation to the conditions.

Red wine in the evening or afternoon is well. Alcohol in other forms, as hard rum, NOT so well. Light wines are very good. Beer NOT good.

28. [Q] What is meant by Red wine?
[A] Means RED wine! Not white wine, not sour wine; not that that is too sweet but any of those that are in the nature of adding to the body the effect of grape sugar...

Foods must ferment, naturally, from acid, the action of acid and alkalin. These passing into the duodenum, especially, become then certain characters of sugars; as produced by the activity of the pancreas juices upon the effect of juices from the liver and the spleen, in digestive forces.

Then the addition of Red wine, which is carrying more of a tartaric effect upon the active forces of the body, is correct; while those that are sour or that draw out from the system a reaction upon the hydrochlorics become detrimental.

Grapes Can Help With Weight Loss

From a statistical standpoint the Cayce system clearly favors the Concord for both dietary and therapeutic applications, but if the Concord is not available any of the darker types are preferred over the lighter varieties. Freshly squeezed juice is often recommended but when this is not practical Welch's is the preferred commercially produced American brand being mentioned in 39 cases. Welch's is also the brand of choice for use in weight loss as the following excerpts illustrate:

1309-3 F 56 OBESITY [This was given in 1940]
4. [Q] Is Welch's Grape Juice preferable to Premier unsweetened? I like Premier much the best.[66]
[A] If that is the more desirable, use same. The Welch's, however, has more of the elements in same that aid in the reduction of the carbohydrates in the system, - and thus tends to supply the food values in a way that is in keeping with that which has been indicated as the purpose for taking same.

---

66   [8] Premier, located in Miramar, Florida, is today part of the Charmer Sunbelt Group

1224-3 F 74 Arthritis:Obesity
24. [Q] Is it important to reduce weight? How much and by what means?
[A] It is more important that an equal BALANCE be kept. As we find, the weight may be reduced some WITHOUT disturbance; and as we find, the better manner would be through the refraining from breads or greases of any kind, of course, and by the taking of Grape Juice, - preferably the juice from fresh grapes, this prepared at the time to be taken, three times each day; taking about an ounce and a half to two ounces [diluted with a little water] half an hour before each meal. If the juice from fresh grapes is found to be impractical, then take the fresh Welch's Grape Juice.

259-10 F 25 Obesity:Tendencies
13. DO take grape juice four times each day [Welch's, preferably]. Stir two ounces of grape juice in one ounce of plain water [not carbonated water] thirty minutes before each meal and before retiring.

Abdominal Grape Poultice

Preference for the Concord is expressed again in this transcript and here the seed is identified as the part most effective against inflammation:

1045-3 F 37 TUBERCULOSIS:FEVER
Keep the poultice, but get the Concord and not the other grapes. If the Concord grapes cannot be secured, then use the seedless white grapes; though the SEED in the Concord grapes are those that take away the inflammation the most.

A general guideline for when the Grape Poultice is used is found in the following:

261-19 M 47
3. [Q] Do you prefer Epsom Salts Packs or the Grape Poultices?
[A] The Epsom Salts Packs are preferable at this time, as indicated. There is not so much inflammation as a tendency for congestion, see? Hence the relaxation by the use of the Epsom Salts; while the Grape Poultices are rather to dissipate inflammation, see?

The following excerpts give excellent directions for how to prepare a Grape Poultice:

261-17 M 47 PTOMAINE POISONING
4. Make application of a Grape Poultice; raw grapes, mashed in a form so they will be at least half to an inch thick across the whole of the abdomen; preferably the Concord Grapes.

5. Be well in preparation for it that there be taken internally orange juice mixed with the grape juice; the fresh, not that preserved or put up, but the fresh - about half and half. Take little sips of this.

6. Keep the pack on for about an hour, and then change and put on a second one. Leave the second one on for an hour.

303-35 F 56 DEBILITATION:GENERAL
5. In the present, while the body rests, we would have the Grape Poultice applied over the upper and lower abdomen. Just crush the grapes on gauze, or old cloth, sufficient in size to cover the upper

and lower abdomen; covering same so as to keep absorption, with the heat from the body, to give strength. Use the Concord grapes, preferably; though if these are not available, use the larger variety [dark grapes, preferably].

In the following case the lady had contracted the flu which had settled in the abdominal area affecting her intestines. She was suffering from severe painful constipation, a condition often described by Cayce as having the potential to turn malignant. A preference for the darker variety of grape is emphasized again:

5280-1 F 59 COLITIS:SPASTIC COLON
6. As we would find, first there would be the application of crushed grapes over the abdomen. Preferably these would be the Concord variety. None are available at present except the preserved or California grapes. Hence the next best would be those of the purple variety. Crush them, place on gauze and apply on the abdomen. Let remain, then, until apparently these have almost dried on the body. This would require an hour and a half to three hours.

An interesting end note is found in the next to the last paragraph of the same transcript:

15. [Q] What doctor would you advise to apply these treatments?
[A] Most of this may be applied at home, if it is desired so. Don't need a doctor. Few people do.

The following are some typical ways grapes and grape juice is used:

352-2 F 24 Food Poisoning
9. For at least three days [and rest during the period] we would eat only grapes, or fresh grape juice. Do not eat the seeds in the grapes, of course.

757-6 F 45 Urethritis
4. We would be mindful that the diet is that which is easily assimilated. Not too great quantities of starch foods, but sufficient to aid in creating the proper balance in those periods of assimilation necessary for proper fermentation. We would not have too great quantities of sugar. Or the body may, under the existent circumstances, go on an entire grape diet - see, ENTIRE grape diet, for at least three day periods; then to the regular normal diet that has been indicated. Quantities of grapes! And should there appear any disturbance in the stomach and duodenum through those periods, make a poultice of the grape hull and pulp – between cloths and apply over those areas; or over the abdomen and liver area, you see. Make this about an inch and a half thick - that large a quantity, you see, all over. Plenty of water, but just grapes for three days - QUANTITIES - all that the body may eat.

In this last excerpt given in August of 1935 the Concord may not have been locally available. The directions call for any kind of grape available - practical advice at any time.

977-1 F 43 Adhesions:Lesions
11. Then we would put the body entirely on a MILK and GRAPE diet! Milk of mornings and evenings. Grapes only for about three days. Milk and grapes for three days as the diet.

12. Also we would use a grape poultice across the abdomen and across the whole of the lower portion of the body. Crush the grapes and put between cloths. Do not heat these. Leave the hulls and pulp

together, of course; just crush, and it would be well to sew same or baste into a bag, you see, so that it may be put over the body; make the pack at least an inch thick with the crushed grapes. Change these about every thirty to forty minutes or an hour. Do this until there is a RELIEF of the pains in the head and the body is more quiet, you see. For these will tend to relieve the body, together with the eliminations set up through the use of the colon evacuation as indicated.

21. [Q] Any particular kind of grape?
[A] Those that may be had on the market.

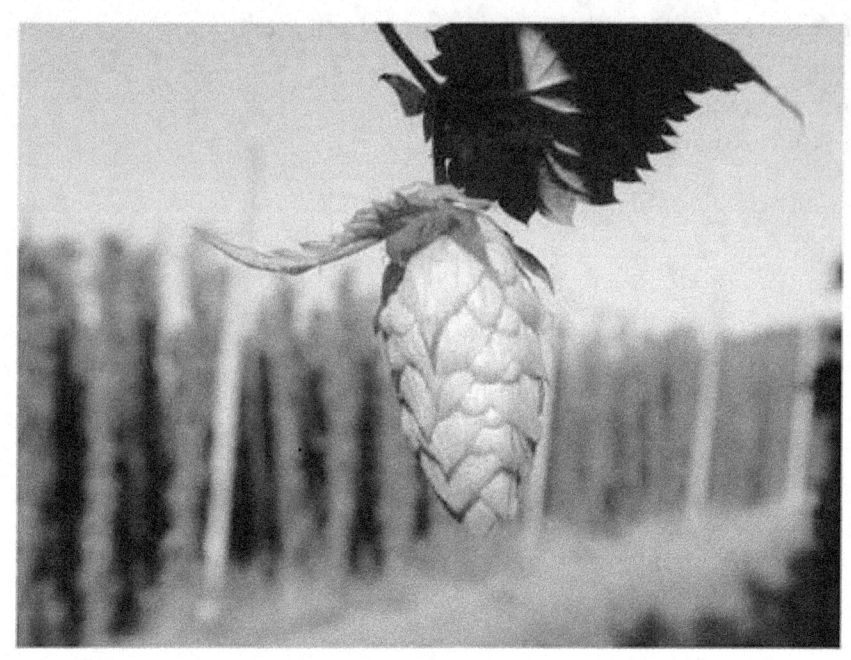

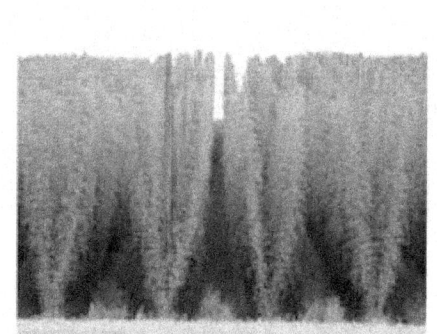

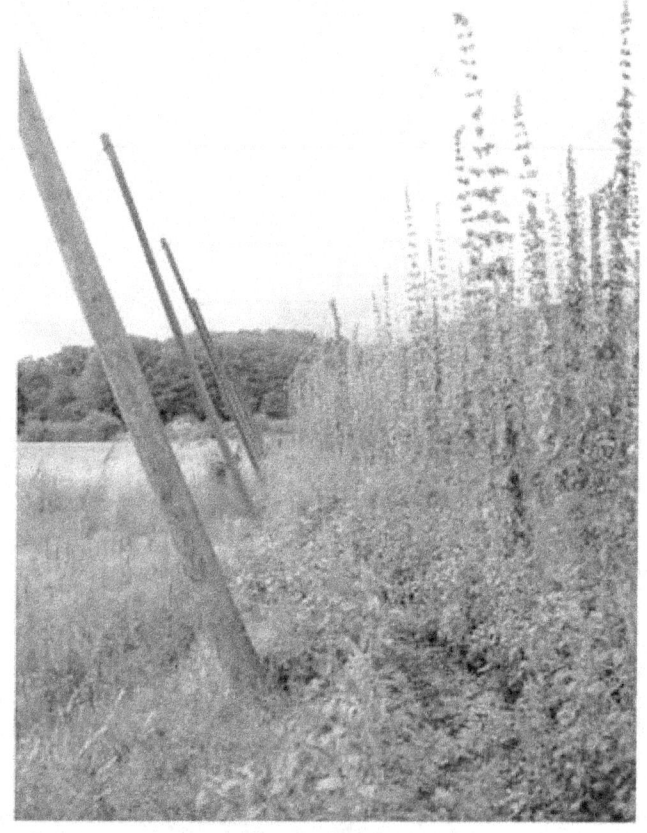

HOPS
Humulus lupulus, Fam. Moraceae

Common and Regional Names
None

History and Common Usage

The hop is native to Europe, Western Asia and North America. It is believed to have originated in China where all three species of the genus still occur in the wild. Pliny mentions the plant but does not give it a significant place either medicinally or as a source of food. He writes: *"plants which grow spontaneously"* and goes on to mention *"In Italy, however, we are acquainted with but very few of them; those few being… the meadow parsnip, the hop, which may be rather termed amusements for the botanist than articles of food.*[67]

Today the hop is almost completely identified with the beer and ale brewing industry but in former times it was used mainly in folk medicine as a tea or decoction. The vines, flowers, fruit and leaves were steeped and drunk as a mild sedative. It was used to treat insomnia, sometimes to quell bouts of alcoholic delirium tremens or as a digestive aid. Today only the female flowers called cones or strobile are used as the leaves and vines are not readily found on the market. Hops contain approximately 1 percent volatile oil and approximately 100 other compounds including polyphenols, tannins and flavonoids. While a great deal of research has been done on the plant the research has not been on its use in healing. It should be noted that taking a tea or decoction of hops together with sleeping pills, alcohol or sedatives is extremely unwise, as the potential chemical interactions are not known.

One folk remedy application for the hop is best identified with medieval times in Europe with a "hop bag" - made today with only the stroibles. Originally the vine, flowers and strobile were stuffed into a pillow to induce sleep. The stroibles used today are moistened with water laced with a small amount of glycerin to prevent rustling and used in cases of headache and insomnia. Some individuals are known to respond very well to this remedy. Local application of a "hop bag" used as a fomentation or poultice on the face is still recommended by some herbal practitioners as a pain reliever in cases of facial neuralgia and to induce healing sleep. Sleep inducing pillows using the hop and other aromatic herbs such as lavender are a significant cottage industry.

Alcoholic beverages have been fermented since the dawn of civilization. In regions where grapes were available wine was made and where grapes did not grow various grains were used such as rye, barley and corn. The oldest records of beer making are found with the Sumerians and the Babylonians. Sumer lay between the Tigris and Euphrates rivers, as did the ancient cities of Babylon and Ur. A record dating to 4,000 years ago records a "Hymn to Ninkasi" the Sumerian goddess of brewing and records a recipe for a fermented drink made from barley. The Babylonian King Hammurabi established the amount of a daily beer ration according to the social standing of the individual. Beer was used as an item of barter and could be considered as money. Laborers received 2 liters and administrators and high priests were entitled to 5 liters per day. The modern word "booze" comes from the Nubian word "boosa or bouza" after one of the many beer styles developed by the Egyptians who brought beer making to a high art. They also made a fermented drink from corn called zythum, which in Greek means a drink from barley. The Greeks and Romans, who had for millennia made wine from grapes, looked down on beer referring to it as an inferior and barbarian drink.

---

[67]   Book XXI, Chapter 50

The high rate of spoilage of fermented beverages plagued the makers of wine and beer from the very beginning, especially in the hot summers. Spoilage represented not only a considerable risk to health but a great financial loss. Beer could not be stored for any length of time and the motion of transportation hastened spoilage. Beer is brewed by a mashing-fermentation process which was originally flavored not with hops but with gruit which imparted not only flavor but fragrance. Gruit is old German, a name given to a blend of herbs and spices by which individual beer makers, in medieval times, would flavor their beer and ale and identify their brand. Some herbs used in early gruit recipes include peppermint, mugwort, fennel, betony, ground ivy and sweet gale. These herbs usually grew on land owned by the local governing authority – usually the crown - and slowly "gruit rights" developed as a royal privilege later granted to early churches giving monasteries and churches the power to collect taxes for brewing rights.

The discovery of the antibacteriostatic qualities of the hop can be credited to the Roman Catholic Church some time between the 7th and 8th centuries. The first recorded use of hops in beer is found in a book written by Hildegard of Bingen[68] entitled Physica sacra. Hildegarde of Bingen was well acquainted with the art of brewing.

Between the 10th and 11th centuries the Roman Catholic Church controlled the lucrative brewing industry in Europe and the stage for conflict between economic interests was set. By the 12th century the economic inducements had proven too great for the ruling classes and brewing rights, long held by the church, began to be undermined by the nobility. Eventually the crown [Emperor Frederick II] began to seize control and the economic advantages of the use of hops to reduce spoilage slowly changed ale to hopped beer.

Hops were not much appreciated when they were first used in Germany and many questions were raised about the effect they would have on health. The bitter taste they imparted was not well liked, but its bacteriostatic properties made it highly desirable to the brewers. When they discovered beer in which hops were added would last longer and would not spoil from the motion of being transported, they began to think only of their purses. Finances and not taste began to drive the beer and ale market but hopped beer was born in a long and bitter controversy. Most sources cite the Netherlands in the early 14th century as one of the first places where commercial brewers used hops as a preservative but the acceptance of "hopped beer" there was also slow. At first hops were banned from being used in the beer and ale industry in England. During the reign of Henry VIII Parliament actually petitioned against the hop as *"a wicked weed that would spoil the taste of the drink and endanger the people."* Hops were grown in England during the reign of Edward VI and came into commercial cultivation in the United States in the colony of Virginia as early as 1648. The brewing of "non-hopped" beer is making a comeback in recent times with a proliferation of various gruit recipes and perhaps with the development of refrigeration and the discovery of pasturization old fashioned beer and ale will make a healthy comeback.

Hops are grown both for their flavor and a preservative substance called lupulin. There are over 160 USDA named hop varieties recognized in the United States alone. Hops are grown commercially in most all temperate regions of the globe with Australia, South America, Germany, England and the United States as the leaders in hop production.

Hops was listed as an official drug plant in the pharmacopoeias of the Cayce era described as an aromatic

---

68   Benedictine abbess. 1098-1179 A.D.

bitter used as a sedative in cases of *"hysteria, restlessness, insomnia and the like."*[69]

Description

Humulus lupulus is a perennial trailing vine of male and female plants which can grow to 30 feet or more in the wild. Only the female vine produces the cones or strobiles so commercial growers will often cut down the male vines after pollination. Hops have the habit of growing in a spiral direction from left to right and clings easily to any support by means of strong hooked hairs on its stems which coil around any available surface. A few people suffer from contact dermatitis when they handle or touch these hairs. The vine climbs readily on any available upright structure including other plants and can easily be trained to wind around stout twine or wire supports for ease of harvesting the heavy cones.

The leaves are deep green, extremely rough, and deeply lobed in 3 to 5 oval parts with serrated edges. The flowers are different in appearance between the male and female plants. The male flowers are greenish in color born in loose panicles between 2 and 7 or 8 inches in length. The female flowers are called strobles. They are leafy cone-like catkins somewhat reminiscent in shape to small pinecones, yellowish green and about 1 1/4 inches long. Each strobile produces from 1 to 3 small, reddish purple seeds.

Growing Conditions and Propagation

Hops are best grown from rootstock purchased from commercial suppliers but can also be easily grown from seed. They do best in zones 3 to 11 and when growing conditions are right they put on length at a phenomenal rate. The root of the plant is often found at a depth of 15 feet or more making well drained subsoil essential. They prefer good, rich garden soil in full sun or semi-shade and once the root is established the plant will come back each spring. To keep the vine healthy and under control the suckers, which develop each spring, should be cut back.

Propagation from rootstock or root cuttings is done in rows between 7 and 8 feet apart and the roots should be planted in "stools" of 2 to 6, depending upon their size. From each "leg" of the imaginary stool the emerging vine can be trained to grow on a pole, arbor or on a trellis. Commercial growers train hops by stringing them to the wires of 18' high trellises. The supporting structure should be strong enough to support heavily laden matured plants. The vine will take one to two years to come to maturity before it will produce a sufficient number of flowers to produce a good crop.

Harvesting

The cones can usually be harvested the last of August or the early part of September. Often 2 or more inches long, they are a bright yellowish-green, loose, crisp and papery to the touch. Their bases are covered with a sticky, yellowish, granular powder containing the valuable lupulin. If allowed to ripen on the vine too long the cones become darker yellow and shatter or break very easily. These are unsuitable for use in flavoring beer and ale because much of the lupulin is lost.

Hops can be picked by hand or by machine. They must be carefully dried to reduce their moisture content down to 10% to 12% so as to avoid mildew or souring. Since hops will spoil very rapidly, they should be moved from the vine to drying as quickly as possible. Drying in large quantities usually requires artificial heat sources. Low drying temperatures are critical and for best results the temperature should be at 100° F, never exceeding 105° F. Hops can be air dried in the sun in climates where humidity is low or dried on trays in a home oven. If dried by an artificial heat source they should be allowed to cool over a period of

---

69   21st Edition United States Dispensatory

6 to 12 days, stirring occasionally to equalize the moisture content. During this time they become tough and pliable and ready for storage in air tight containers kept out of direct sunlight.

Use in the Edgar Cayce Readings
Hops are not recommended therapeutically in the Cayce system but questions raised by a number of individuals resulted in valuable information about them and their action in the body. They are mentioned 40 times. The references to hops are always in relation to beer and whether or not it is injurious to drink.

Consistently Cayce advises against any beverages containing hops because they have a tendency to dry the intestines, disturb the lymph system and in some cases individuals are unaware they have an allergy to hops, the accumulative and long term effects of which are detrimental to the liver. The following excerpts are typical examples of questions and answers about hopped beer:

257-199 M 45 Diet:Acidity
30. No large quantities of beer especially, or of any hops-formed products that cause a strain or a drying. Though it may be a liquid it may produce drying effects through the jejunum and the whole even of the alimentary canal; thus stimulating a condition in the hepatics that produces for the alimentary canal disturbing conditions that may become aggravating to the system.

416-18 M 38 Alcohol Not Recommended
5. [Q] Skin eruptions on back and arms? Cause and treatment.
[A] Warnings have been indicated to the body of diets, especially as related to carbonated waters and hard drinks and hops in drinks. Eliminate these, this will disappear.

6. [Q] Is the moderate use of alcohol injurious to this body and what is moderate for this body?
[A] Occasionally if you took a drink - once a year, it wouldn't be too bad - but wouldn't be too good either. Not that one becomes a total abstainer, but when in Rome, do as the Romans, but needn't get drunk over it, nor become so that ye seek too much of those things. Light wines will do very well, the rest you'd better cut out, not good for this body.

1023-1 F 49 ADHESIONS ANEMIA Toxemia
35. [Q] Is alcohol injurious to the body?
[A] As indicated from the suggestions to not consume sweets and starches at the same meal, such a form of alcohol becomes detrimental. Wines - and even rum at times - are helpful, if taken AS a body-BUILDING meal; that is, a small glass - preferably in the afternoon - WITH black or sour bread. But those forms that are of the hop nature are detrimental, for they produce - to a disturbed condition in the system - activative forces that are harmful.

2596-1 F 28 NEURASTHENIA:CURED
24. These are the DON'TS: DO NOT take carbonated waters or drinks of ANY character. DO NOT take any drinks the basis of which is from hops or from yeast.

3147-1 M 61 ANEMIA DEBILITATION:GENERAL
11. Then keep the mind young, but the body activities of its own age. These will be better for the body. DO NOT take carbonated waters, nor any of these drinks made from hops or of that nature.

3534-1 M 61 HEMORRHAGE:INTESTINES:AFTER EFFECTS

8. In the diet keep close to those things that are more easily assimilated. Refrain from any of carbonated waters or strong drinks of any kind, especially anything with hops. For the body is allergic [so-called] to such. For these tend to produce a filling of the lymph through the alimentary canal, as well as the lymph flow in throat. Don't use these things.

Out of the 40 cases only one individual was advised to drink beer. In this one case the information indicated that hops would make a beneficial change in the katabolism in the assimilating and digestive system.

243-22 F 56 ASTHENIA

6. But Malted Milk with egg would be MOST helpful. Malted Milk with beer, of EVENING, will be helpful. But THIS ONLY, though [the beer], during the days when the Yeast is NOT being taken, see? for it is the hops that makes for a change in the katabolism in the assimilating and digestive system.

It would seem the Cayce system is in agreement with famous English Botanist, John Evelyn [1620-1706] who was opposed to the use of hops turning good English ale into beer. In 1670 in his work on fruit growing for cider making entitled "Pomona," Evelyn wrote the following:

"Hops transmuted our wholesome ale into beer, which doubtless much alters its constitution. This one ingredient, by some suspected not unworthily, preserves the drink indeed, but repays the pleasure in tormenting diseases and a shorter life."

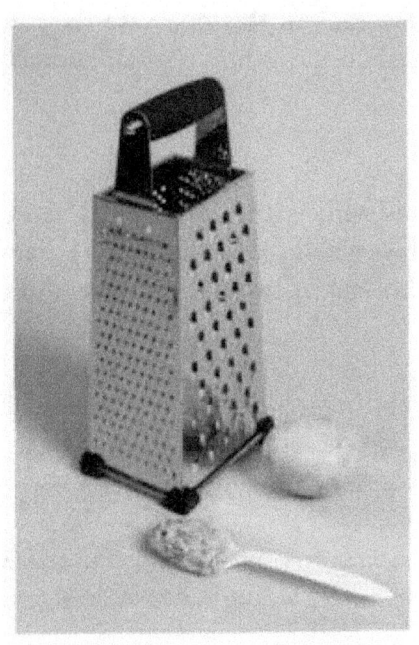

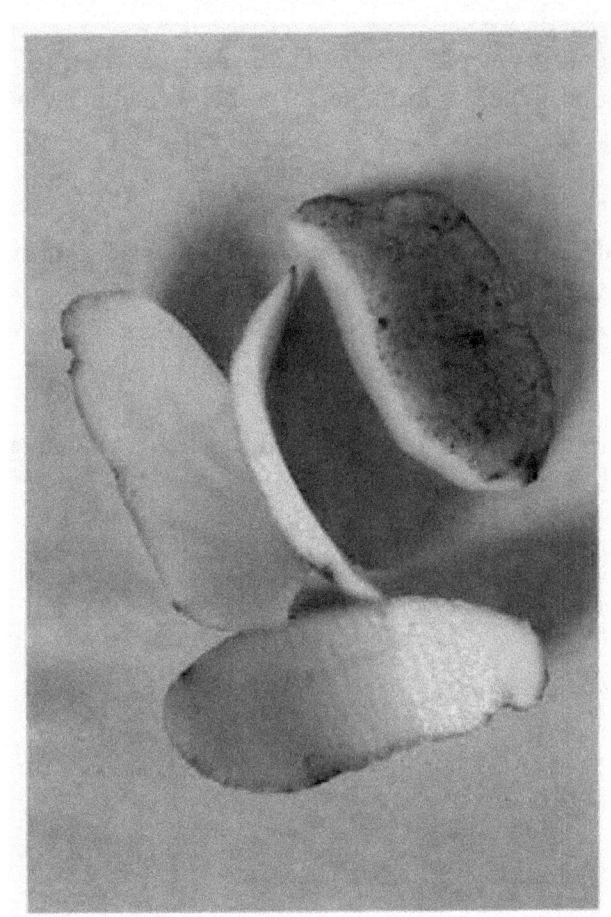

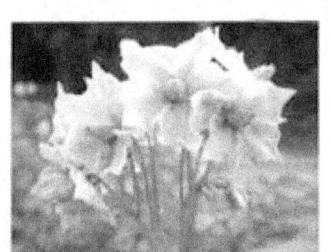

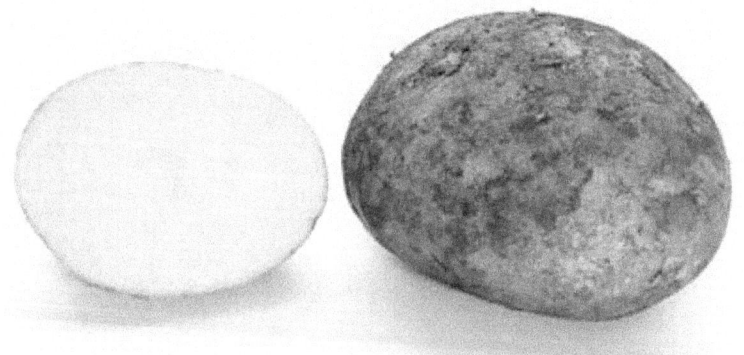

IRISH POTATO
Solanum tuberosum, Fam. Solanaceae

Common and Regional Names
White potato, spuds, common potato, Pomme de Terre

History and Common Usage
The potato is cited by most botanists as having originated in the temperate valley regions of the Andes Mountains in Peru and Bolivia in South America. Close relatives of the modern potato, one of which is *Solanum andigenum*, can still be found growing between 4,000 and 6,000 feet, adapted after eons to the short growing season and harsh, dry conditions. The name is thought to have come from the original Indian name: "Batatas."

As the fourth largest food crop in the world the potato is cultivated in 150 countries with 95 known genera and a reported 2,400 species. There are 160 wild or indigenous varieties catalogued and 20 commercially cultivated varieties. All are frost sensitive and come in a modest variety of colors. Skin colors range from red to pinkish-red, tan, bluish purple, and from brown to bluish lavender. The flesh comes in a variety of colors including white, buttery yellow, pale gold, red, pinkish-red, purple, purple sometimes streaked with white, and blue to nearly black.

The modern history of the potato is difficult to trace due to confusion caused by the name being used over centuries for many different kinds of plants. There is the sweet potato, [*Ipomoea batatas*, actually a member of the morning glory family] the yam [*Dioscorea*] and many other unrelated plants also called potato. The Spanish are certainly credited with the discovery of the vegetable during their early explorations in Peru beginning in the year 1524. It is known the plant was taken to Italy in 1585 and was introduced into Germany, Austria and Belgium two years later in 1587. The Belgian Prefect of Mons, one Philip de Sivry, is credited with a colored drawing of the potato dating to sometime around 1588 which is thought to be the first European illustration. The original is on display in the Plantin-Moretus Museum at Antwerp, Belgium. Potatoes were cultivated in France soon after 1600.

John Gerarde created considerable confusion as to the origin, history and proper identification of the potato by giving the plant a misleading name, *Batata virginiana*, whereas the potato was actually introduced *from* Europe to the new world sometime during the very early settlement period. The official botanical designation, *Solanum tuberosum*, was first used in 1596 by Swiss botanist Kaspar Bauhin. Linnaeus, in publishing his SPECIES PLANTARUM in 1753, adopted this name by which the plant is known today.

Sir Francis Drake is often credited with introducing the potato to England and Ireland sometime in 1586; however the six rooted or tuber forming plants he described in his writings, and in the subsequent descriptions by Thomas Heriot,[70] one of the survivors of Raleigh's Colony on Roanoke Island, do not even remotely resemble the now well known potato.

Sometime between 1650 and 1840 the potato was established as a staple in Ireland. During the Great Potato Famine of 1845 it began to be known as the Irish Potato. When blight wiped out the crop hundreds of thousands died of starvation and thousands of Irish were forced off their land by their

---

70   [1560 -1621] Astronomer, scientist and mathematician. Author of *A BRIEF AND TRUE REPORT OF THE NEW FOUND LAND IN VIRGINIA*.

British landlords. The stench of rotting potatoes hung over mile after mile of fields and for over four years crop failures decimated the population. Forced migrations from Ireland to America and other countries finally focused international scientific attention on the lowly potato.

The susceptibility of the plant to blight was caused by *Phytophthora infestans* and the disease was overcome 30 odd years later through a fortunate combination of two events. First a blight resistant strain of potato was developed in the United States by Luther Burbank in 1871 and second an effective fungicide was found in 1883 by the French botanist, Alexandre Millardet. This gradually restored the potato to its former prominence as a staple food crop, but it was too late to restore the Irish population or to redress the financial wrongs they had endured.

The potato of commerce today is a relatively young cultivar called the Russet Burbank or sometimes simply an "Idaho." It was developed 130 years ago in Lancaster, Massachusetts by Luther Burbank.[71] The pedigree of the Russet Burbank can be traced to the "Rough Purple Chili" first introduced to the United States from Panama in 1851. In fact the pedigrees of approximately 25% of the ten most important varieties grown in North American can also be traced to the original Rough Purple Chili.

A rather famous use of potatoes is in the distillation of a fermented high alcoholic content beverage called vodka. Originally considered the traditional "spirituous drink" of Russia, the Baltic States and Poland, vodka is now manufactured internationally made mostly with rye and malt from various grains.

In the past 200 years the potato has become a food staple around the world but there are only few citations for its use as a medicinal plant. Some herbal medical sources cite the potato as effective in preventing infection in treating burns and wounds. Many folk medicine traditions call for simply cutting a raw potato in half and rubbing it on sunburned skin or an infected eye.

Both the American and British Pharmacopoeias of the 1920's through the 1930's list *Solanum tuberosum* as an important source of starch but it is not listed as being used medically.

Description
Solanum tuberosum is classified as a dicotyledonous[72] annual although the plant will re-grow from tubers left in the ground from year to year. The smooth and hairless stems of the plant bear dark green alternating leaves. The plants grow 12 to 18 inches high and up to 4 feet wide. The flowers vary in color from white, to stippled white and purple and sometimes lavender with yellow stamens.

Potatoes contain low levels of a poisonous alkaloid called solanine. Solanine is present in the greenish tinge on the skins of potatoes that have been exposed to sunlight. Solanine, quite toxic if ingested in a more pure form, is also present in the leaves and stems.

Growing Conditions and Propagation
The potato propagates by rhizomes and seeds. The rhizomes or stolons form an underground system of vines that produce the potatoes and underneath that a true root system that nourishes the plant. This root system penetrates to considerable depth. Seeds develop from the flowers in small fruiting bodies which resemble little green tomatoes. These fruits should never be eaten as they are poisonous.

---

71   Luther Burbank, American horticulturist, born March 7,1849. He died April 11, 1926.
72   A plant that has two leaves developed by the embryo of the seed plant.

Potatoes can also be grown by planting "seeding eyes" which are known commercially as seed potatoes. Seeding eyes that are too old or too dry may develop plants but no tubers, so the factors of age and correct harvesting, storage and handling of seed potatoes are very important. When purchased from reputable local supplier's seed potatoes will be of the right chronological age to produce healthy plants and tubers, certified disease free, and will be a variety appropriate to the area.

Most potatoes bought in western supermarkets are engineered hybrids and will not produce tubers. Heritage varieties will reproduce from eyes and seed. The home gardener can save Heritage seed from year to year and can also save tubers with "good eyes" for the next year's crop. The following spring the gardener uses a sharp, clean knife to cut the seed potatoes into pieces containing 2 or 3 eyes and then plants them immediately

Planting time is temperature dependent. Generally potatoes should not be planted in excessively wet soils [the seeding eyes will rot] and soil temperatures should not be below 45°F or above 70°F, which is much too hot for good germination. In the southern United States potatoes are planted from November to February and in the middle zones March and April. In the north and in Canada the planting time is usually April to early June.

Potatoes do best in rich, well drained and loose, friable soils. Consistent moisture levels throughout the growing season, whether through watering or adequate rainfall, are important. Potatoes require full sun and a soil pH of 5.0 to 5.4. The soil should be prepared to a minimum depth of 24 inches to accommodate the deep rooting system. The eyes are planted 2 to 3 inches deep, about 11 to 14 inches apart, in soft, well worked trenches or rows about 30 to 36 inches wide. Hilling, or mounding the soil around the plants during the first six to eight weeks of growth is crucial in creating a soil space for the tubers to develop.

Sprouts will emerge within two weeks. When they are between six and eight inches tall and side shoots or vines, more accurately called stolen, begin to develop gently scrape the soil from both sides of the row mounding it up around them, leaving only half of the emerging vine exposed. New potatoes form between the seed piece and the surface of the soil. Two more hillings are necessary, one after 2 to 3 weeks, and a final one 2 weeks after that. The last two hillings should only add an inch or two of soil to the hill to make certain that the new potatoes are never exposed to the light. Mulching the hills with straw also reduces competition for water and nutrients from weeds and further protects the young tubers from the light. Potatoes require four months to grow from planting to harvest.

The plant is subject to the common potato bug. Adult beetles are about 1/3 of an inch in length, black bodied with yellow stripes. Their heads are orange-red. Their larva attach to the underside of the leaves. Hungry chickens are the best solution to the problem but this is probably not an option for most city and suburban gardeners. In a small plot gardeners may avoid using pesticides by removing these pests by hand.

Since potato beetles winter over in the soil alternating planting beds is critical. Potatoes should not be planted in the same bed year after year and should at a minimum be rotated every three years. Preventing soil contamination by disease-causing pathogens as well as the common potato bug through alternating beds will ensure healthy, pest free crops in the future. It is necessary to have twice the amount of garden space so that alternating beds can be more easily managed. It is best to have potatoes planted on opposite ends of the garden from year to year, leaving a strip of ground between for other vegetables. The resting bed can be enhanced with rotted barnyard manure or other soil amendments or planted with a rotation crop such as clover, soybeans or other "green-manures" during the fallow year.

Harvesting

Potatoes are alive when they are taken from the ground and continue to live and breathe throughout their lifecycle. They are tender skinned when first pulled and must be handled gently, cured properly and stored correctly. Without enough air potatoes will suffocate. Too much light and they will turn green, their skins becoming toxic. If too cold they will freeze. Too warm and they will begin to sprout.

Potatoes are ready to harvest 10 to 14 days after the plant has completely died back. Their keeping qualities are enhanced if they are kept in the ground until after the first frost. This ensures that the skins have thickened properly which decreases the risk of bruising and increases storage life. Potatoes can cure in the ground after the tops have been completely removed or can be cured on top of the ground if they are covered with burlap to keep them from the sunlight. Potatoes must be handled gently to avoid spoilage from bruising.

There are two types of bruises which occur: blackspot and shatter. Blackspot is a bruise that is not visible until the potato is peeled and looks like a slight uniform discolored area beneath the skin. Blackspot is a low impact contact bruise which occurs when potatoes are bumped or rubbed together, skin to skin, or when they rub against other surfaces while being moved. Hand rubbing of freshly dug potatoes to remove the soil, if done too vigorously, can cause blackspot. Shatter is an actual fissure, often discolored around the edges of the fracture, which may penetrate into the center of the potato. Shatter occurs because of tossing or dropping during harvesting.

A great deal of research has been done in determining the best harvesting conditions so as to avoid bruise losses during harvesting. Harvesting, as with planting, is also temperature dependent. There will be less chance of bruising if harvesting is done between 11:00 AM and 11:00 PM. Soil temperatures should be above 45°F.

Potatoes are dug by hand or by using a spading fork or pitchfork being careful to place the fork well outside the hill to avoid damaging the crop. The potatoes are mounded in piles [under a makeshift roof to protect them from rain] covered in burlap to protect them from any exposure to the sun, and left to "sweat" or cure in temperatures between 57 to 70 degrees for one to two weeks. They can also be left in a warm dark room to cure, such as a garage, which for the home gardener lacking a shed roof in the backyard may provide the best option for a rain free curing period.

During the curing period a waxy, fatty compound called suberin is produced by cells just below the surface of any cuts or bruises. This seals any breaks in the skin and prevents shrinkage through evaporation and spoilage from invasion by pathogens. Suberin is produced within 4 to 7 days. Next, a specialized tissue called periderm forms developing protective cells to replace the damaged skin destroyed by any wounding. The periderm process is complete in about 17 to 21 days.

At the end of the 2 to 3 week curing period they are ready for cold, dark, long term storage in an area where air is circulated freely. They can be gently cleaned of soil but should not be washed until they are used. The crop should be sorted over to remove bruised or cut tubers as they will rot and spoil other potatoes stored with them. Use these damaged potatoes within 2 weeks. Burlap bags and wooden crates are ideal for storage as they allow for circulation of air. Always temperature sensitive, the potato can tolerate 70°F for the two week curing period but, when they are placed in long storage they require high humidity [90 to 95%] and temperatures near 40°F in order to remain dormant. If stored below 36°F they may become sweet and then need to be stored at ordinary room temperatures for a few days to restore their natural flavor. Most potato varieties will remain dormant in storage for 160 to 210 days at 40°F; 95 to 160 days at 45°F and 60 to 150 days at 50°F. If the tubers start to sprout during storage, the eyes should be rubbed off as the sprouts contain high levels of solanine and should never be eaten.

Local state Cooperative Extension offices as well as Rodale Press and Storey Publications are good sources of information in the United States for the serious home gardener on growing potatoes and on food storage structures.

Use in the Edgar Cayce Readings

Mentioned over 800 times, the potato is not a companion plant in the Cayce system. When used therapeutically it is used alone. The skin is grated for use as a poultice in the treatment of cataracts and eye infections. Potato peelings are recommended as a dietary item and, combined with other modalities, are used prepared as a tea or tonic to treat hair loss, tone the thyroid and to restore hair color.

Potato Eye Poultice

The Cayce system is very specific as to the condition of potatoes used for eye poultices. This is to insure that the toxic alkaloid solanine is not present in the skin of the potato although there are probably other unknown factors involved. Consistently the information states that it is the common white or Irish potato that is to be used. It is always to be fully matured, sometimes described as "old" and preferably of a larger size. It can never have been frozen, or begun to sprout and never one that shows any green. These stringent conditions are important to follow. A potato that has been frozen or shows signs of budding or greening is one in which adverse chemical changes have taken place and should not be used.

Note: Whenever the potato eye poultice is used in nearly every case chiropractic or osteopathic treatment of the spine is also required as are dietary changes for a successful result. It is also very important to follow the instructions precisely when selecting potatoes to use for these poultices as irritation can be caused even by the age of the potato as the following excerpts illustrate:

774-2 F 76 BLEPHARITIS
2. ...Do this for two to three days, or two or three evenings; then rest by leaving it off for two or three days - if it makes for too great an irritation, which at times it would, dependent upon the newness or oldness of the potato, you see, that is used.

5451-3 M Adult CATARACTS
2. In the applications for conditions for the vision, we would NOT operate - for this must at least mean the full loss of sight to the one eye. While the vision has gradually faded with the constant accumulation of tissue thickening over a portion of the ball, there is NOT the atrophy of the optic nerve. There IS the pinching of the central nerves as LEAD to the optics. These need STRENGTHENING, and - as has been INDICATED - would there be the application [this simple, yet effective in this particular condition] those of the Irish potato - scraped; not the peel, but that of the larger the better - this scraped, and of evening cake same over the eye socket - eyes closed, to be sure. Then, of morning, when this is removed, CLEANSE same with a weakened solution of an antiseptic that will aid in the CLARIFYING of the MUCUS from the system.

Staph infections are common and known to be resistant to conventional treatments. The following suggests some cases may yield to this old fashioned home remedy:

5391-1 R6. 11/19/73 Letter from Bette Nelson, R.N.: "I was reading Health Hints sent to me by the Cooperating Nurses Unit. The article on Irish Potato poultice was especially intriguing, as my mother, who was 1/2 Irish, raised five children on a farm and used no other treatment for anything except Irish potato poultices. We were never sick, and I never met a doctor till I was 19 years old.

"Last year my friend's new born baby contacted Staph in the nursery, along with several others. I kiddingly told her to use the Potato Poultice. It cleared it up in 3 days. The infection was a severe one and not responding to any other medicine. Another girl friend used it on conjunctivitis and it cleared up beautifully."

Dietary Recommendations

From the standpoint of statistical generalities the Cayce system heartily endorses making the skin or peelings, and not so much of the pulp, as a regular part of the diet. It is often difficult to separate a general dietary recommendation from a treatment specific recommendation but the peel of the potato with a little of the pulp is clearly considered by Cayce to be the healthiest and most nutritious part of the potato, containing salts that are helpful to the thyroid. The information is quite specific about how the skins should be prepared:

337-24 F 50 Thyroid:Hair:Baldness
9. [Q] What is causing the hair to fall out and what can be done to restore it?
[A] This arises from impoverishment of forces or influences to the activity of the glandular system from which there are the secretions to keep such portions active in the body.

9...A great deal may be gained from the use in the diet of the Irish potato peel and that portion close to same. However, the thyroid extract taken in small quantities would be beneficial. The salts in the potato peel, though. Prepare the potatoes so that the jackets may be eaten. If these are desired boiled, it is preferable to boil them in Patapar Paper, so that the elements may be preserved. If the body prefers them roasted or baked, these may be taken, - but do not burn the peel so that the skin and that close to same - for at least an eighth of an inch - is destroyed by being so charred as to drive out the salts necessary for activity in the system.

The following advice leaves no confusion as to which part of the potato Cayce favors in the diet:

1904-1 F 42 Thyroid:Hair:Baldness
12. Then as to the diet: Add to the diet the Irish potato PEEL, but not the pulp a great deal. It would be better if the nice potatoes are cleansed, peeled and only the PEELINGS cooked and eaten! Throw the other part away, or give it to the chickens, or distribute it in some other manner besides eating it!

This case illustrates how the pulp affects some people:

404-7 F 49 LUMBAGO
20. [Q] Even a teaspoonful of potato affects the liver, causing a hardening for 24 hours or more. Why is this?

[A] Then leave 'em off! Just don't take 'em! Should know better! Anything that comes from below the ground almost, save such as carrots OR the oyster plant, will affect the body near the same way; and these don't try to eat them cooked eat the juices or the raw!

These cases illustrate only 3 of the hundreds of recommendations for eating more of the skin of the potato than the pulp:

842-1 F 50 Glands:Thyroid:Hair
19. [Q] My hair has always been thin. How can I make it grow thick and glossy?
[A] These baths will be beneficial. Of course, the diet is the greater activity. Oranges and Irish potato peels are the better elements that carry the forces for activity with the thyroids when they are working normally - which, of course, as indicated, are not; and these treatments will make for the better activity of these portions of the body.

1398-1 M 38 ARTHRITIS
22. Beware, then, of white bread, spaghetti, white potatoes - save those that may be roasted and principally the portion only eaten that is close to the jacket and the jacket of same [as the salts from same will be helpful in keeping the proper balance through the body].

1000-22 F 50 Prescriptions:Teeth
19. [Q] The enamel on my front teeth seems to be wearing away. Is there any special treatment for this, or is there a special diet?
[A] A diet that will carry more of enamel-building foods would be well; or the Calcios, or calcium foods, - as well as the SKINS of Irish potatoes; not so much the bulk of the potato but the peel.

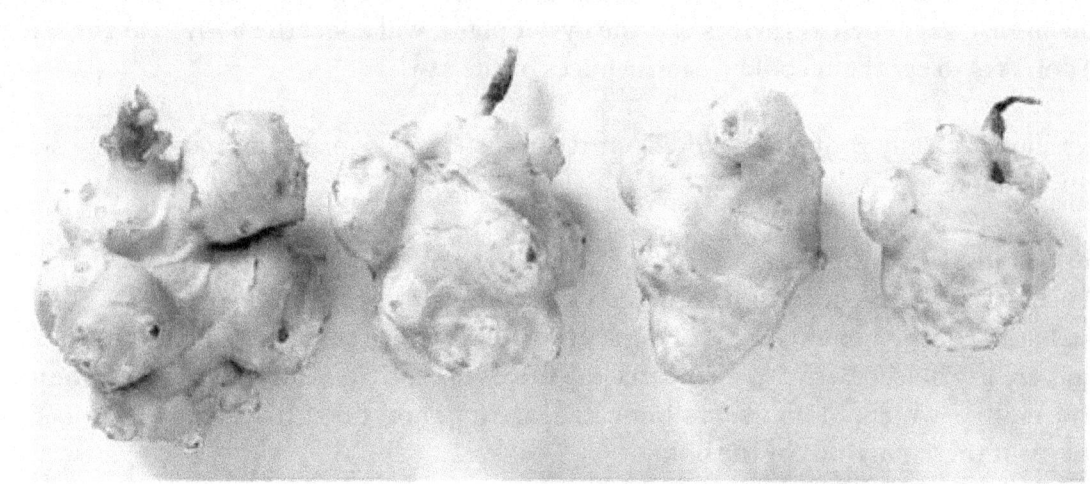

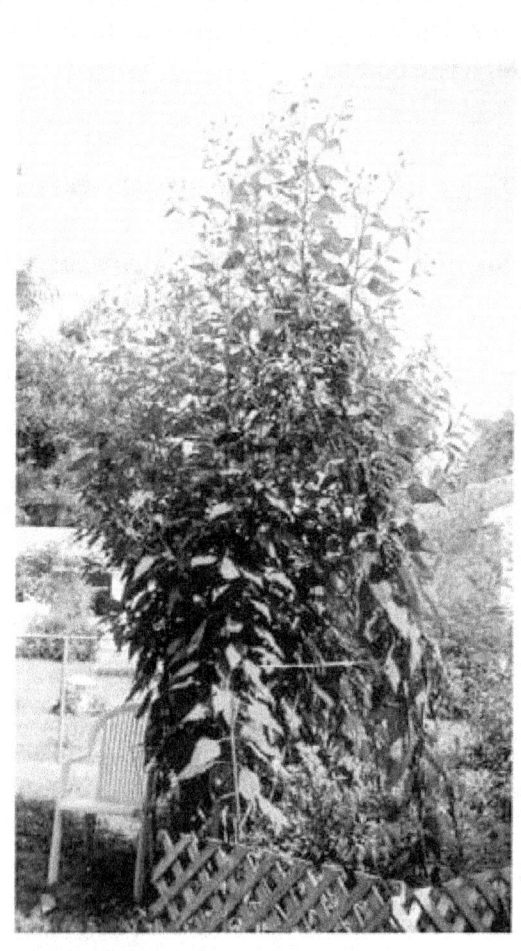

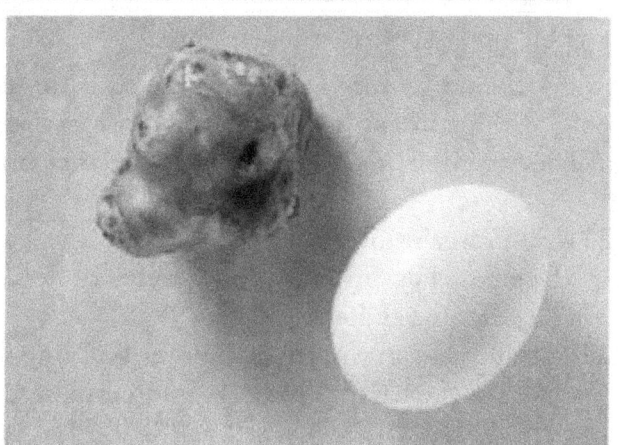

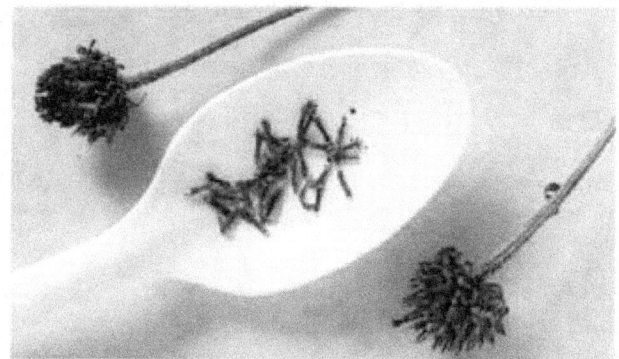

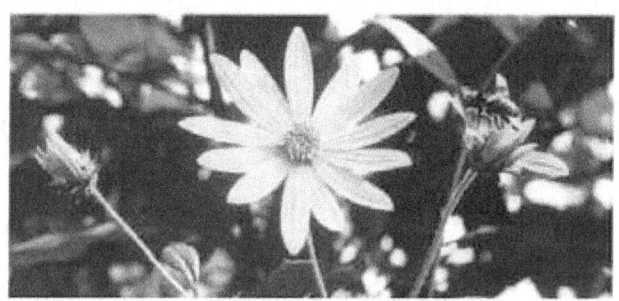

Jerusalem Artichoke
Helianthus tuberosus, Fam. Asteraceae

Common and Regional Names
Sunchoke, Girasole [Turning to the sun], Sunflower Artichoke, Potatoes of Canada

History and Common Usage
The Jerusalem artichoke is believed to be a native of North America. Early settlers discovered it originally growing in the plains states. It occurs naturally in what is today the Canadian lake region to the west in Saskatchewan and south to Arkansas and in the central region of Georgia. The roots or tubers of the artichoke were used as a food plant by the Native Americans long before the earliest settlers arrived and it is recorded that in 1805 early explorers Lewis and Clark ate the tubers prepared by Native Americans when they were traveling in what is now North Dakota.

One of the earliest published citations on the Jerusalem artichoke dates from 1629 in Gerarde's <u>Herball</u> and since that time the plant has been imported to Europe and India. The French are said to have obtained the plant through their Canadian explorations and it is now grown extensively in England and France both as a vegetable for table use and as stock feed.

A University of North Carolina agricultural bulletin states: *However, unlike most starchy vegetables, the principal storage carbohydrate in sunchokes immediately after harvest is inulin rather than starch. When consumed the inulin is converted in the digestive tract to fructose rather than glucose, which can be tolerated by diabetics*[73].

The 21st Edition of the United States Dispensatory lists the Jerusalem artichoke as an unofficial drug plant containing an abundance of inulin. Inulin is a polysaccharide, a simple sugar, found in plants and used as a natural form of insulin.

Description
Jerusalem artichoke is not to be confused with the globe artichoke [*Cynara scolymus, L.*] of which only the bud is edible.

Jerusalem artichoke is a large plant reaching heights of 7 to 15 feet. Bright yellow flowers up to three inches across appear in early to mid-summer on rough branching stems which can grow to 1 to 4 feet long. The leaves are medium green, larger towards the bottom of the plant, and somewhat smaller and more slender toward the top. In the earliest stages of growth the young plant is sometimes confused with its much larger cousin the common sunflower. The edible parts are tubers which grow below the ground. They are irregular in shape, sometimes knobby, thin skinned, light tan in color and white inside. Eaten raw their taste is similar to water chestnuts. They are also cooked and eaten like Irish potatoes.

Growing Conditions and Propagation
Jerusalem artichoke is pollinated by insects and wind. It is an extremely vigorous, cold hardy perennial which can quickly become invasive. It will grow in any climate where corn and potatoes can be grown.

---

73   Jonathan R. Schultheis, Extension Horticultural Specialist, Department of Horticultural Science. *Growing Jerusalem Artichokes.* The University of North Carolina Department of Horticultural Science. Revised 1/99 – Author Reviewed 1/99 – HIL-1-A

They do not perform well in extremely hot climates and the tubers will soon die out because *Helianthus tuberosus* requires a winter dormant period.

The plants are propagated by seeding and through their underground roots. Planting whole tubers or a portion containing an "eye" or a bud will develop into a new plant in a similar fashion to that of the Irish potato. Plant the tubers as early as possible in the spring. For optimum results plant them no deeper than 3 to 4 inches. Given the slightest chance of sun, adequate water and good soil even the smallest roots will send up new plants.

Neglected or crowded plantings will exhaust the soil resulting in tubers considerably diminished in size and quality. Unless the plants are thinned regularly, mulched and fertilized it is best to dig up a few roots and re-plant them in a new location every three years, allowing 18 to 24 inches of space between plants in rows a minimum of 4 feet apart.

The plant spreads rapidly from its rooting system. To maintain a small degree of control over unwanted growth remove the bottom of a large heavy gauge plastic pail and bury it in the garden keeping about 2 to 3 inches of the rim above the level of the soil. Plant one healthy root in the soil space inside the pail and at harvest time dig the tubers and sift through the soil by hand discarding even the smallest pieces. Large plastic pails are available from restaurants, building contractors etc. and can often be had at no cost.

The stalk of the Jerusalem artichoke is woody so in areas subject to high wind it is best to grow them along a fence. The stalks can also lean from their own weight and tip very easily. Although the plant will continue to grow and produce, bent and half broken stems are unsightly and make it difficult to weed and maintain the garden.

Harvesting
The tubers are ready to be harvested in the fall. Waiting until after the first frost produces a much crisper and sweeter tuber. North Carolina State University research referenced above states: *The crop should not be harvested until after frost. Tubers dug later in the season are sweeter but have less levels of inulin.* In warmer areas where winters are milder harvesting is done after the plant has died back.

Jerusalem artichoke is not an "easy keeper" and does not store well. The tubers can only be kept for a few days after digging. They can be stored for a few months at 32° if humidity is maintained at 85 to 95% humidity. Some home gardeners report successful winter storage [in areas of deep frost] using containers of clean moist sand or sawdust with the tubers buried, kept moist but not too wet, and out of the light approximating their conditions in the ground. The tubers may not spoil but their therapeutic value may be reduced by these methods. It is best to leave them in the ground and dig them as needed.

To find the plant in deep winter after heavy snowfall the stalks of the plants can serve as natural makers. Mulch the ground heavily to prevent frost from penetrating and trim the stalks down to 2 or 3 feet depending on how deep snowfall is in the area. Remove all dead side branches, leaves and small stems.

Use in the Edgar Cayce Readings
The Jerusalem artichoke is not a companion plant in the Cayce system. Diet is a major treatment modality both in prevention and health maintenance and Jerusalem artichoke is recommended in nearly 200 transcripts as a specific treatment food in cases ranging from arthritis to diabetes to vitiglio.

When using Jerusalem artichoke therapeutically, questions are always raised about fresh tubers, which can sometimes be difficult to obtain vs. convenience of prepared or dried. That same question was asked in December of 1940 by a 45 year old woman who asked the question on behalf of her husband Mr. 470. The answer below increases the desirability of having the fresh tubers available in the garden when needed:

1100-30 F 45 PRURITIS
[Q] Is the Bragg dehydrated artichoke all right for [470] to use, instead of the fresh artichoke?
[A] Not as efficacious or efficient in its activity in the system as the fresh. For, dehydration - especially of artichoke - is to lose not only the vital forces of its activity upon the system, but to produce an effect in the functioning of the system such that it requires a continued usage of same, or it becomes something upon which the body is dependent, rather than attuning the functioning of the organs, - as the liver, pancreas and spleen, - to the needs, or to the ability to produce - through the activity of the glands through these - that necessary for keeping a balance in the body.

Use the fresh, rather than the dehydrated.

This warning, given for a 37 year old male makes a point in paragraph 20 of specifying the fresh vegetable and not a prepared extract:

2772-1 M 37
19. And here [in the physical] the body should take care the more towards those things and tendencies in the physical that have to do with the heart, the liver and kidney circulation, and beware of those tendencies towards too much sugar in the body-forces. [See 2772-1, Par. R1.]

20. These may be tempered by the chemical forces as combined in the Jerusalem artichoke; not as an extract but the use of the vegetable itself. Don't neglect this!

The following two excerpts describe what the Jerusalem artichoke does in the body.

2094-2 M 70 DIABETES
32. [Q] What was the Jerusalem artichoke given for?
[A] An activity upon the pancreas. It carries - it is the greatest source of insulin that may be assimilated by the body.

1937-2 M 17 LYMPHANGITIS
6. In the diet we would add occasionally the artichoke, preferably the Jerusalem variety - if this is practical. This is to aid in the activity of the glandular force as related to assimilation. This should aid in stimulating better eliminations through the kidneys and a better coordination of the activity of the pancrean forces by the assimilation of the insulin from same.

In the following, taken from a life reading, the subject - a dentist - was warned about developing a sugar problem in later life and was told not to neglect using the Jerusalem artichoke to avoid developing diabetes:

2772-1 M 37 Diabetes Tendencies

19. And here [in the physical] the body should take care the more towards those things and tendencies in the physical that have to do with the heart, the liver and kidney circulation, and beware of those tendencies towards too much sugar in the body-forces.

20. These may be tempered by the chemical forces as combined in the Jerusalem artichoke; not as an extract but the use of the vegetable itself. Don't neglect this!

The following 4 excerpts are typical dietary recommendations:

2406-1 F 78 DIABETES:TENDENCIES

17. Also include in the diet the Jerusalem artichoke. Do not give injections of insulin, but DO give the nervous shocks to the system by the use of these properties from which it is often extracted, - that is, the Jerusalem artichoke. Give one of these [about the size of a guinea egg] EACH day for three successive days, leave off a week, then give for three successive days again, and continue it in this manner as a part of the diet, you see. This should be prepared by boiling it in Patapar Paper, not overcooking nor undercooking it, but about as an Irish potato would be cooked. Let this be prepared and eaten with the meal, you see. And this shock, - as from the activity to the pancreas and the general nervous system, - WITH the other applications, - will aid in better activity through the body.

470-14 M 47 DIABETES:TENDENCIES

13. Precautions in the diet; not an excess of CANE sugars. Use rather the raw sugar, or preferably beet sugar; whether in the drinks or foods; or resort MORE to the sugars from fruits and vegetables in the diet. But include at least twice a week the artichoke; [Jerusalem Artichoke. See 470-14, Par. R3] the bulb as well as the root. The root may be used as in soups or cooked as potatoes. These carry the greater quantity of an active force upon the adrenals, that may be created through the activity of the glandular system - and will keep a normal balance for this particular body, if the other precautions are taken.

1904-1 F 52 GLANDS:CHEMICAL IMBALANCE:BALDNESS

13. Especially we would have in the diet all forms of artichoke, - the American, the bulbular, as well as occasionally the Jerusalem artichoke. Not so often either of these, but about once or twice a week, - this preferably boiled [the Jerusalem artichoke] as you would boil an Irish potato, but the WHOLE of this would be eaten, you see. When it is boiled, boil it in Patapar Paper, and the juice which comes from same would be saved to be mashed with the pulp of the artichoke; and it should be mealy or crumbly just as the roasted or baked potato, see?

1855-1 M 31 KIDNEY INFECTION

17. The Jerusalem artichoke should be a portion of the diet each day. This would be taken preferably cooked, but it may be taken raw if preferable. The insulin from same - as it is easily assimilated for the activities not only of the pancreas and spleen and liver activity but - will aid in reducing the inclination for the inflammation and pus activity in the kidney itself. One artichoke the size of a duck egg or turkey egg, or thereabouts, should be taken each day, - that is, the tuber of the Jerusalem artichoke, see?

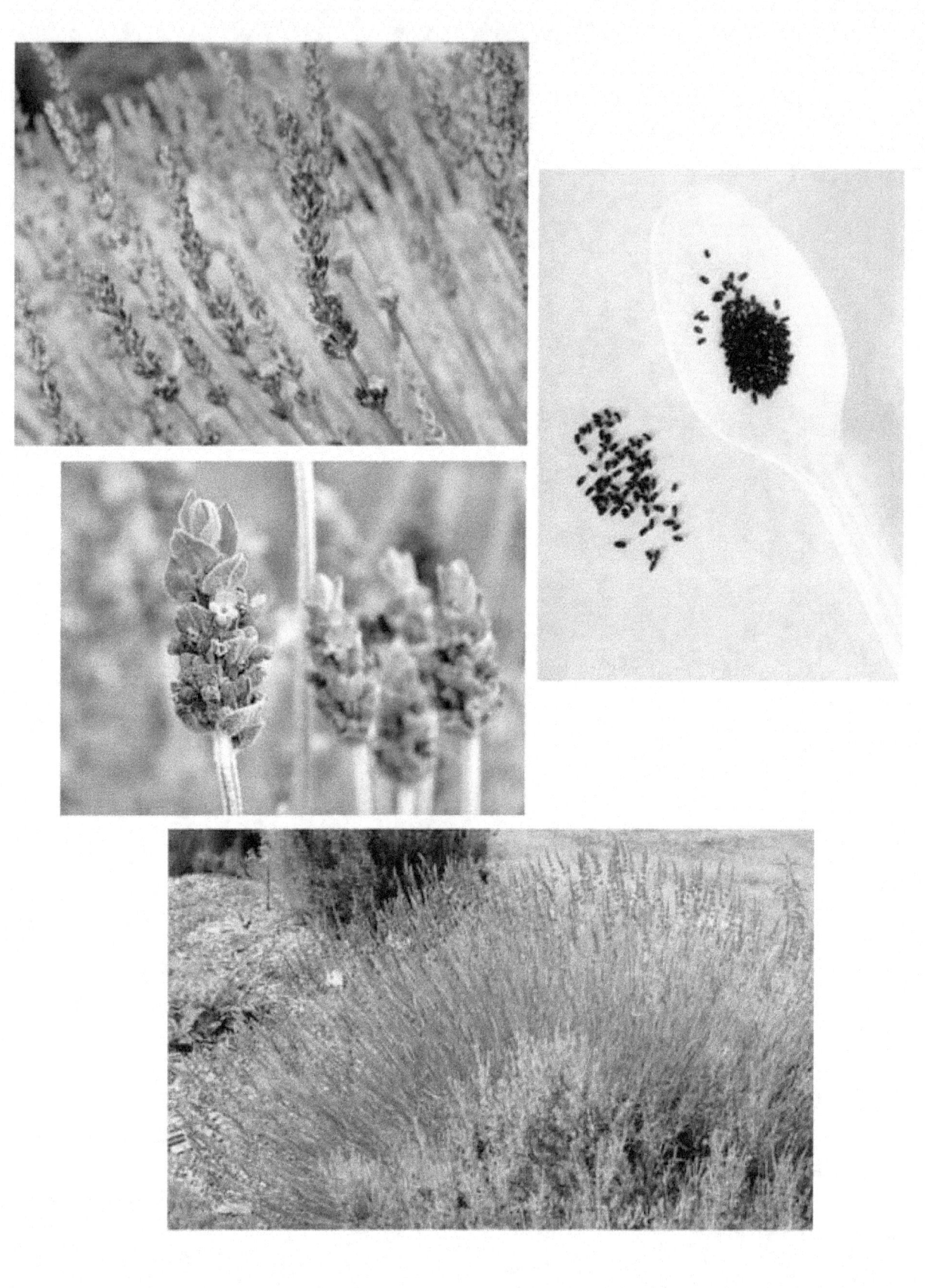

LAVENDER
Lavandula officinalis, Fam. Labiatae
Synonyms*: L. angustifolia* P. Mill. *L. Spica* [Linnaeus], *L. officinalis* [Chaix,
L vera [DeCandolle]

Common and Regional Names
English Lavender, Spanish Lavender, French Lavender

History and Common Usage
Most plant historians agree that this delightfully fragrant plant originated in the western regions of the Mediterranean, Southern Alps and in the dry and barren regions of Spain, Italy and the South of France.

Lavender does not hold a significant place in ancient medicine and does not enter written records until about the time of the Greeks and Romans. The current history of lavender begins with the Romans and their famous baths as the name lavender comes from the Greek word for wash, "lavare." It is known that the Romans brought the plant with them during their conquest of the British Isles where it soon entered into cultivation emerging as what is known today as English Lavender. It was officially listed in the British Pharmacopoeia in the 18th century. There are hundreds of hybrids and varieties today, and all can and have been used medicinally in the form of tinctures, compound tinctures, oils and essences.

Lavender has always been prized for the beauty of its foliage and fragrance, and in addition, it has held a place of importance as an insect repellent to deter flies, mosquitoes and fleas. Some medical historians suggest that in regions where periodic bouts of plague were not as devastating were areas where herbs with insect repellent properties such as lavender were in use on floors as a strewing herb and stored in clothing and other household linens as a deterrent to fleas. Lavender has a long history of use in bathing, in scenting soaps and the oil applied to the temples has traditionally been claimed to soothe headaches. It has a minor medical presence for use in salves and as tinctures to expel worms. It is immensely popular in potpourris and sachets, and the flowers have been, and still are used - sparingly - as a condiment.

There are many unsubstantiated claims in circulation for the use of lavender among various early civilizations and cultures. One such claim is that lavender is the spikenard mentioned in the Bible and was the ointment used by Mary Magdalen to pour over the feet of Jesus. As dramatic a claim as this may be it cannot be historically or scientifically substantiated. Scholars have long agreed that this costly aromatic ointment, ever so carefully preserved in alabaster boxes to preserve the fragrance, was derived from a member of the *Valerianaceae* family [Valerian] by the name of *Nardostachys grandiflora* [or *N. jatamansi*]. It is known as "sinbul Hindi" or "Indian spike." This plant grows in Nepal, Bhutan and the valleys of Tibet. An essential oil is extracted from the root and hair stems of *N. jatamansi* for use as a costly perfume and as a hair tonic. It is very sweetly scented and of a rose red color. Wealthy Romans used it for anointing the head and as an emollient. It was long held that the use of the ointment increased hair growth and turned the hair black. The historical use of *N. jatamansi* is well documented.

Botanists have struggled since the time of Linnaeus to arrive at the right names for the different species of lavender and to come to agreement as to whether or not a particular hybrid is a species or a variety. Much confusion exists even today among sources as to which name to use. In general there are three major species: English, Spike and French.

English Lavender [Synonyms *L. vera* and *L. officinalis*] probably leads the world in commercial production. English Lavender is prized because its oil is considered by many to be of the finest and most fragrant.

Spike Lavender [Synonym *L. spica]* produces a higher volume of oil than the English, but again purists claim the English fragrance is of a better quality.

French Lavender [Synonym *L. stoechas]* may be the one variety that can be traced to times of antiquity. It is sometimes referred to as "wild lavender" and occurs naturally in the Southern Alps. It is scientifically impossible to determine if this is the "original" lavender, but if it is, it means that *L. spica* and *L. vera* have adapted in their individual environments, evolving their unique qualities into two separate species over the past 400 or so years.

Lavender has a significant presence in the world of modern commerce but there is no established lavender market which provides an infrastructure to connect production of lavender to other industries. Growers create and market their own products from field to consumer which means the signature of an individual company has retained its uniqueness and this has perhaps contributed to the enduring high quality of the product. Lavender is of extreme importance in Provence, France, very nearly defining its culture. It appears on its coat of arms and an entire tourist industry has developed encouraging visitors to explore "lavender routes." The lavender products of Provence are marketed around the world.

Norfolk Lavender also enjoys an equally significant international reputation. Originally established as a plant nursery in Norfolk, England in 1874, an entire industry has grown around the marketing of soaps, sachets, potpourris and honey all from plants grown in the region, including a dazzling array of unique lavender theme gift items.

Oil of lavender was official in the American and British pharmacopoeias during the time the Cayce information was being given. The designations in the 21st edition of the US Dispensatory are given as *L. Spica* [Linnaeus], also *L. officinalis* [Chaix], and *L vera* [DeCandolle]. Oil of lavender is described as being distilled from the flowers and is described as a clear or yellow liquid with the strong, fragrant scent of lavender. It is cited as being used chiefly as a perfume although it has some digestive and stimulant properties. It was recommended for use in cases of *"nervous languor and headache.[74]"*

Description
Lavender is a shrubby, perennial evergreen that appears from a dwarf of approximately 10 inches to 4 feet high. Older plants [they are considered mature at 3 years of age] become bushy and spread to 3 or 4 feet in diameter. It has soft green-gray rather short thin leaves which are a little fuzzy or wooly on young plants. The leaves vary a little in size and width according to the species or variety. The flowers form at the tip of the four sided spikes [also called wands] which make up the body of the plant and vary in color from white through pink, pale lavender to deep bluish lavender and on to rich deep purple. The French tends to be darker in color. All parts of the plant are aromatic.

Growing Conditions and Propagation
Lavender can be difficult to grow. In order to be successful it is wise to consult area growers and nurseries to determine which species or varieties are locally adapted. Because of their origins, most lavender will grow in poor, coarse and rocky soils and prefer warm growing conditions in full sun. It does best in

---

74   United States Dispensatory. Wood-LaWall.. 21ˢᵗ Edition.. J.B. Lippincott, Co. 1926. [762]

neutral pH. It cannot survive long, harsh freezing winters and will not survive in hot climates. In the United States it can be grown in zones 5 through 9, although some gardeners report success in zone 10. Lavender does not like wet feet and is very susceptible to root rot.[75] It needs good drainage and once established does not need much watering. It is best to let the soil dry completely leaving the plant to Mother Nature. If the soil is healthy and friable, fertilizer is not needed.

Lavender is an enthusiastic hybridizer which makes cutting the best method of propagation. In most climates cuttings can be taken in May through mid-August by selecting a not too green and not too brown stem. Pieces are cut in lengths of 3 to 4 inches, the leaves trimmed from the bottom and the stalk inserted into a rooting medium. Stalks need to be kept moist [never allow them to remain in standing water] at about 70 to 75 degrees in dappled or filtered light. The young plants will be ready for transplanting by the following spring.

Propagation can also be done by layering. This is best if begun in the spring. Choose a stem with between 6 or 8 inches of leaves near the top. Bend the stem to the ground being careful not to break or crack it at the base. Notch the stem slightly and pin that area to the ground. Cover the notched area with soil and hold the tip with the leaves above the ground using either a forked stick or a small stone. Water the notched area lightly. Leave the notched stem in place undisturbed and check for signs of continued growth at the tip. The following spring the stem is cut from the mother plant and re-planted.

Lavender propagates by seed but is a reluctant germinator. Plants are difficult to grow from seed, and because of their propensity for hybridization, seeds will often not produce true to the parent stock. Germination can take up to a month and unless conditions are ideal seedlings do not often survive. Seeds can be started in pots in February in most areas and transplanted to the garden when soil temperature is warm enough to ensure survival.

Serious growers advise pruning immediately after blooming so that the plant has time to recover before winter. This is in addition to cutting any stems for drying. Any stems that do not produce flowers need to be cut back to maintain vigor and encourage new growth, but do this carefully. The plant needs leaves to survive and should not be cut back to the woody stems. In very cold climates mulching is necessary. Again, it is best to consult local growers and nurseries for the best variety.

Harvesting
The stems are cut just as the first flower buds begin to open. It is important to cut the stalks before the buds open completely as their fragrance weakens as they mature. The flowers and stalks can be used fresh or dried for later use. For drying the stems are bundled and tied with string or rubber bands and hung in a warm dry, dark place. When dry the flowers can be either stripped from the stalks, or the whole stalks can be stored. Airtight containers are necessary to retain the fragrance as long as possible.

Use in the Edgar Cayce Readings
Lavender is used alone and also as a companion plant. It is mentioned in 19 transcripts. The recommendations are mixed between the use of the color and fragrance and its use as a fume bath additive and massage oil.

---

75   Phytothphora

Both the color and odor of lavender are generally described as an aid to meditation and a helpful influence in keeping a spiritual focus. A 61 year old podiatrist was told that the color purple should be kept close to her body and that the odor of lavender would make for "attunements." In another case the parents of a young child were told that their child would be especially gifted if trained *"in connection with the spiritual through music,"* and influenced by the odor of lavender and shades of green. [4137-1 F Child] In another case a 37 year old woman was simply told it would be better to change the odors used in her room from almond to lavender but no further information was provided.

A 20-year-old young lady concerned about her complexion was advised to change her diet, take some hydrotherapy treatments including colonic irrigations, and a series of osteopathic treatments of the spine. She was then told to make a lotion to use on her face, hands and arms:

2154-2 F
30. To 2 ounces of Grain Alcohol, add - in the order named:
> Rose Water.................4 ounces,
> Oil of Lavender..........30 minims,
> Pure Olive Oil........1 1/2 ounces.

Two other ladies were told to have a dry cabinet sweat finishing with a steam treatment with one teaspoonful of witch hazel and 10 drops oil of lavender.

Oil of lavender was only recommended as massage oil in 2 cases. The first combined oil of lavender with olive oil and rosewater. The second is a little more complex and refers to some of the ingredients as being part of the anointing or sacred oils. This case is one of many where the treatments were not able to be followed; however since this is the only such reference in the Cayce collection to the sacred oils it is included here:

Background 3372-1
B1 9/2 1943…Dear Mr. Cayce, …I will try and make my story very brief, when [3375] was born she suffered a brain injury in the course of the delivery which developed into a spastic condition and also affected her speech so that today she can neither talk or run as other children of her age and believe me Sir, it is most heart breaking. She is at present taking orthopedic treatments but unfortunately I see little improvement and the various specialists give me very little encouragement.

3375-1 F 3
11. … During such periods use not merely the corrective measures for the structural portions, but do so with oils - that are partially the anointing oils, the sacred oils - in this combination; adding these in the order named:

Olive Oil......................   2 ounces,
Tincture of Myrrh [heating
the Oil to add the Myrrh]... .2 ounces.

12. Beat thoroughly, then add:

Calamus Oil....................2 minims,
Oil of Lavender.................1, 2, 3, 4, 5 drops.

13. These if combined in their correct proportions will aid in alleviating any strain in the muscle and tendon forces, and also aid at the base of the brain, by assisting the nerves to be normal in their reflexes - internally as well as externally - and thus gaining control of the locomotory centers [and these will come first in upper portion of body], and the reflexes to the auditory centers; as speech, hearing, vision. For, all are partially hindered in the present - some more than others.

A 37 year old young man working as a chemist in a perfume laboratory was given information on the importance of the sense of smell, and the physiological, spiritual and emotional responses to various odors, a field of inquiry largely neglected by the scientific community. The information stated that the parent stock of various plants had been given the ability to produce their individual odors as an expression of the "Creative Forces." The information went on to indicate that synthetic odors had been accepted but to do so was much like *"accepting shadows for the real thing!"* Of lavender the young man was told:

274-10 M 37
13. ...Did lavender ever make for bodily associations? Rather has it ever been that upon which the angels of light and mercy would bear the souls of men to a place of mercy and peace, in which there might be experienced more the glory of the Father.

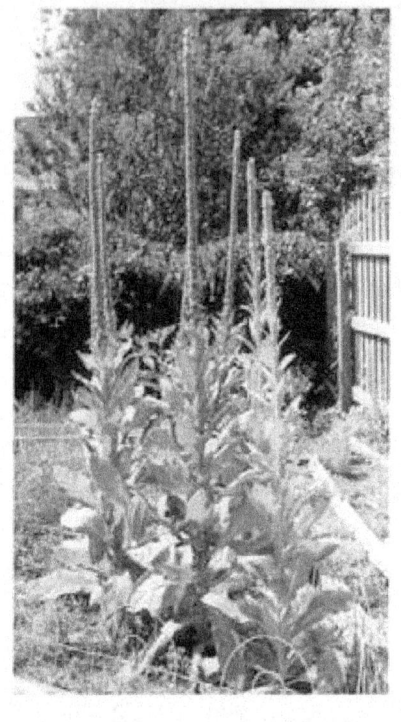
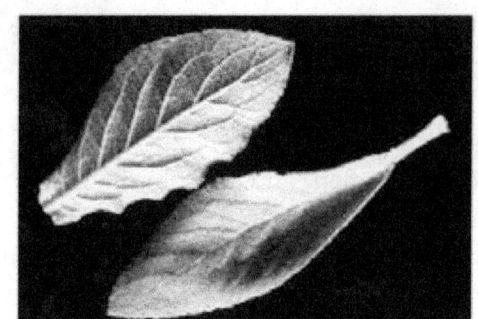
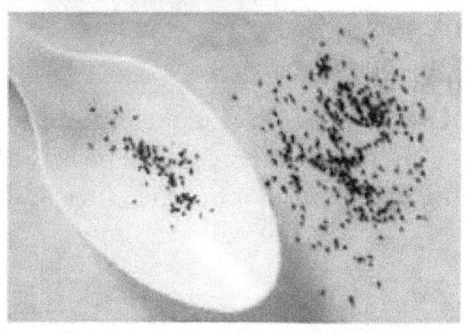
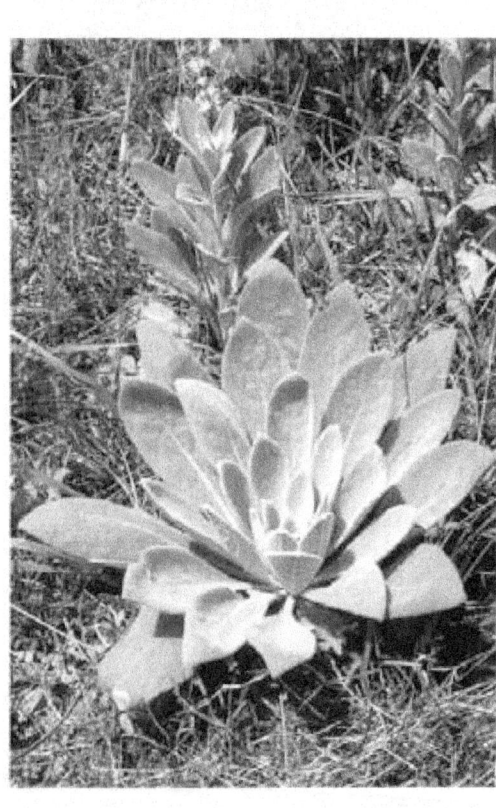
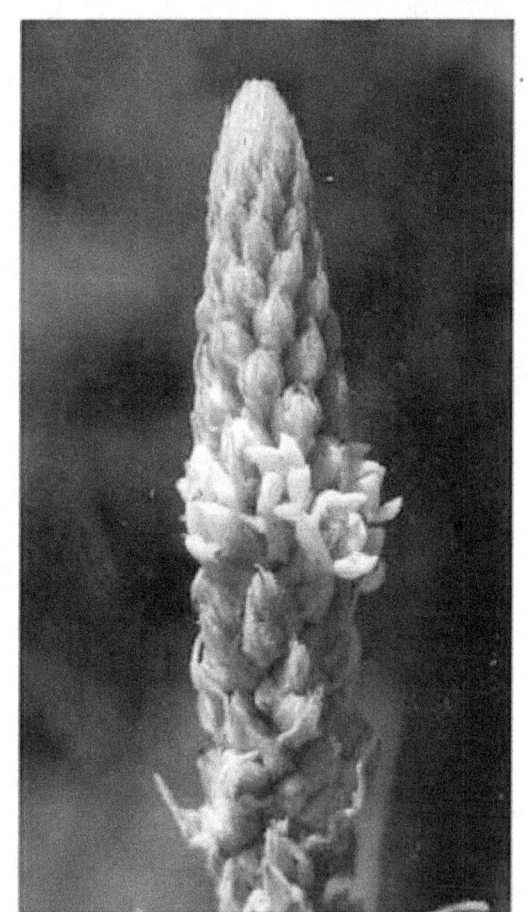

MULLEIN
Verbascum Thapsus, Fam. Scrophulariaceae

Common and Regional Names
Aaron's Rod, Donkey's Ears, Bunny's Ears, Bull's Ears, Velvet Plant

History and Common Usage
Originally believed to be native to Europe, northern Africa, Egypt, Ethiopia and Asia mullein is now naturalized in all temperate zones of the world. An important medicinal plant used by the earliest indigenous peoples, it is presently found in Hawaii, New Zealand and Australia where in some areas it is classified as an invasive weed. There are approximately 125 species of the genus in Europe and Asia.

Mullein leaves, bruised by hand or in hot water, have been applied to the body to relieve pain and reduce swelling for millennia. Mullein oil is used for ear, gum and mucous membrane infections and as a local application for hemorrhoids. The oil is easily made at home by filling a small jar with flowers and pouring in enough olive oil to cover. Seal the jar and place it in the sun for 2 weeks to infuse. Pour the oil through a sieve and store in a glass jar. While the storage life of the oil has not been scientifically determined, it should keep for a year at which time a fresh batch should be made.

Mullein has been used for centuries in the Ayurvedic system in the treatment of respiratory problems. Teas made from the flowers and leaves are used in any number of folk medicine traditions in cases of bronchial and lung infections. The leaves are rolled into cigarette shapes, dried and smoked, lending their slightly sedative properties for relief of asthma and to ease the symptoms in tuberculosis of the lungs. Some scientific credence can also now be given to age old claims for the antiviral properties of the plant. In recent clinical studies conducted by Julie Serkedjieva at the Institute of Microbiology at the Bulgarian Academy of Sciences, in Sofia, Bulgaria, an infusion of the flowers has been found to be effective in reducing influenza viruses in studies of various tissue cultures.[76]

Mullein is officially described as a demulcent and an emollient in both the United States Dispensatories and the national formularies during the time the Cayce information was being given.

Description
Mullein is a biennial. It forms a rosette pattern low to the ground in its first year of life, and the next year it sends up a compact spike which often branches into multiple arms tipped with flowers. When adverse conditions are present mullein has been known to remain dormant for two to three years before coming to flower. The plant can grow 8 feet high or more. The leaves tip downward in an alternating fashion from the spike, larger at the base and smaller towards the top. They are woolly, light green; often well over a foot in length and between 4 and 8 inches wide. Small bright yellow flowers appear at the tip of the spike, blooming in an incremental fashion between June and as late as September in some areas. The flowering tips can be between 6 to 12 inches long.

Growing Conditions and Propagation
Mullein is pollinated by insects, wind and is also self pollinating. It propagates by natural seed casting. The plant loves full sun and is often found in harsh conditions in poor soil but can also occur in thick,

---

76   Phytotherapy Research. Volume 14, Issue 7, Pages 571-574, Wiley-Interscience. October 23, 2000. © John Wiley & Sons, Ltd.

tall grass. The very tiny black seeds are easily gathered from the mature spikes by hand stripping in the fall and can be simply scattered in the garden on top of prepared soil.

An easy way to obtain a plant is to transplant one during its first year of growth. A dormant plant - one in the rosette stage - will transition easily provided enough soil is taken so as not to hurt the roots which are very shallow. Transplanting may cause the plant to remain dormant only coming to flower in the third year of its life cycle but once established it will self seed and soon a balance between dormant and flowering plants will be self-sustaining.

Harvesting

The best time to harvest leaves is in the morning before the sun gets too hot and preferably after a heavy rain the day or night before. Plants in the garden can be cleaned by watering or sprinkling the afternoon or evening before harvesting decreasing the shock to the plant. Leaves are used fresh or spread to dry and will be ready for storage in two or three days. They can be crushed or pulverized and stored in sealed glass jars or plastic storage bags.

Freezing fresh mullein leaves can easily be done for off-season use. The leaves are "bruised" or blanched in boiling water for a few seconds and then immediately dipped in ice water. They are gently dried [paper towels work best] and placed flat between two pieces of plastic cling film, patting the edges to exhaust as much air as possible so as to prevent freezer burn. Stored in freezer bags they can be frozen flat or rolled.

The flowers are picked in the early morning over a number of days and used fresh or dried. After drying in a warm dark place and sealed in plastic bags they can be stored on the pantry shelf or in the freezer. Dried or frozen mullein will keep for a year.

Use in the Edgar Cayce Readings

Mentioned in approximately 141 transcripts, mullein is used both alone and as a companion plant. The leaf, flower and seeds are used variously as a tea, as poultices and as syrup in compound formulas for the relief of coughs.

The action of mullein is described in case 988-7: *the very nature of the Mullein is to absorb poisons from the body itself; relieving pain and causing the accumulations to be thrown off through the respiratory system.*

On rare occasions the seeds are to be smoked as a hypnotic for temporary relief combined with using the leaves in topical applications:

849-5 M 21 Veneral Disease:Gonorrhea:After Effects
4. About those portions of system - in the testes, and in those portions where the pain or the acute attacks occur, or reoccur [urethra - swollen right knee, etc., gonorrheal synovitis?] - well were these kept with mullein lotion, or stupes of mullein or mullein with the leaves bruised and in hot applications applied to the body, and these would bring relief. As would the smoking of seeds from those of the mullein or of ginseng - these would also bring relief for this PARTICULAR condition; though are not curative forces, but only as a hypnotic for the condition. By following those as has been outlined would bring the better general physical forces for this part of the body.

The Cayce system makes extensive use of mullein packs [also called fomentations or stupes] in the treatment and relief of a great variety of physical ailments, often combined with suggestions for drinking mullein tea made from the leaves. This is often seen in the treatment of varicose veins. Fresh tea is clearly preferable but in 457-14 shown below it was made very clear that which ever was available, dry or fresh *"use the same all the while."* Take note of the rather pointed remarks in paragraph 18.

Tea

457-14 F 36 Prescriptions:Mullein Tea:General

17. [Q] Would the Mullein Tea be good for body now also? If so how much?
[A] Not unless there is trouble with varicose veins or the tendency for a dropsical condition through the pelvic areas. This taken occasionally is not bad for anybody and it will be very good for you.

18. [Q] Does it make any difference whether the Mullein is dried or fresh?
[A] Does it make any difference whether cabbage is wilted before it is boiled? It should indeed be fresh, not as in people, but as in the vegetable kingdom; not applying to people being fresh, but plants used for medicinal purposes, the fresher, the more active the better. And there is quite a variation between green Mullein and dried Mullein, but whichever you use, use the same all the while.

The advice below helps a young woman avoid developing varicose veins during pregnancy:

457-13 F 35 Pregnancy:6 Months Varicose Veins:Tendencies

3. As we find, in the main, conditions are developing nominally. However, the body should take those precautions about being on the feet so much and not using them. Standing is hard on the body, as is being indicated by the swelling in the limbs - which will tend to make very bad circulation, and produce varicose veins unless there ARE some activities taken to prevent same. Either WALK or DON'T STAND ON THE FEET SO MUCH! Walking is the best form of exercise for the body.

4. If there will be the walking, and not merely standing or resting, and the taking of a small quantity of Mullein Tea every other day, these will disappear - and this disturbance will disappear. The therapeutic reaction is to better circulation - through the kidneys, especially as related to the lower limbs.

5. Prepare the Mullein Tea in this manner: Bruise the fresh Mullein Leaves and some of the flower, especially at this period of the year. Use about two ounces [in quantity, not in weight] to about a quart of water. Let this steep as tea. Take two or three ounces every other day; it may be taken twice during that day, but this is the quantity to be consumed during the day, see? Keep it in a cool place, and make fresh almost each time it is used, see?

Stupes and Packs

Case 2332 is included here because of its severity. This woman's feet were in such bad condition that she was unable to work and could barely able to walk without extreme discomfort. Cayce called for at least 8 osteopathic treatments, dietary changes and the use of mullein. Miss 2332 describes her condition as follows:

B1. Breaking out and terrible swelling and rawness of feet; breaking out on neck, arms and legs. Some doctors say it is athlete's foot, some eczema; none seem to know what is causing it or what to do; been to Dr. Dormire and Dr. Taylor at Virginia Beach. It occurred last summer also; been off my feet several weeks now, unable to work.

2332-1 F 40 ECZEMA:CURED
17. Each day, - preferably just before retiring, - take internally about an ounce or ounce and a half of Mullein Tea. Prepare same in this manner; preferably gathering the Mullein Leaves AND the flower fresh - at this season: Cut these very fine, and put about two ounces of same [by measure, not by weight] in a quart of water. Let this steep as tea. Do not attempt to keep this longer than two days, even with keeping same on ice, for it will not keep, you see. Hence it should be made fresh every third day, you see.

25. The glandular forces, of course, are in the adrenals. Thus the Mullein Tea will relieve the pressures upon the kidneys, as well as the bladder disturbance that at times causes some anxiety.

27. If the feet and limbs give a great deal of trouble, apply Mullein Stupes also to the limbs - which will reduce the disturbance. Bruise the leaves, pour boiling water over them to wilt them, and then apply to the limbs as a poultice.

28. [Q] Is beer harmful?
[A] Very harmful for the body. For, the hops act upon the glandular forces that are disturbing to the body; especially the NEW - and so little is aged at present.

Especially the combinations of ale and beer are harmful.

Keep free from ANY carbonated waters, for the carbonations cause an effluvium in the blood. To be sure, Coca-Cola is helpful to the kidneys, but if taken, use the Coca-Cola syrup in plain water - and this to the body will not be very palatable.

Treatment information was given August 27, of 1940. Three months later in November her doctor sent this note to Mr. Cayce:

R1. 11/11/40 Letter from Dr. C. W. Irvin to EC: "...Miss [2332] was one of the most remarkable cases I have ever treated. You remember, of course, the condition of her feet and I am frank to tell you that I was skeptical when I started treating her, but after the fourth treatment her feet were entirely well and up to a week ago, the last time I saw her, they were perfectly normal..."

The two excerpts below contain typical directions for the preparation and topical application of mullein leaves for edema and varicose veins:

Stupes and Packs
304-45 M 83 EDEMA:Physiotherapy Applications:Mullein:Edema
6. First, in the preparing of the Mullein Stupes - put the Mullein into lukewarm water and let come almost to a boil; not on a fast or hot boil but rather a slow fire. When prepared for the Stupe, do not wring it too dry but place between a thin layer of cotton, so the cotton becomes moist with the

fluids as come from the Mullein by the Stupes as well as from the wet Mullein itself. And this should become, of course, thoroughly heated, thoroughly saturated - that is, the Mullein in its preparation - or should come to a boil and yet allowed to set after turned off until it is sufficiently cool to put the hands in same, see?

7. Then this upon a gauze cloth; that is, the thin layer of cotton, then the cotton over same, see, and this applied. This allows the moisture [not too much of same, but the heat or the moisture] to take up the poisons or to act upon the exterior portions of the body.

3523-1 F 54 Physiotherapy:Packs:Varicose Veins

19. Over the areas of the varicose veins we would apply the Mullein stupes. If the dried Mullein is used, this may be used in a very strong Mullein water. Do not attempt to have these veins removed by surgery. For, when these have been reduced by the activities of the osteopathic adjustments, later - when Spring comes - there may be used the mullein Tea - made from the fresh tender leaves of the Mullein that will be very helpful in this respect; keeping up the Mullein stupes, however, about once a week along on the varicose veins.

20. Do use an equal combination of Olive Oil [heated] and Tincture of Myrrh to massage in knees, limbs and feet, right after these have been bathed in hot water. Massage these oils well into them.

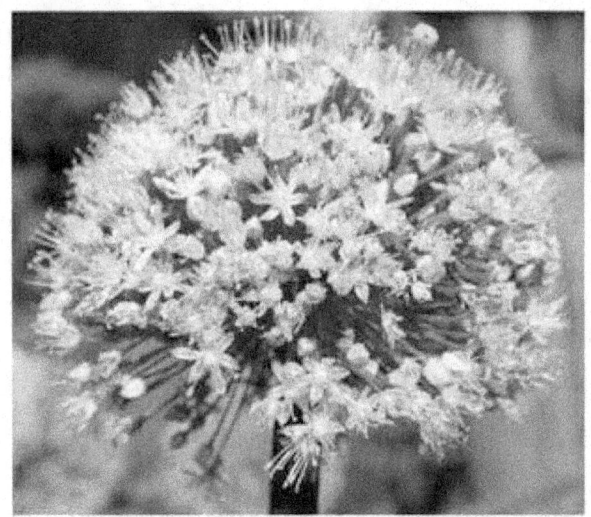

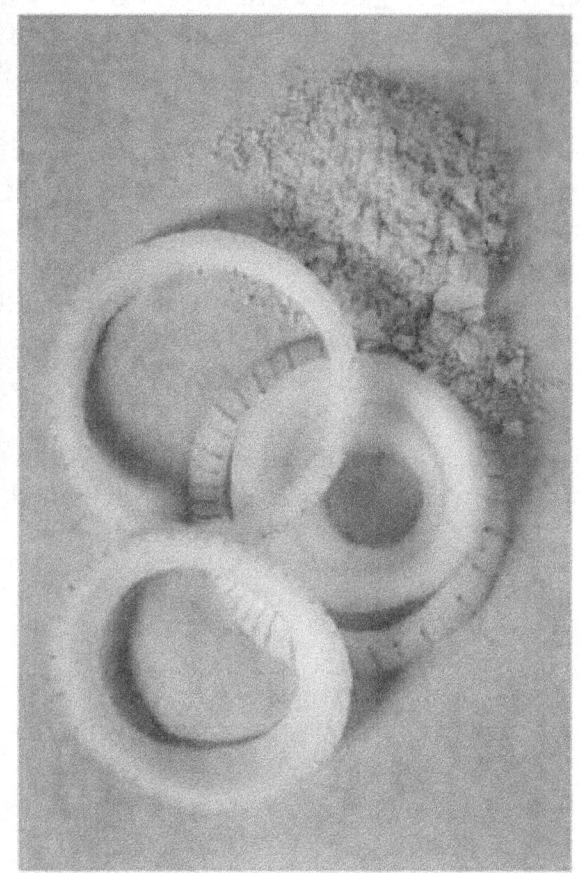

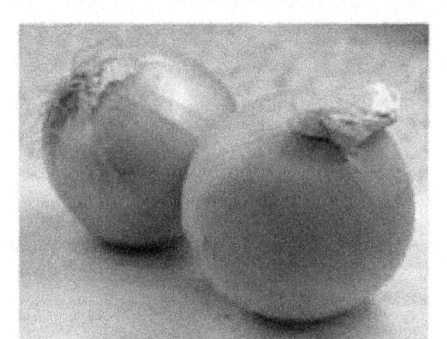

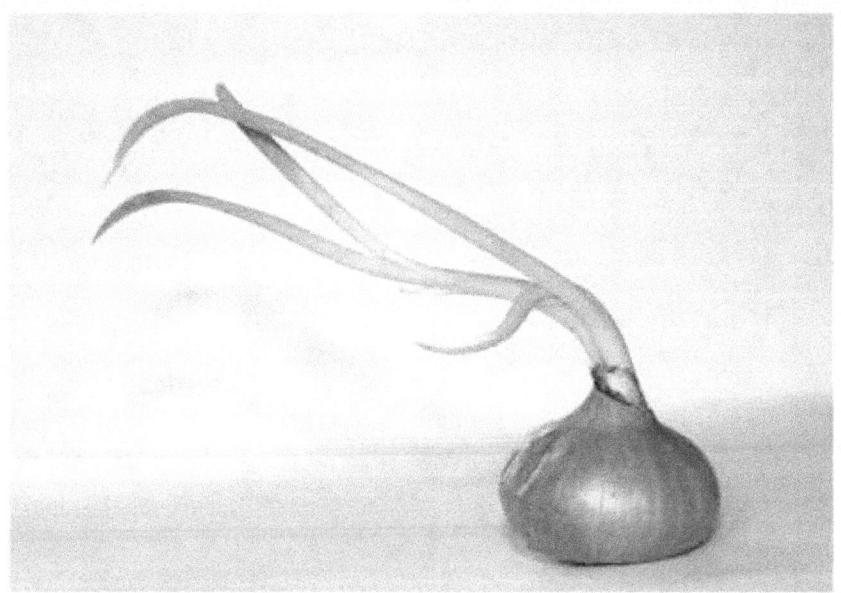

ONIONS
Allium cepa, Fam. Lilaceae

Common and Regional Names
Common Onion, Bulbing Onion,

History and Common Usage
Onions are referenced in some of the oldest Vedic writings and are known from existing records to have been cultivated in China for at least 5,000 years. Seeds have been found in Egyptian tombs dating to 3200 B.C. Some Egyptian mummies have been x-rayed revealing small onions placed in the eye-sockets, including the mummy of King Ramses IV who died in 1160 B.C and onions are often found stored in jars in tombs as food for the afterlife. Most authorities cite the onion as having originated in a region ranging from present day Israel to India to Asia, and all agree that the onion has been an important food source since Mesolithic times. Their flavor would have certainly inspired the early selective cultivation of the largest and tastiest bulbs.

Egyptians are known to have taken onions so seriously that some swore oaths upon them as evidence of good faith. Their encircling layers are said to represent eternity and they have long been used as religious offerings and appear in various art forms dating to both the Old and New Kingdoms. Onions were grown in Sumer and a Sumerian text dated to about 2400 B.C. records the unhappy event of the accidental plowing of the city governor's onion plot. The Book of Medicines lists over 15 prescriptions using onions distinguishing between the red and the sweet.

They were grown in the garden of Ur-Hammu, King of Ur in 2100 B.C. The Israelites are recorded in the book of Numbers in the Judeo-Bible as mourning the loss of onions and leeks from their diet when Moses led them on their long journey to the land of Canaan. Esteemed by Pliny, grown in Pompeii, and used by Roman gladiators as a massage agent to firm up their muscles,[77] the onion has been eaten raw, baked, roasted, fried, caramelized and boiled by every civilization throughout recorded history.

A final sad historical note regarding this vegetable is found in a small legal note from World War II. It is a decree published by the Minister of Agriculture of the Protectorate of Bohemia and Moravia[78] [Nazi-occupied Czech lands] dated November 8th, 1941.

Paragraph 1: *"The procurement of fresh, edible Onions [hereinafter referred to as "Onions"] can only be conducted, in the political districts and communities in which potato ration cards [23] have been issued, on the basis of ration coupons."*

Paragraph 6: Article 3 reads: *"Jews are excluded from the procurement of said Onions."*

They have long been recognized as having antiseptic qualities and because of this they have an important presence in folk medicine. A roasted onion, bound over an infected ear, was often the only remedy in the days before modern antibiotics. They have been used medicinally to alleviate headaches and the juice of

---

77   Tanya J. Fell, Director of Public and Industry Relations, *Onions Historically Healthy,* National Onion Association, Greeley, Colorado.
78   Sammlung der Gestze und Verordnunen des Protektorates Boehmen und Maehren. Druckerei des Protektorates Boehmen und Maehren in Prag. 1941 [Apples and garlic were also denied. Within less than a year, the majority of Jews from the Protectorate were deported to the camps.]

onions has long been used on open wounds to ward off infection. This last is now attributed to their allyl sulfides, which are responsible for the tearing response when peeling and slicing raw onions.

The 21ˢᵗ Edition of the United States Dispensatory lists the onion as an unofficial drug describing them as a dye plant stating further on page 1406: *"The Onion is sometimes used in domestic medicine as an expectorant in subacute bronchitis, and the Onion poultice is sometimes employed as a mild irritant."*

Description
The onion has edible, cylindrical, dark green, hollow leaves and an enlarged bulb that develops underground nourished by small, whitish-tan, short roots that grow in a crown–like-fashion from the bottom of the bulb. They are commonly found in three colors, red, white or brown [yellow] and come in a great variety of flavors ranging from very strong to very hot, and from peppery to mild to sweet.

There are two kinds of onions determined by day length which is the number of hours of sunlight required for them to develop and mature. There are long-day onions and short-day onions. Long-day onions require between 14 and 16 hours of daylight. Short-day onions will produce a bulb in areas where there are 12 to 13 hours of daylight.

Within these two major groups are three species: *Cepa, Aggregatum* and *Proliferum. Cepa* includes the large, familiar bulbing onion which is propagated by seeds. The *Aggregatum* includes the multiplier onions and last but not least, the top-setting group called *Proliferum*. There are hundreds of cultivars, all differing in day-length requirements and some known by intriguing names. Among the most interesting are the Potato Onions [also called multiplier onions] and Tree Onions [also called the Egyptian or walking onions] that produce small bulblets at the top where flowers are usually found. There are shallots, which seldom form seeds, are delicate in flavor and which divide into multiple sections after the fashion of garlic. There are Welch Onions, also called Japanese Bunching Onions which never form rounded bulbs but only white scallions and are favored as green onions. The mild flavored leek, delicate chives and pungent garlic are all cousins of the common onion.

When they flower to produce seeds the inflorescence develops on the tips of the stalks as a rounded body of tiny, greenish-white flowers from which the tiny seeds are developed. Sometimes flowers do not form and only tiny bulbils are present.

Growing Conditions and Propagation
Onions are pollinated by wind and insects. The *Cepa* group is propagated by seeds, transplants or sets. The *Aggregatum* propagates by multiplying bulbs. The *Proliferum* is propagated by planting the bulblets from the previous spring or late fall, or by root division every 3 years.

Onions prefer moderately cool temperatures, sufficient sunlight and adequate moisture. While they will grow in almost any type of soil, they do best in dark, rich, well drained loam in direct sunlight. Heavy clay and silt loam often prevent the full development of the bulb, so loose, well-worked, friable soils are best. To encourage the development of the largest bulbs possible the soil should be high in organic matter, and should fertilizer be necessary use one high in phosphorus and potassium. They do best in a soil pH between 6.2 and 6.8. How close they are planted is determined by their intended use. If green onions are desired they can be planted very close together. If grown for large storage bulbs 4 to 5 inches should be left between plants. Some gardeners will plant 2 inches apart and harvest every other plant for green onions allowing the rest to reach maturity. Allow 18 to 24 inches between rows for ease of garden maintenance.

Onions should be planted as early as the soil is dry enough in the early spring so that standing water will not kill the crop. Young plants can quite hardily withstand light freezes. Planting before May 15th in most areas is necessary in order to have the largest possible bulbs at harvest and to ensure they will store. The planting months of choice are March or early April in prime regions for producing storage onions. The long-day does best in the north and short-day varieties perform best in the warmer southern regions. Green onions can be planted anytime during the growing season.

Growing onions from seeds requires patience. They must be started indoors 2 months prior to planting time. Adequate lighting is necessary to encourage continued growth once the seedlings have emerged. They need to be kept moist but not wet and are ready to be transplanted in the garden as soon as they have reached 2 to 4 inches. Nurseries also supply transplants for the garden and there will be varieties suitable for storage or use as green onions.

Onion sets are used to produce green onions because bulbs from sets do not always mature and store well. Sets are small bulbs, usually no larger than ¾ of an inch in diameter, which have been pulled and dried forcing them into dormancy. When they are replanted and supplied with water they "come to life" continuing their interrupted growth cycle. Onions grown from sets are more subject to bolting [they go to seed quickly] than transplants or those grown from seeds. Plant sets about 1 inch deep and let them touch one another, as they will be pulled before crowding becomes a problem. Since onions have very shallow roots, keeping them free from weeds is important.

Harvesting

Storage onions are varieties within the *Cepa* group. They are brown [or yellow], white or red. The sweet are not good keepers and should be enjoyed fresh soon after harvest as there is no storage method which will keep them in peak condition for very long. Green onions can be pulled at any time after their tops have grown to at least 6 inches in length although most gardeners wait until the tops are 12 to 18 inches long.

High temperatures and low humidity produces the best bulbs for long-term storage. These conditions are also very important during the curing process. Onions are ready for harvest when the tops begin to fall over and the neck of the bulb begins to show signs of drying. Do not break or tie the tops before all the leaves have fallen over and dried as this is a sign of full maturity. If the tops are prematurely broken or tied too soon growth is interrupted resulting in smaller bulbs which will not keep well in storage.

When fully matured and ready for harvest, onions are pulled in the early morning and allowed to remain on top of the soil to dry until late afternoon and taken in before nightfall. They must not be allowed to get wet or be out in the dew. If the sun is extremely hot they should be shaded to avoid sun-scald.

At the end of the same day they are pulled they can be braided by their tops and hung in a dry, sheltered area with good circulation to cure. The dried tops can be cut back and they can be stored in crates with open sides or on slats or screens which allows for free and generous circulation of air. Complete drying and curing takes 2 to 3 weeks before the skins reach the "papery stage." The "dry wrapper scales," or outer skin of the onion must be completely dry. Do not try to store bulbs that have cuts, bruises or green tops. They will only spoil in a short period of time so use them immediately. Ideal storage conditions are at 32°F which is not usually available to the homeowner; however they can be stored until at least late winter in most areas. They should be checked frequently and any soft bulbs should be discarded.

Use in the Edgar Cayce Readings

The onion is used alone and as a companion plant. They are recommended in over 190 transcripts in a dietary context and the juice is prescribed for internal use. Sliced or chopped raw onions, combined with a small amount of yellow corn meal, are applied to the chest as a poultice in cases of cold and congestion.

As an important dietary item they are frequently recommended to be eaten green, tops and all, for their beneficial effect upon the kidneys and, as the following suggests, to help the circulation, lungs and eliminations: *Fresh Onions if possible; if not, those that are well preserved - or the Spanish variety. These properties will act upon the circulation and the whole of the pulmonary reaction, as to produce a better elimination. [909-2]*

In 308-2 boiled onions are recommended for their benefit to the digestive and assimilative processes: *"And each evening let a portion of the meal be of BOILED Onions, that are boiled in their OWN juices; not in water. Those eaten before retiring preferably should be raw; not large quantities, but small quantities, for these carry a vitamin and the elements necessary for the dilation of not only the pulmonary activity but for the juices - gastric juices of the stomach and assimilating forces of the body."*

Raw onion juice is recommended to be taken by mouth to *"act upon the digestive forces"* [326-10] and also that it *"would be most helpful in relaxing the body for sleep…"* [1208-13]

In cases of chest congestion a poultice of raw sliced onions, mixed and heated with a small amount of corn meal, is applied either directly to the chest or on cheesecloth and then to the skin. The onion poultice, perhaps more accurately described as an onion cataplasm[79] is found in nearly 70 cases in the treatment of various kinds of lung or bronchial infection, inflammation, cold and congestion, including in those days the potentially fatal pneumonia.

It is important to note that deaths from bacterial infections in the United States alone are only 1/20th what they were before even the limited availability of penicillin beginning in 1943. As newer strains of bacteria become increasingly antibiotic resistant perhaps some of these older remedies may take on new importance.

The following are samples of some of the ways the onion is used in the Cayce system:

2148-1 M 2 Months COLD:CONGESTION
7. Almost immediately, or as soon as practical, apply an Onion Poultice over the chest, as well as between the shoulders. Do not make the poultice too strong, else it would be too severe for the developing body. Chop the onions very fine, heat them - or cook them until they are about half done, you see; keeping most of the juice with same, - preferably cook them in Patapar Paper, this would be the better way. Then mix just sufficient raw corn meal with same to make into a poultice, not too thick but just sufficient to allow the poultice to be applied - between gauze - directly to the body. For this body, preferably use the YELLOW corn meal.

---

79   Cataplasm – chopped, grated or mashed vegetable matter applied to the body.

Apply the poultice while it is still warm, you see. Leave it on for at least thirty minutes. Then if there is not a change in the congestion, in twenty-four hours, put it on again, - making a fresh poultice, of course.

243-37 F 62 PNEUMONIA:TENDENCIES

3. As we find, conditions are rather serious in the present. The cold and congestion, combined with the fracture, has produced a stoppage in that side of the lung. [Pneumonia?]

5. Prepare an Onion poultice. This should be full, but cut Onions, heat them, mix then with a little meal - yellow corn meal, preferably; and apply on gauze over the area where the injury is indicated from the fall. This should cover both front and back of this side, see?

6. When this has been on about an hour, change and apply another.

391-4 M 21 Eliminations:Incoordination

15. For that tendency at times in evenings for the little disturbance or irritation in the throat, which arises from the gastric juices of the stomach, especially when the body retires, we will find that if there will be taken the juice pressed from half-boiled Onions, or the syrup from same, with a little sugar - or preferably honey or saccharin, this will allay the condition even if only a few drops are taken at a time.

17. [Q] What can I do to keep my throat from clogging up every morning, when I don't have a cold?
[A] We have just given it! We got ahead of you!

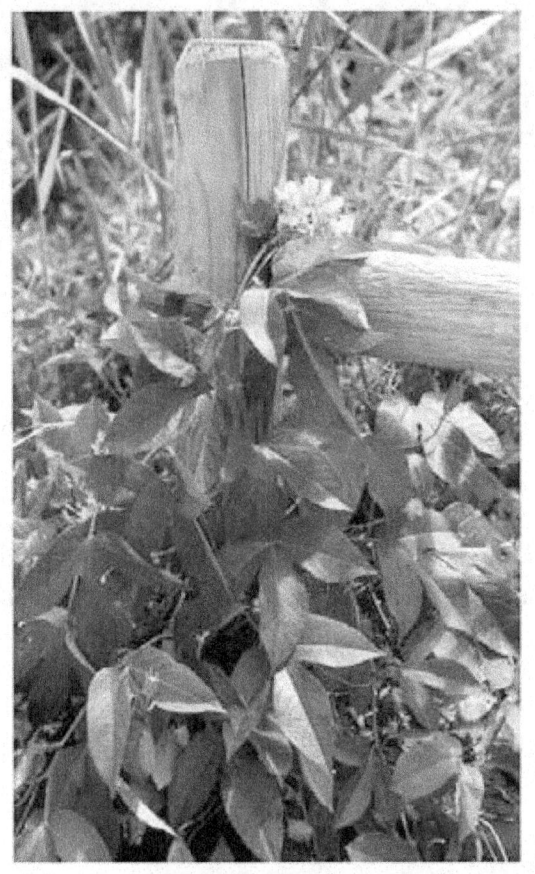

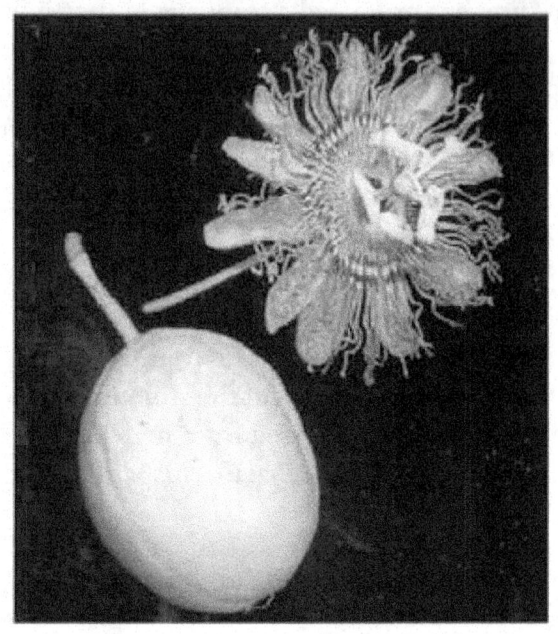

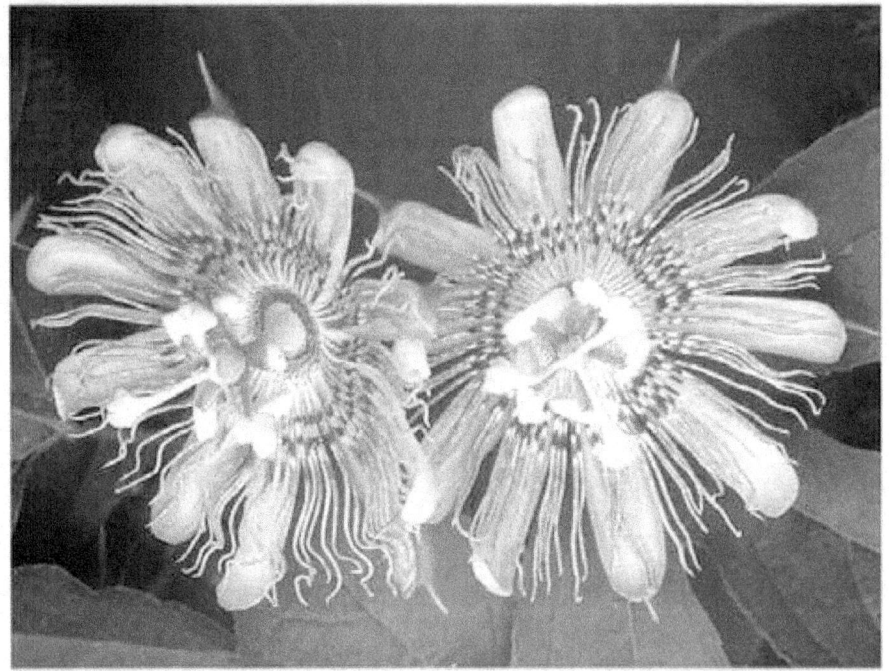

146

Passion Flower
Passiflora incarnata, Fam. Passifloraceaea

Common and Regional Names
Maypop – Apricot Vine

History and Common Usage
The genus *Passifloraceae* boasts over 400 varieties and is found throughout South and Central America and parts of North America. More than 55 species are grown for their edible fruits, the most widely grown being the *Passiflora edulis* originally found in the Amazon region. The fruit of other varieties is edible but bland and tasteless. Most yellow skinned varieties are grown for juice. Wherever passion flower grows it has been used in local herbal medicine.

One of the first European records of the plant dates to 1569 when it was discovered in Peru by Spanish explorers. After being described by the Seville physician and businessman Nicolas Monardes it soon became used as a favorite herb tea throughout Europe. One of the early references to medicinal use of the plant in the United States is found in Schoepf's *Materia Medica Americana*, a Latin work published in Germany in 1787 which mentions its use in the treatment of epilepsy of the elderly. Another of the earliest citations in American medicine took place about 1840 by Dr. David Lewis Phares of Mississippi when the plant was used as a nerve sedative to allay general restlessness, to relieve insomnia and in the relief of certain convulsive or spasmodic disorders.

Glycosides, alkaloids, phenolic compounds and other volatile constituents have been found in *Passiflora incarnata* but early efforts to separate and isolate these chemicals to produce a synthetic were not successful. Recently the University Institute of Pharmaceutical Sciences, Punjab University, Chandigarh, India published a study reviewing the historical uses of *Passiflora incarnata* in an effort to explore the potential uses of the newly isolated benzoflavone as a central nervous system depressant.[80] Advances in technology may soon result in the scientific determination of the therapeutic value of the plant but in the meantime the natural plant [fresh or dried] must be used.

A gentle tea or tisane of passion flower is made by pouring one cup of boiling water over one freshly picked flower [or one teaspoon of dried flowers] leaving it to steep for 10 minutes straining before drinking. However, because contraindications have not been determined, passion flower should never be used by pregnant or nursing women or mixed with any other medications without first consulting a doctor about possible harmful interactions.

The 21st edition of the United States Dispensatory lists *Passiflora incarnata* as an official drug plant citing its use as a nerve sedative used as a pain reliever in neuralgia. It states: *"While there is considerable evidence that this drug possesses some therapeutic virtue, it has not been carefully studied."*

Description
Passiflora is a rapidly growing perennial vine, with medium to dark green three lobed leaves. The flower is named for the passion of the Christ. The lavender to purple flowers are very exotic in appearance, the rays and sepals are shaped in such a way that their Catholic discoverers were reminded of the crucifixion. The length and thickness of the vine varies from species to species but can reach 30 feet in length. The

80   Journal of Ethnopharmacology. Volume 94, Issue 1, September 2004. Pages 1-23.

147

flowers range in color in shades from red or blue to rose to palest lavender and on to a deep and vibrant purple.

Growing Conditions and Propagation

Passiflora should be considered as a warm climate perennial. It grows in tropical and sub-tropical areas and will not survive frost. When cultivated in cooler climates mulching is necessary and it can also be grown as a houseplant if a method of allowing it to climb can be managed. As a wild vine it can be found growing in ditches along the edge of roadways climbing over taller shrubs and smaller trees to spread its leaves in full sun. It is often found in areas characterized by poor or sandy soil. *Passiflora* does not like wet feet so good drainage is essential. It will die back in the fall and reappear in the spring.

Passiflora incarnata can be difficult to propagate but once established will self-seed or come back the next year from the established root structure. The easiest method is to buy one from a nursery or find a wild plant and transplant it in an area where it will receive full sun. It is necessary to get as much of the root as possible and unlike some other wild plants, the more native soil taken the better.

Other methods of propagation are by layering or cuttings. To propagate by layering the leaves are carefully removed from a section of vine in late summer, and that portion of the vine is tucked under the soil, with the leafy end of the vine out of the ground. If kept watered roots should develop, but since success depends upon development of a full root system, plan on leaving the layered section through the dormant or winter season and only cut and transplant in the following spring if healthy new leaves have appeared.

Propagation by cuttings is time consuming and is subject to a high mortality rate. Sections of the vine, 4 to 6 inches in length, are cut in the fall [September in most areas of the southern United States] and dipped in a rooting and fungicide compound. Planted in perlite peat pots they are left in a warm place in low light for 2 to three weeks. As the cuttings establish themselves they are then re-potted, peat pot and all, in larger peat pots until they are well enough established to survive the move to the garden. Because *Passiflora* does not like to be disturbed peat pots should be used from beginning to the final placement in the garden.

Propagation by seed requires *"time, space and patience"* [262-114] as the *Passiflora incarnata* seed will germinate only in its own good time. Gather seeds from the mature seed pods in the fall. [Since squirrels will eat the pods as quickly as they appear, cover a select few with wire mesh.] Remove the seeds from the pod, dry them and store in a cold, dry place over the winter. They should not be frozen. The following spring plant them directly in the garden or in prepared pots filled with light sandy soil and cover the seeds lightly. Keep the pots moist but not wet and in a sunny location. Germination takes place in late summer although some seeds have been known to stubbornly wait until the following spring and others have been known to take a year.

Harvesting

The leaves, flowers, seedpods and vines are all combined for use in teas and tonics. Gather the materials early in the morning before the sun gets too hot and while the vine is still in blossom. The flowers will open from the bud in 30 minutes and are spent in the first hours of bloom. Because they are very delicate they are best picked and dried separately. Spread in a single layer on trays or clean paper toweling they will be ready for storage in 1 or 2 days.

Rinse the vines, fruit and leaves in cool, clean water. Remove the fruit to dry separately either whole or cut into pieces. The vines and leaves can be dried whole or cut into pieces before drying. Keep materials in a warm, dark place [70 to 80 degrees F] on fine screening or trays.

Many people prefer to use just the flowers. They are best if they are picked each day just as they are fully opened. They can be collected and dried incrementally in small batches throughout the summer.

Passiflora does not freeze well and it is only used fresh or dried. Drying methods should be gentle, no artificial heat source should be used, and the materials should be kept out of the light. When everything is dry, it is mixed for storage in plastic freezer bags from which as much air as possible has been exhausted. Store the material in the pantry out of the light and use within 12 months.

Use in the Cayce Readings
Passion flower is a true companion plant. Mentioned over 90 times it is used in a variety of teas and compound formulas. Often the terms passion flower and maypop are used interchangeably. The use of a compound formula containing *Passiflora incarnata* is cited in roughly 63 epilepsy cases and in three cases indexed as tendencies to epilepsy. A non-habit forming sedative, this formula is also referred to as Maypop Bitters, fusion of Passiflora or green tonic. There are, of course, other equally critical modalities in the treatment of epilepsy such as osteopathic treatments of the spine, olive oil by mouth and the regular use of abdominal castor oil packs.

A few excerpts illustrating the various formulas using *Passiflora incarnata* are shown below beginning with a standardized formula referred to as Maypop Bitters which was given for Miss [543] as follows:

543-5 F 21 EPILEPSY *[Author's Note: Standardized Maypop Bitters Formula]*
4. In the compounding of the Maypop, take one gallon of the vine, leaf, fruit, flower, of Maypop. To this add 2 gallons of distilled water. Reduce by slow boiling to 1 quart. Strain, and then add 6 ounces of 85% alcohol, with 1 ounce tincture or elixir of the Wild Ginseng. The dose would be a... half a teaspoon three times a day, taken half an hour before the meals - half an hour before retiring, and retire EARLY enough for those of the proper reactions of body through the evening or night. Ready for questions.

5. [Q] How much should be taken at each dose?
[A] Half teaspoonful each dose. This may be taken in water or plain.

6. [Q] What should be done to control an attack once it has started?
[A] Apply ice at base of brain.

Following 5 excerpts are just a few of the many ways *Passiflora incarnata* is used:

1495-1 F Adult EPILEPSY
10. These should be specific adjustments; coccyx, 4th lumbar or lumbar axis; 1st, 2nd, 3rd and 4th cervicals. These would require at least twelve to fourteen adjustments of such natures.

11. Then take the juice or a tonic made from the Passion Flower. Put about 12 ounces of the Passion Flower, with the leaves and the like, in a gallon of water and reduce to about a pint. Add sufficient

alcohol to keep same. The dose would be a teaspoonful at least four times a day. This is not habit-forming, as are the drugs that are used as sedatives for the system.

14. [Q] Should the Passion Flower prescription be begun at the same time as the other treatments? [A] As indicated, this is begun AFTER the osteopathic treatments. This tonic would be taken for periods of a month - every day; left off for a period of three to four weeks, then begun again. Twelve ounces to the gallon of water reduced by slow boiling, but do not put in aluminum kettle; rather in enamel or glass ware.

3790-1 F 23 EPILEPSY

6. Taking [all of this to come after the operation, see?] *[Author's note: tonsillectomy]* those properties in medicinal manner of Maypop Tea or Bitters, see? that as is prepared in the same way, or that as may be prepared in this manner: Take Maypop Root and the Maypop Bulb or Fruit when just ripe - the root and the fruit at the same stage, see? To 6 ounces of the root and of the fruit add 32 ounces of distilled water, and reduce to 16 ounces, see? by simmering. Strain off. Cool. Then add sufficient of the alcohol to preserve same, which would be, to the 16 ounces, 6 ounces of the grain alcohol, see? The dose would be [and this must be kept constantly taken for at least ten month], 4 times each day, teaspoonful in half a glass of water, before each meal and before retiring.

521-1 M 20 EPILEPSY

16. There should be also taken, as an internal reaction to those portions of the system that are affected in the nerve pressures, properties prepared in this manner - that may be prepared in quantities and a small quantity at a time also:

17. Take sufficient Maypop [this includes the vine, the fruit, the flower of same; preferably of that which is seasoned] *[Author's note: This means a mature vine where the seed pods are ripening.]* that when it is reduced by simmering the specific gravity of same is six and a half, see? This is preferably made with distilled water, and would be about the proportion of one gallon of the dried vine or vegetable to two gallons of water, see? and reduce until by specific gravity or hydrometer test it is six to six and a half. So, if it is reduced to where the gravity is much higher, simply add water to make same; or if lower, simply boil longer to produce same.

18. After cooling, add sufficient grain alcohol to make a preservative for same, which will be about the proportion of two and one-half ounces to each sixteen ounces of the solution.

19. The dose of this would be a teaspoonful after each meal and before retiring at night.

5232-1 F 25 EPILEPSY CURED

2. EC: Yes, as we find, there has long been a lesion in the coccyx area of the cerebrospinal system. There are the after-effects of shocks to the system. There are the results of indiscretions of parents of the entity. *[Author's note: Spanking too hard.]*

3. These are, then, partially karmic conditions. But if there are the spiritual attitudes and aptitudes, the breaking up of the lesion in the coccyx area and those tendencies for adhesions in the lacteal duct area, the relaxing in the upper cervical areas, these gradually worked together, osteopathically, these as we find can change the periods of these convulsions, lapses of memory, lapse of coordinations.

4. There will come 1 or 2 very severe periods with some of these changes. When these occur we would administer a heavy fusion of Passion-Flower. That would be the fruit, the leaves, the vine, a gallon by measure. Put this in a 2-gallon container and fill with water. Reduce by slow boiling to a quart and a pint. Add sufficient grain alcohol to make a preserving of the solution; then this would be strained off, of course, or filtered off.

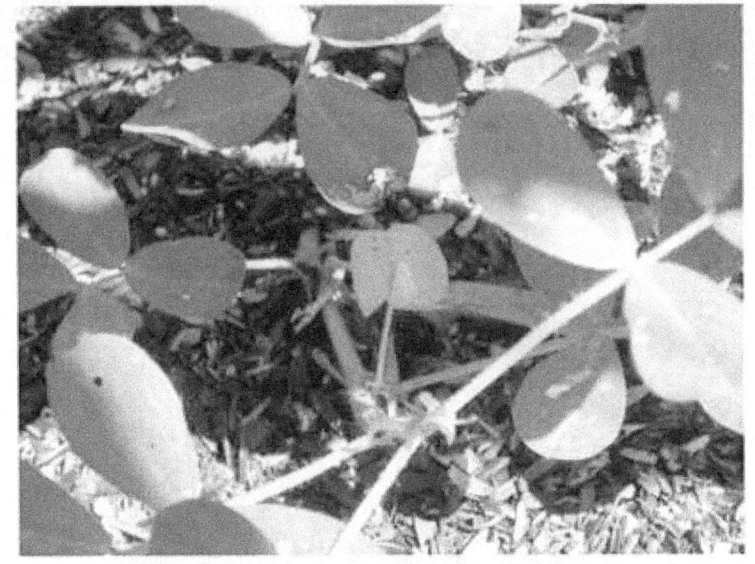

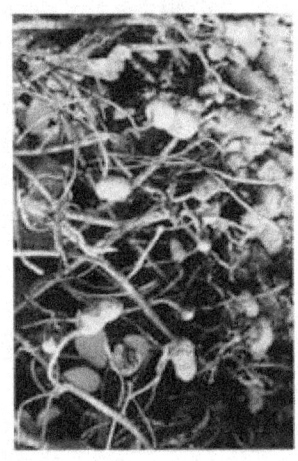

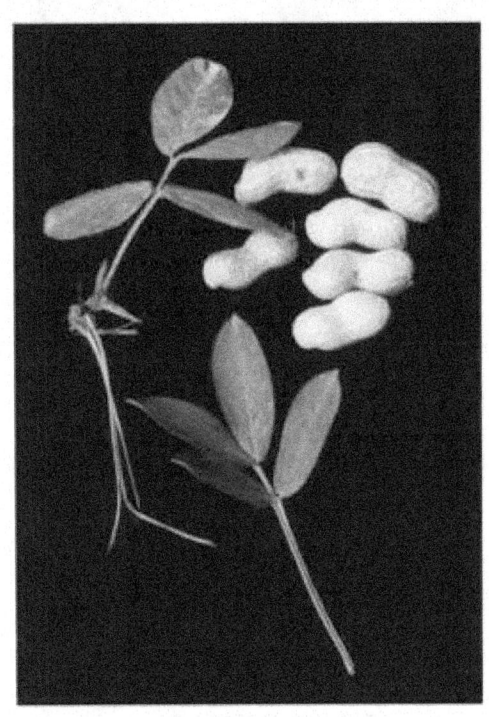

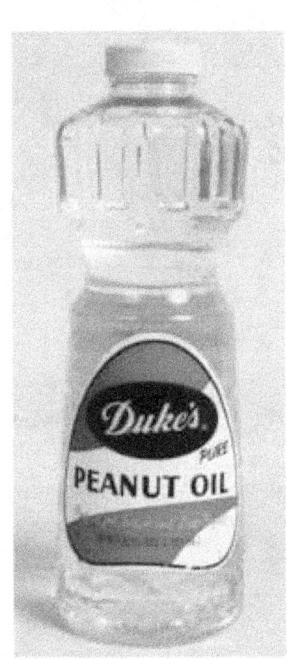

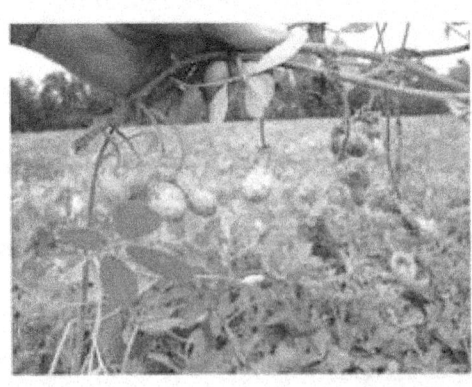

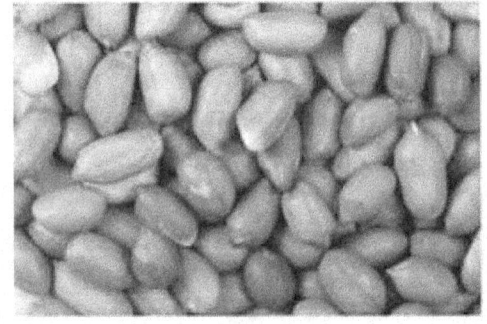

PEANUTS/PEANUT OIL
Arachis hypogaea, Fam. Leguminosae

Common and Regional Names
Groundnut, goober, goober peas, pinder, earthnuts, ground peas, Manilla Grain, Chinese Almond

History and Common Usage
The modern peanut has always been thought to be a native of South America originating in Peru and the area between what is known today as southern Bolivia and northern Argentina where it was first discovered by the early Spanish explorers. Recent findings challenge this long held theory. A wild type of peanut found in hearths and floors of buried sites in the Nanchoc Valley in northern Peru have been dated to 7,600 B.C. A squash was dated to 9,000 B.C., and a cotton ball to 5,500 B.C. Archaeologist Tom D. Dillehay, chair of the Department of Anthropology at Vanderbilt states: *"The plants we found in northern Peru did not typically grow in the wild in that area...We believe they must have therefore been domesticated elsewhere first and then brought to this valley by traders or mobile horticulturists."*[81]

The place of origin of the peanut may never be discovered but its identification with South America will not be easily erased. Pottery decorated with peanuts or shaped like peanuts, some dating back 3,500 years is frequently found. Graves of ancient Incas often contain jars filled with peanuts as food for the afterlife. In pre-Columbian times the plant was introduced to the West Indies and Mexico and in the early post-Columbian period the plant was introduced to Africa and eastern Asia. During the colonial period African slaves carried peanuts with them. The name goober comes from the Congo name for peanuts "neguba." The peanut is not a true nut but a legume.

Peanuts were not grown extensively during the early American settlement period because growing and harvesting the peanut was a difficult, slow and labor intensive process. They only began to be recognized as an important food source in the United States during the Civil War when they were eaten by foraging troops of both sides of the conflict. One of the earliest records of the use of peanuts in the United States is in 1890. St. Louis, Missouri food product manufacturer, George A. Bayle, Jr., processed and packaged ground peanut paste as a food supplement for people unable to chew meat. This early form of modern peanut butter was sold out of barrels for six cents a pound.

The first US Patent on peanut butter was obtained in 1895 by Dr. John Harvey Kellogg of Battle Creek, Michigan, mentor of Dr. Harold J. Reilly. Dr. Kellogg was the founder of the Battle Creek Sanitarium. With his brother Will Keith Kellogg they pioneered the development and marketing of modern day breakfast cereals. The Kellogg brand is known today around the world.

It was not until 1903 with the work of Chemurgist[82] George Washington Carver at Tuskegee Institute in Alabama that the peanut rose to economic prominence in both agriculture and manufacturing. Dr. Carver's work produced over 325 products from peanuts. The demand for those products combined with the development of labor saving farming and harvesting equipment turned peanuts into an extremely important cash crop.

The largest producers in the world today are China, the United States and India followed by Africa and Central and South America. Between India, China and the United States approximately 70% of the

---

81   Ancient Farm Transitions. June 29, 2007. Science Magazine.
82   Chemurgist – One who engages in the utilization of organic materials for industrial applications

world's crop is grown, generating employment on the farm and in the areas of processing, marketing and transportation.

The peanut is grown for peanut butter, candy and roasted nuts. There is also great demand for the oil for use in margarine and other foods as well as for use as fuel, such as in diesel engines. Peanuts are grown as feed for livestock, and for 300 derivative products include flour, soap, ice cream, and plastics, all stemming from the pioneering work of Dr. George Washington Carver.

Citations of the use of the peanut in folk medicine are few in number. There are no records of the plant being known to the ancient Egyptians, Greeks, Romans and Chinese or Mesopotamian cultures. The peanut is listed as an unofficial plant in the 21st edition of the United States Dispensatory but there are no medical uses cited.

Description

The peanut is an annual legume characterized by the habit of ripening its seeds underground in a manner similar to that of the potato. It is a medium green oval-leafed plant about 18 inches tall, which develops delicate yellow flowers around the lower portion of the plant. The compound leaves are similar to clover and the flowers are pea-like in appearance. There are two types of plants classified by growth habit described as either bunch or runner. These are either Virginia or Spanish nut types. The Virginia is the larger of the two containing 1 or 2 kernels per pod. The Spanish is smaller often containing 3 to 4 kernels per pod.

The plant is self-pollinating. After pollination each flower develops an unusual stalk-like structure called a peg which grows from the flower into the soil underneath the plant. Fertilized ovules in the tip of the peg develop the familiar peanut pod after the tip is well below the soil. There is also a root system underneath this which nourishes the plant. The pegs function as roots to some degree too because unless the soil is well supplied with calcium peanuts will not develop from the pegs no matter what nutrient is available to the roots of the plant.

Growing Conditions and Propagation

Peanuts can only be grown from seed and the best method for the home gardener is to purchase raw peanuts in the shell from the local grocery store. The nuts are removed from the shells taking extreme care to leave the fragile skin on the raw kernel intact to help deter insects. They are planted about 1 ½ to 2 inches deep about 3 inches apart. The plants will bloom about a month or a month and a half after planting.

Peanuts will grow under a wide range of environmental conditions between 40 degrees south and 40 degrees north of the equator. The ground should be prepared in the same manner as for any legume such as lima beans, green beans or peas. Peanuts do best in sandy loams and a soil temperature of 65°F is necessary for germination. Peanuts are considered "warm season annuals" requiring 120 to 140 days of frost-free weather to reach maturity after planting. Soil testing for calcium levels and the addition of any necessary soil amendments is important to insure germination, vigorous growth and the development of healthy peanuts.

As soon as the plant begins to peg, hoeing for weed control is discontinued. Any weeds that appear after this should be pulled by hand. It takes about 10 to 15 days for the peg to penetrate the soil. Mulching can be of help to control weeds.

Harvesting

The plant will flower and peg at different times throughout the season so all pods will not mature at the same time. When the foliage begins to yellow in the late summer or early fall the majority of the pods should be ready to harvest but it is best to wait until the tops are completely destroyed by frost or have died back. Using a pitchfork or spading fork gently dig the plants lifting the pods to the surface, shaking the vines to remove as much excess soil as possible. Sift through the soil around the plant by hand to collect the loose peanuts. The vines can be hung over taut clothesline in a shed or garage to dry, however this method produces an inferior product. The pods should be separated from the vines as soon as possible and put in shallow trays for drying. They take about two months to cure before they are ready for use and should be turned frequently during this time. A dark warm attic makes an ideal drying area; however, mice and squirrels are very fond of peanuts so care should be taken to protect the nuts from contamination from their urine and droppings.

Approximately two months from the harvest date the shells should be sufficiently dry to store in mesh bags and stored cool dry place. Peanuts can also be shelled and roasted, frozen or packed in ordinary canning jars for long-term storage.

Use in the Edgar Cayce Readings

The peanut, mentioned over 600 times, is used alone and as a companion plant. The Cayce system does not recommend eating peanuts as frequently as the oil is recommended for massage. In 11 dietary citations 6 indicate that peanuts should not be eaten and 5 indicate they should. Massage recommendations number in the hundreds, the oil being used alone or combined with other oils and products for massage. Peanut oil from the supermarket shelf is satisfactory for use:

1158-32 F 51
17. [Q] Is the refined peanut oil satisfactory for massage?
[A] Satisfactory.

The following are a few of the many ways peanut oil is used in the Cayce system.

Peanut Oil in Cooking

The Cayce system favors peanut oil for cooking:

826-14 M 40 Assimilations:Poor
10. Also have fish and fowl, but these prepared with the reinforced vitamins in the flour, the meal or the like. Use not the vegetable oils in the cooking, but either the peanut oil or the Parkay margarine - for this especially carries D in a manner that conforms with these properties in preparation for assimilation by the body.

Peanut oil is used in hundreds of cases for skin care:

2455-3 F 28 Psoriasis

10. For the conditions of hardening, as on toe, we would use a mixture of baking soda and Castor Oil. Do not bind up, but massage this on after the feet AND the lower limbs - from the knees downward - have been massaged thoroughly with the Peanut Oil. Do this at least three to four times a week; and the condition - it will be found - will disappear.

For dry skin and general skin care this lotion is well worth the time to make at home:

1968-7 F 31 Complexion

10. For making or keeping a good complexion, - this for the skin, the hands, arms and body as well, we would prepare a compound to use as a massage [by self] at least once or twice each week.

11. To 6 ounces of Peanut Oil, add:

> Olive Oil.............2 ounces,
> Rosewater.............2 ounces,
> Lanolin, dissolved....1 tablespoonful.

12. This would be used after a tepid bath, in which the body has remained for at least fifteen to twenty minutes; giving the body then a thorough rub with any good soap to stimulate the body-forces. As we find, Sweetheart or any good Castile soap, or Ivory, may be used for such.

13. Afterwards, massage this solution, after shaking it well. Of course, this will be sufficient for many times. Shake well and pour in an open saucer or the like; dipping fingers in same. Begin with the face, neck, shoulders, arms; and then the whole body would be massaged thoroughly with the solution; especially in the limbs - in the areas that would come across the hips, across the body, across the diaphragm.

14. This will not only keep a stimulating, with the other treatments as indicated taken occasionally, and give the body a good base for the stimulating of the superficial circulation, but will aid in keeping the body beautiful; that is, as to any blemish of any nature.

2072-13 F 33 Massage Oils:Skin Care: Peanut Oil

11. [Q] Is it well to remove the matter from the pimples and blackheads that form?
[A] This is very well, provided the areas are rubbed soon afterward with this combination of oils:

> Peanut Oil.......................2 ounces,
> Olive Oil........................2 ounces,
> Lanolin [liquefied]............1/4 ounce.

Peanut Oil used to Diminish Scars

Of the many formulas given to eradicate or diminish scars the following is easily made at home:

2015-10 F 3 Scars
7. [Q] Will continued use of Camphorice gradually eliminate scar on arm resulting from severe burn two years ago?
[A] Camphorice, or better - as we find - Camphorated Oil. Or make the own Camphorated Oil; that is by taking the regular Camphorated Oil and adding to it; in these proportions:

    Camphorated Oil..............2 ounces,
    Lanolin, dissolved.........1/2 teaspoonsful,
    Peanut Oil...................1 ounce.

This combination will quickly remove this tendency of the scar - or scar tissue.

Peanut Oil for Massage

As a massage lubricant peanut oil is highly valued in the Cayce system with hundreds of recommendations describing it as food for the nerves and muscular forces of the body. It is used alone and is also often found combined with grain alcohol, olive oil, witch hazel, oil of pine needles or other oils. The Cayce system states that peanut oil supplies nutriment to the skin, and to the ganglia, muscles, nerves and tissues. Transcript 2642-1 states: "*This oil does not become rancid on [the body]; it does supply nutriment, elasticity and activity to the cerebrospinal system.*" And the information states again in 257-233: "*It is the best rubbing oil if sufficient of it is given for the body to absorb, for it becomes rancid less often than others.*" The information also describes peanut oil as food and a preventive for arthritis: "*For this, as it were, is food – and if the Peanut Oil is kept regularly, there will never be - or need never be any fear of neuritic or arthritic tendencies... 2582-1*" The following two excerpts contain interesting information on the oil from the "*humble peanut.*"

2968-1 F 19 POLIOMYELITIS Physiotherapy:Massage:Peanut Oil:Paralysis
15. Daily, for at least half to an hour and a half, massage the body; not rudely, not crudely, not with the attempt to make adjustments - for many weeks yet. Massage with Peanut Oil, - yes, the lowly Peanut Oil has in its combination that which will aid in creating in the superficial circulation, and in the superficial structural forces, as well as in the skin and blood, those influences that make more pliable the skin, muscles, nerves and tendons, that go to make up the assistance to structural portions of the body. Its absorption and its radiation through the body will also strengthen the activities of the structural body itself.

2563-1 M 52 [Author's note: *Note the use of the words "skin food."*]
36. Then there would be the thorough rubdown, using an equal combination of Olive Oil and Peanut Oil. From the poor superficial circulation there are the natural tendencies for dryness to occur in portions of the body where the circulations are deflected. Hence this skin food should be massaged in, while the body is thoroughly relaxed.

An easy home method to alleviate simple arthritis of the hands or finger joints is to soak the hands in hot saturated salt water [which can be saved and re-used] followed by a massage of the joints with peanut oil. Any kind of salt is used for this simple remedy although Epsom's Salt was usually preferred by Dr. Reilly. An enamel or stainless steel pot large enough to accommodate the hands comfortably should be used, NEVER use aluminum. A salt pack or Epsom's Salts bath followed by a peanut oil massage is very often recommended in the Cayce system. The amount of salt used for a 40 gallon bath varies from 1 pound to 25 pounds. The following four excerpts are typical of the use of peanut oil:

340-43 F 52 ARTHRITIS
4. Then, - at least once in two weeks, or once every ten days until five or six are taken, we would take an Epsom Salts Bath. Have an almost saturated solution; that is, fill the tub with water as hot as the body can well stand, and stir in same about eight pounds of Epsom Salts. Lie in this for at least thirty minutes; gradually massaging the joints in the lower limbs, joints in the hands and arms and shoulders with the solution while in the Bath.

5. Sponge off thoroughly, and massage thoroughly with plain Peanut Oil [not other things added] - over the arms and shoulders and limbs, and across the hips.

6. Do not do this too often, but do it at least about every ten days for the first three or four times; then it may be done once a month or the like.

2288-1 M Adult Osteopath ARTHRITIS
13. Then, - on the eighth day in the second series, - take an Epsom Salts Bath; almost a saturated solution, and lie in same in same until there is the absorption of same through the system. Let it be as warm as the body can well stand, having sufficient water to submerge the body in same. In a large tub that would hold fifty gallons of water, put at least twenty pounds of Epsom Salts.

14. Have a thorough rubdown afterward, massaging especially the cerebrospinal system, and through the joints of the extremities, with Peanut Oil.

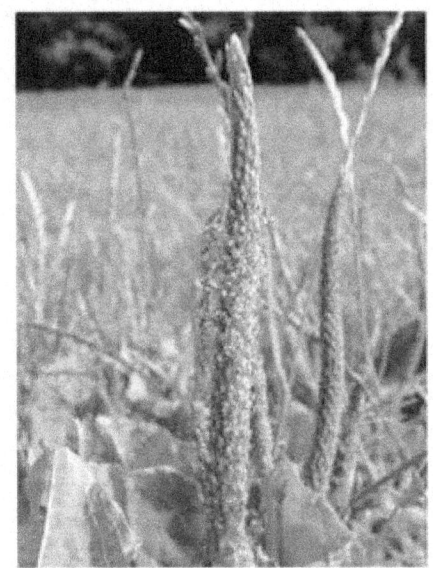

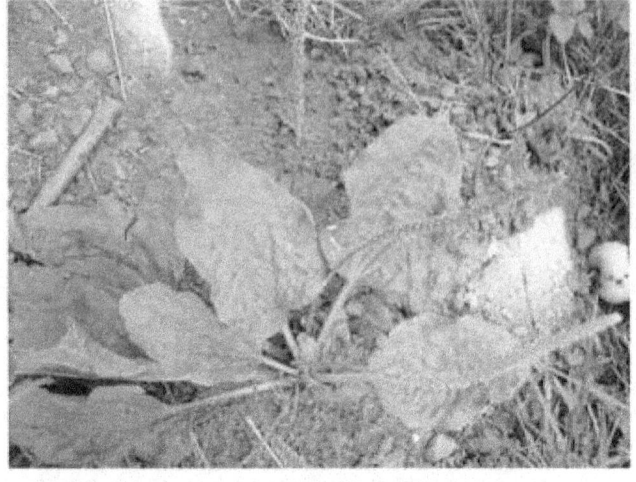

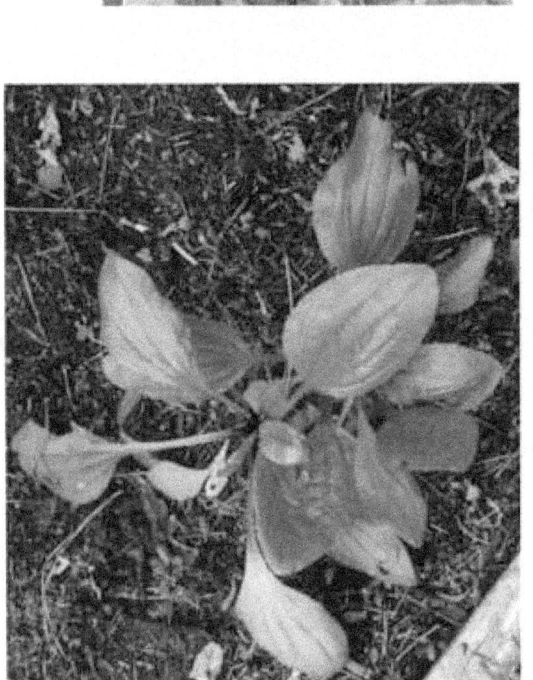

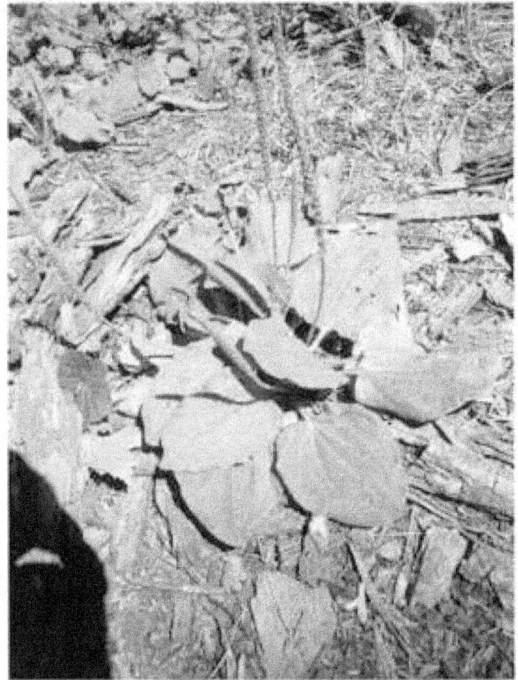

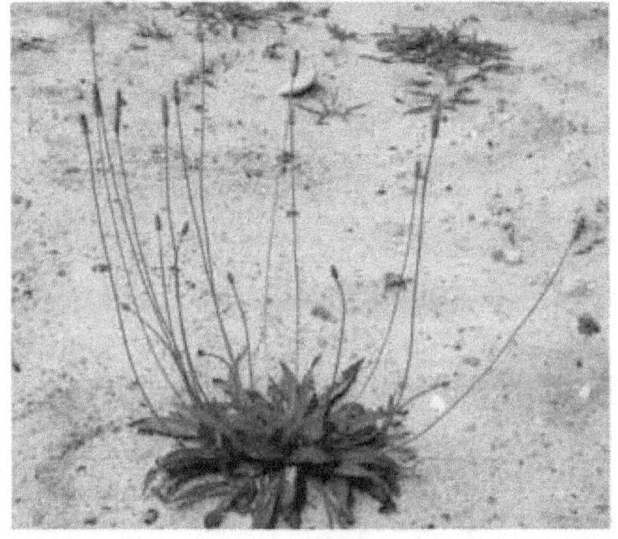

PLANTAIN

Plantago major and *Plantago lanceolata, Fam. Plantaginaceae*

Common and Regional Names
The major: broad-leaved plantain, Great Plantain, Ripple Grass, Waybread, Waybroad, Weybroed, Snakeweed, Englishman's Foot, White Man's Foot, Slan-lus, Ribwort.

The lanceolata: Lanceleaf Plantain, Ribwort, Buckthorn Plantain, Buck's Horn, Buckshorne, Hartshorne, Herba Stella, Herb Ivy, Cornu Cervinum, British Plantain, English Plantain

History and Common Usage
Evidence of plantain has been found in many ancient Egyptian gardens but is not an official plant identified in their pharmacopeia. It is mentioned in early Syrian records but some scholars believe these references are to *Plantago psyllium* or *Plantago ovata* and until additional records come to light this confusion is quite likely to continue without resolution.

Pliny the Elder mentions the use of plantain for ulcerations of the mouth describing both the broad and narrow leaf and makes a clear distinction between psyllium and plantain. Erasmus [1466-1536] the Dutch humanist, remarks in his Colloquia on the use of plantain in a manner that assures us the plant had a place in the healing arts during this time. It is mentioned in the writings of fourteenth century English poet Geoffrey Chaucer and seventeenth century English apothecary/physician Nicholas Culpepper. It is listed as one of the nine sacred herbs in the most ancient source of Anglo-Saxon medicine, a manuscript entitled the Lacnung.[83] "Waybroed [Grows along the way and is broad of leaf] is among "the nine sacred herbs." It is frequently cited as being a native British herb but most sources agree that since it was known to Pliny and other early Greeks and Romans that it was also originally native to Europe.

The most common use of the plant in traditional herbal lore is as a topical application in the treatment of minor wounds, sores and ulcers and as an antiseptic or astringent. In 1650 a decoction of plantain was considered good for the kidneys and was frequently boiled with celandine, elder buds, angelica, black currant leaves, dock, comfrey or other plants in recipes for various complaints. The young leaves of lanceolata are used in some cultures as a salad green and some herbal enthusiasts harvest the young seed spikes of both varieties for pickling.

In Germany plantain appears in the official pharmacopeia and there are specific areas set aside for the *P. lanceolata* to be grown.[84] The plant is prescribed as a tea and for mouth washes and gargles and to suppress coughs, treat bronchitis and to reduce skin inflammation. *Plantago major* is being used in the United States today as a primary ingredient in homeopathic remedies to deter smoking through means of a spray under the tongue to address tobacco cravings.

Description
Plantain belongs to a group of more than 200 species. It is a low growing plant characterized by medium green leaves which grow directly from the root. The leaves of the *P. major* are broad, oval, medium to

---

83   11th Century manuscript from an earlier translation of indeterminate date. The Lacnunga or "leech knowing" is known as Harley 585 and is presently in the custody of the British Museum

84   EEC Regulation 1765/92.

dark green and ribbed. In the *P. lanceolata* the leaves are thin and narrow, of a medium to dark green and also ribbed.

Both plants send up one or more long cylindrical spikes during the flowering stages which are characterized by small greenish to pale purplish flowers near the top of the stalk. The *P. lanceolata* flowers appear fuzzy as they mature. The seeds of both are tan in color.

The 21st Edition of the United States Dispensatory lists the narrow and broadleaf as unofficial plants stating they were "held in esteem" by the ancients and that the plants have been used in domestic medicine to treat sores.

Growing Conditions and Propagation
Plantains are opportunistic and vigorous perennials thriving in areas wherever grass grows. They can be found in meadows, parks, the cracks in sidewalks and in between cobblestones. Where grass is subject to regular mowing the plants adapt by growing flat to the ground often with only two or three tiny leaves to betray their presence. Where grass grows to longer lengths their leaves reach 8 to 10 inches in length. The broadleaf can produce leaves as wide as 3 to 5 inches wide on stems between 8 to 12 inches long.

In the spring *P. lanceolata* is easily recognized by a few narrow, dark green leaves closely resembling grass. They develop into the shape of a star around the root base, accounting for one of its common names, "Herba Stella." These green spears, darker than the surrounding grass, were thought to resemble the horns of the male deer giving it another of its common names buck's horn, or buckshorne.

Propagated by seed plantain is easily established and will enthusiastically self-seed year after year producing whole colonies of helpful plants.

Harvesting
The leaves, stalk, seeds and roots of the plant are all used and are harvested at different times of the year according to the requirements of use. The leaves are picked when young and tender. The leaves, stalks and roots can be used fresh or dried.

The leaves and stalks are best gathered during the blooming season and unless otherwise directed the root is best gathered in the fall of the year. The small roots are washed, cleaned of their tiny hairs, cut from the leaf base and spread to dry. They are then stored in airtight containers. The fully ripened seeds are stripped by hand and stored in the usual manner.

Use in the Edgar Cayce Readings
Plantain is used alone and as a companion plant. All fresh parts of the plant, root, stalks, seeds, and leaves are used. It is recommended as a tea, a poultice and as an ointment or salve in over 90 cases.

Plantain tea is recommended as an internal astringent in cases indexed as injuries, cancer, abrasions, varicose veins, boils, gangrene, and dermatitis. Plantain salve or ointment is used for abrasions, ulcers, abscesses of the spine, hemorrhoids, skin cancer and to treat sarcoma nodules.

Frequently the admonition is given that the salve must be made fresh every few days and that no preservatives are to be used: *As we have given, it is necessary that this plantain salve be made fresh at least every few days, for to use the preservatives in same would hinder the effects that may be had or created for the system by the use of same, see? [325-45]*

Equal amounts by weight or volume of the freshly gathered, tender green leaves, and either oil of butterfat or what was called in Cayce's day "top cream" – [today half and half will do] are brought to a low boil in a glass or enamel pot. [The simplest method is to use half a cup of the leaves to half a cup of half and half or light cream] The directions caution that after the mixture comes to a gentle boil not to cook it over too high a heat because long cooking and high heat destroys the medicinal properties. The length of time recommended varies from one minute to fifteen minutes. Stirring constantly the mixture is gently cooked into the consistency of a thick cream or salve.

The mixture is then placed in a small glass bowl, sealed with plastic wrap and stored in the refrigerator. The information suggests that it to be made fresh every two or three days. The plant material does not completely dissolve and the salve will have a slightly "weedy" smell. Instructions were very clear that the salve is not to be applied directly over any open places, just around the edges of any sores. Gradually the open area becomes smaller and smaller healing over without incident.

When a plantain stupe or poultice is called for the fresh leaves are prepared by bruising the leaves between the hands to help release plant fluids and then put them in boiling water. They are then put directly on the skin, the area is then covered with plastic and heat is applied. When larger areas of the body are treated the plant material is placed on gauze, such as cheesecloth, and then placed on the skin.

Plantain tea can be made with anywhere from a tablespoon of fresh leaves (stalk and seed may be included) to half a cup, steeped in boiling water from ten to thirty minutes. Strain and drink without adding a sweetener of any kind. This "astringent" can be drunk as often as a cup three times a day to as little as a tablespoon per day.

The following excerpt contains excellent directions for the preparation of a tea, a poultice and a salve.

4074-1 F 30
5. The Plantain tea and also the plantain poultice should be prepared fresh daily. Obtain the tender leaves of plantain just now beginning in this area to indicate itself. Use not the roots but the leaves. Cut these fine. Put a level teaspoonful in a teacup and fill with boiling water. Cover with a saucer or glass top and let stand for thirty minutes. Strain off and drink the tea. Do this once each day.

6. The poultice would be prepared in this manner, to be put over the pubic center:

7. Mix a tablespoonful of the tender leaves (cut fine) with a tablespoonful of thick sweet cream that rises to the top of the milk - not the heavy cream, not that soured, but the pure fresh cream skimmed from the top of milk. Mix these together and let come almost to a boil - using these properties, you see, to make the salve for the poultice. Spread on gauze and apply over the area. Do this daily.

The following are only 4 examples of the 90 odd recommendations for plantain:

3370-1 M 1 ½ TUMORS:KIDNEYS:WILMS
9. Once each week do give the body internally a small quantity of Plantain Tea. Use the tender Plantain leaves, and make the Tea fresh whenever practical. Give a teaspoonful of this once each

week. It would be prepared in this manner: Put two pinches of the Plantain leaves [between thumb and forefinger] in a cup and pour a tablespoon of boiling water over same and let stand for thirty minutes. Then strain and give a teaspoonful. The rest may be kept for another teaspoonful the next week, but don't let it stand longer. Keep in the icebox or frozen, when this is being kept for the next dose.

3121-1 M 39 SARCOMA

17. But to purify these from the body-force, we would also take internally a Plantain Tea, made from the tender top leaves of the same plant, with - at this season, especially - the seed of the Plantain - about half and half. Fill half a pint cup with these, and add to one quart of Distilled or Rain Water - using only an enamel or glass container, not metal. Cook until reduced to about half the quantity, or half a pint of the liquid. Take this as a tea, a teaspoonful four times each day; after each meal and at bedtime. Keep this where it is cool, and if the quantity tends to turn a bit sour, discard it - but this whole quantity should be taken before it would sour. It is not so good to add a preservative for this particular material, for it changes this.[85]

3187-1 M 39 CANCER:SARCOMA

12. Also each day we would drink at least two ounces of Plantain Tea, made in this manner:

13. Gather the fresh Plantain leaves, - not the heavy dried ones, but with the seed and the Plantain. Pour a pint of boiling water over half a pint of the Plantain cut up, and allow to stand for twenty to thirty minutes [in a teapot or crock container, covered]. Strain, cool and drink - two ounces of this each day. This may be kept in the ice box for two days, but make fresh every other day.

3532-1 F CANCER:SKIN

12. As an ointment for the place on the head, we would prepare Plantain Cream. Cut the green Plantain, the tender shoots; cut in fine pieces, as with the scissors or the like, and not too tight but pressed in. Then to this add, in an enamel or glass boiler, the same quantity of thick fresh cream - not sour cream, but that settling on the top of milk. Let this come to a boil. Skim, and set aside. Use this as an ointment on the head. This will heal, yet will not cause other than segregation, and - with the properties taken internally as indicated - when the operation is necessary, the place will be able to heal clear, clean, and not cause deterioration through other portions of the body. For this is of a stony nature[86] internally.

---

85   Author's note: please note the admonition NOT to add a preservative.
86   Nineteen kinds of cancer are described in Cayce transcript 1242-6.

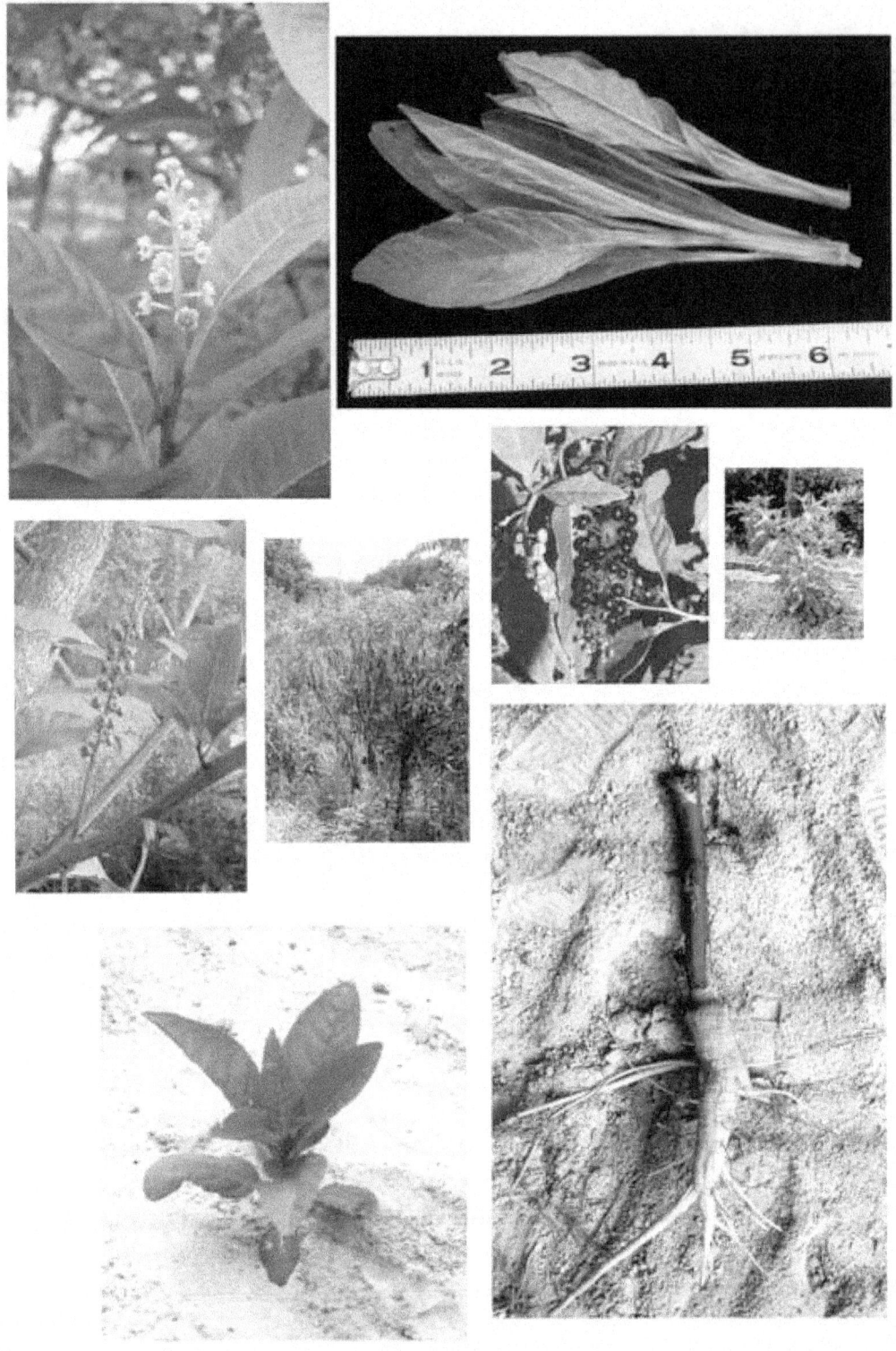

POKE
Phytolacca Americana, Fam. Phytolaccaceae

Common and Regional Names:
Pokeroot, Skoke, Red Plant, Pocan, Pakon, Puccoon, Polk, Pokeweed, Pokeberry, Inkberry, Garet, Pigeon Berry, Bear's Grape, Cokan, Chongras, Virginian Poke

History and Common Usage
Poke is found in northern Africa, southern Europe and throughout North and South America. The Americanized name poke is thought by most scholars to have been derived from the Algonquian Indian word "pakon" or "puccoon." This comes from their original use of the plant as a dye source for staining as the juice of the poke berry yields a fairly permanent but primitive dye. In spite of being poisonous poke was used as a medicinal plant by the Native Americans long before the arrival of European settlers.

Poke is an ingredient in a controversial formula that came to the attention of the greater American public in 1956 with the publication of <u>You Don't Have To Die, The Amazing Story of the Hoxsey Cancer-Treatment</u>, by Harry M. Hoxsey[87], N.D. The Hoxsey regimen for cancer was unequivocally rejected by the AMA and the Hoxsey treatments were never fully or objectively investigated. Cayce scholars find it of interest that in 1924 Cayce gave an internal formula outlined in transcript 4695-1 [shown below] for an adult male diagnosed with cancer of the throat that contained the same ingredients as the Hoxsey formula.

In 1969 a song entitled "Poke Salad Annie" was popular describing a poor southern girl who picked a wild plant called pokeweed. The Allen's brand of cut leaf Poke Salet Greens advertising "no preservatives – organically grown" may still be available in some supermarkets in the United States.

Poke root is cited in early dispensatories and formularies for use as an "alternative" in *"chronic rheumatism, granular conjunctivitis and even in cancer."* There are also directions for the use of the young spring shoots cooked and eaten as a fresh green vegetable, calling for 4 changes of water. Cooking the leaves in several changes of water destroys and removes the *Phytolacca* toxin which is present in all parts of the plant. The berries are eaten by wild birds and free ranging domestic fowl and if eaten in great quantities the berries impart an unpleasant flavor to the meat, and can actually cause purging when eaten. The plant is unpalatable to grazing animals so it represents no danger to livestock. The 21st edition of the United States Dispensatory lists poke as an official drug plant describing the root as the active part, and describing it as an emetic but *"not fit for use as such."*

Description
Poke is a large herbaceous perennial best recognized in its mature state by its unmistakable dark reddish stalks. It has branching limbs with alternating leaves and a carrot-like tap root which contains the active principles. All parts of the plant - stalk, leaves, root and berries - are poisonous. By degrees the plant can cause purging, spasms, convulsions and sometimes death due to paralysis of respiratory organs. Saponin and lesser amounts of the alkaloid phytolaccin are the active poisonous principles. Even small amounts of the berries [10 or more] can cause serious poisoning in adults. Children can die from the consumption of only a few berries. The symptoms begin with burning of the mouth followed by severe gastroenteritis. Vomiting should be induced immediately and medical attention sought as soon as possible.

---

87   1901-1974 See also http://www.tldp.com/issue/166/166hoxs.htm

The plant flowers in June through September and often reaches heights of 12 feet or more in a single growing season. The plant dies back in the autumn and in the following spring re-grows from the roots, first putting out tender shoots which, when prepared correctly, are tasty and nutritious.

Growing Conditions and Propagating
Poke is pollinated by insects and wind. It propagates by natural scattering of the ripe berries containing the seeds, through bird-borne seeding, and from spreading through its root system. The young plant can be dug in its native habitat and transplanted to yard or garden in the very early spring; however care must be taken to obtain the whole taproot to ensure the plant will live. Once established its vigorous habits will bring it back year after year.

Harvesting
To collect young shoots the location of the mature plants should be marked in the fall and the area re-visited in the spring. Shoots are leaves that have not yet developed a stem and this is when they are at their tender best. They are gathered when they are between 4 to 6 inches in length and can be easily snapped off by hand or cut with a knife or scissors. Harvesting the shoots at this stage will not harm the plant and will often result in re-growth which can be collected a second and even a third time. Sources from the 1920's through the 1940's call for bringing the leaves to a boil, discarding the water, boiling again in fresh water for a total of 2, 3 or, in the case of one cautious source, even 4 times. The Cayce system calls for only 1 "boil and discard" of the liquid in the cooking process stating the water will be somewhat greenish and the leaves drained in a colander. This difference can probably be attributed to the size and age of the shoots recommended by Cayce. Once properly cooked they can be served in the same manner as spinach or any other greens.

Poke root is harvested in the fall after the plant has died back, which is November in most areas of the United States. Where the ground is hard the roots should be dug up rather than pulled [which will result in only part of a root] and then cut from the stalk. They are washed very carefully under clean, cool running water using a soft vegetable brush, removing any small hair roots. The fresh root can be processed immediately or it can be dried. For drying the root should be allowed to air dry over night before slicing. The next day cut the root into as thin as possible transverse slices and dry. The root is tough, woody and hard and large roots require a very sharp knife or a clean hatchet. In some areas a gentle heat source may be necessary. The fresh roots are pale ivory in color, often branching with small rootlets. They are odorless when dried and they turn to a light tan or medium brown during the drying process.

The dried slices can be stored in plastic bags with as much air as possible exhausted and stored in the pantry. In areas of high humidity they can also be double bagged and frozen. Frozen or dried roots should be labeled as to date and used within twelve months.

Use in the Cayce Readings
Poke is used as a companion plant and as a dietary item. An extract, tincture, fusion or essence of the root is used in compound formulas for internal use and the shoots or greens are recommended as a vegetable.

Dietary recommendations are found approximately fifty times however the directions for preparing poke are at variance with directions given in other sources such as cookbooks and the U.S. Dispensatory as discussed above.

Dietary Recommendations

3331-1 F 36 Diet:Asthma:Vegetables:Poke

9. In the matter of the diet, - do include leafy vegetables such as red cabbage, spinach, all forms of leafy greens - as mustard, lamb's tongue, as dock, as poke - as this is very tender, but be careful how it is prepared. Put the tender poke leaves in plain water and allow to come almost to a boil, pour off the water or drain and then the leaves can be mixed with any other greens. The activity of these would be purifying, in such a way that will be found in few other such greens or vegetables.

2985-1 F 45 GLANDS

16. In the diet, - keep away from too much of starches. In this period, especially, we would take much of the foods that act as clarifiers or purifiers to the blood supply; such as poke salad. We do not mean pork meat, but poke salad - the plant. Cook the very tender leaves, allow to come almost to a boil and pour off the first water, then put in fresh, clear, cold water, and cook a few minutes. This taken about twice each week for three to four weeks will make a great deal of change in these periods of irritation from the superficial circulation. If three to four stalks of the Irish Potato tops are put with the poke salad, it will be most beneficial.

601-27 F 52 Cancer:Tendencies

10. Also those foods that are purifying and cleansing in nature would be well; such as the GREENS [the tops, of course, not the roots]; as mustard, lambs' tongue, poke [not pork meat, but poke greens] [pokeweed] and their combinations.

11. Not too much of turnips - either the greens or the bulbous part; but those other greens which carry HEALING and cleansing forces are well.

2948-1 F 11 Poliomyelitis

24. At least three times a week have either carrots or beets, or beet tops, as a part of the diet. These should be cooked, even the beet tops - very soon cook with the tender shoots of poke; not, however, without the poke having been first prepared, but these are especially blood purifiers, adding to the body-forces. Prepare the poke by first putting in cold water, letting it come almost to a boil; then drain, as through a colander - the water will be rather greenish. Then it may be cooked with the beet tops. And these are excellent, at least two to three times each week; as are the carrots. These may be cooked with fresh peas, and diced for the body, if desired.

5300-1 F 65 COUGH: CHRONIC ICTHYOSIS

8. Then the diets: Stay to those things which are thoroughly cleansing. Do use through the season when obtainable, and obtain it for the full season in the various territories where it may be obtained, a great deal of poke salad. In preparing this, put it in water, say all that can be put in a half gallon container in a gallon of water. Let it come to a boil, then put in a colander and strain off. This water will be green, very green. Then put in fresh water and cook. This will aid in purifying the system. This would be good for anybody. This especially early in the spring, but for this body it should be kept more than in the spring, but it changes as it comes through various portions of the country from Georgia to Manitoba - that's Canada.

Used Internally

The Hoxsey formula mentioned above is shown here as it was given by Cayce in 1924.

4695-1 Adult Male

12. These conditions may be assisted and the condition brought to that of little effect in system if cared for in proper manner. Then do this: We would take first in the system these properties:

Tincture Wild Cherry Bark................1/2 ounce,
Tincture Valdalia [Stillingia]..........1/2 ounce,
Tincture Yellow Dock Root...............1/2 ounce,
Tincture of Poke Root...................1/2 ounce,
Tincture of Burdock Root................1/2 ounce,
Iodide Potassium........................3/4 ounces.
Sufficient simple syrup to make...........6 ounces.
[See GD's note at end of Reading.]

Shake solution well to-gether until all is dissolved.

13. The dose would be half a teaspoonful four times each day, letting one dose be just before retiring, and apply to the body through the solar plexus center, and at the second cervical, the plates or vibrations that will be found in the Abrahams Osculator [Abram's Oscillator] for sarcoma germ. This will, within three to five weeks, reduce the condition to that of almost nil. Then the general health afterwards must be kept.

[GD's note: See pp. 45-46 of YOU DON'T HAVE TO DIE, The Amazing Story of the Hoxsey Cancer-Treatment, by Harry M. Hoxsey, N.D. [Milestone Books, Inc., N.Y., 1956], listing all of the above prescription ingredients as basic medication by Hoxsey "in all cases of cancer, internal and external."]

A year later a second formula minus Iodide of Potassium and containing other ingredients was given for the same gentleman:

4695-2 M Adult

4. To 6 ounces of Peptotol, or Simple Syrup, add:

Syrup of Sarsaparilla.............4 ounces,
Tincture Valerian.................2 ounces,
Tincture Stillingia...............1 ounce,
Tincture of Poke Root............30 minims,
Tincture of Yellow Dock Root....1/2 ounce,
Tincture of Wild Cherry Bark......1 ounce,
Elixia Calisaya...................1 ounce,
Elixia Celerina...................1 ounce.

5. Shake solution well together before each dose is taken, which would be taken four times each day, before meals and before retiring. Half a teaspoonful in half a glass of water, or taken plain and water taken afterward.

Sadly as in so many instances no follow up information is recorded on the outcome of this case. Other internal formulas are shown here:

303-7 F 48 Eliminations:Incoordination

2. There needs to be, as we find for the physical forces of this body in the present, the better coordinations through those activities in the eliminations; making for coordinations of the eliminating centers of the body, where the stiffness occurs and the headaches and those reactions for the digestive forces.

3. A tonic made in this manner to be taken by the body will be found to be most helpful:

4. To a pint of Spirits Frumenti or good whiskey as the base, add:

> Elixir of Calisaya...................1/2 ounce,
> Fluid Extract of Yellow Dock Root...1/4 ounce,
> Fluid Extract of Poke Root, or a
>   fusion of same....................10 minims (no more),
> Essence or Tincture of Stillingia...1/2 ounce,
> Tincture of Capsici.................10 minims.

5. Take this about four to six times a day; half a teaspoonful. It'll be bitter and hot, but it will do good!

140-1 F Neuritis

13. Then, to give the necessary relief to the body, we would take these properties in system that would give the correct incentives to the functioning of the system - correct osteopathically by manipulation with applied heat, conditions in upper dorsal region from sixth to the first dorsal and in the lumbar region.

14. To one gallon of rain water, add:

> Sarsaparilla root................2 ounces,
> Yellow dock.....................2 ounces,
> Burdock.........................2 ounces,
> Poke Root.....................1/2 ounce,
> Calisaya Bark...................1 ounce,
> Elder Flower....................2 ounces.

Reduce by simmering, not boiling, to one quart, strain well. While warm add three drams balsam of Tolu cut in four ounces of grain alcohol. The dose would be a teaspoonful four times a day, before meals and before retiring.

42-1 F Adult Prescription:Circulation

11. Then to bring the normal conditions to this body, we would first take in the system those properties that would bring the correct incentives to the whole system, taking then this:

> Syrup Sarsaparilla...............1/4 ounce,
> Fluid Extract Wild Cherry........1/2 ounce,

Fluid Extract Stillingia.........1/2 ounce,
Fluid Extract Poke Root..........1/2 ounce,
Fluid Extract Yellow Dock Root...1/2 ounce,
Iodide Potassium..................20 grains.

12. Mix well together and add sufficient simple syrup to make 8 ounces. The dose would be half teaspoonful 4 times each day.

4370-1 M Adult Prescriptions:Eliminations
3. Then, to bring, to give, to affect those conditions that would give the better relief and bring the near normal functioning of the system, we would leave off some of those conditions that have been applied to the system and use these.

4. We would first make these properties for the body:

Syrup of Sarsaparilla..........2 ounces,
Tincture of Wild Cherry Bark...2 ounces,
Tincture of Valerian...........1 dram,
Essence Yellow Dock Root.....1/2 ounce,
Essence of Polk [Poke] Root...20 minims,
Elixia Calisaya................1 ounce,
Capsici.......................2 minims.

Add to this sufficient simple syrup to make 12 ounces. Shake solution well. The dose would be teaspoonful night and morning, morning before meals, night before retiring.

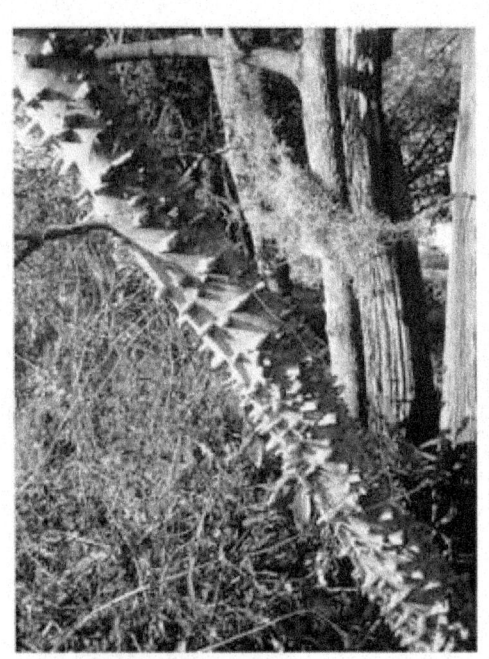
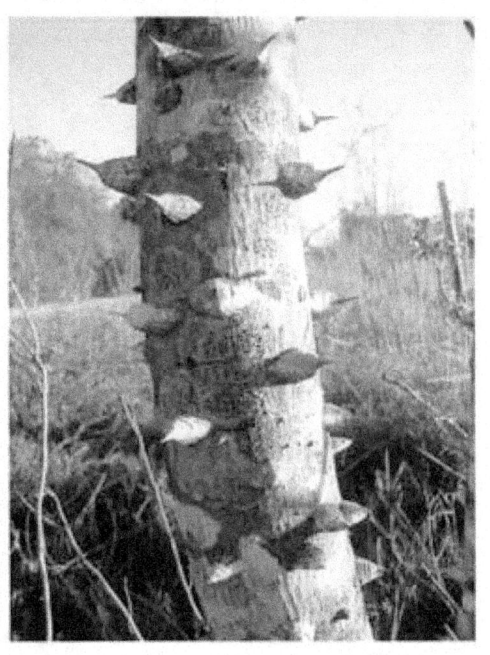
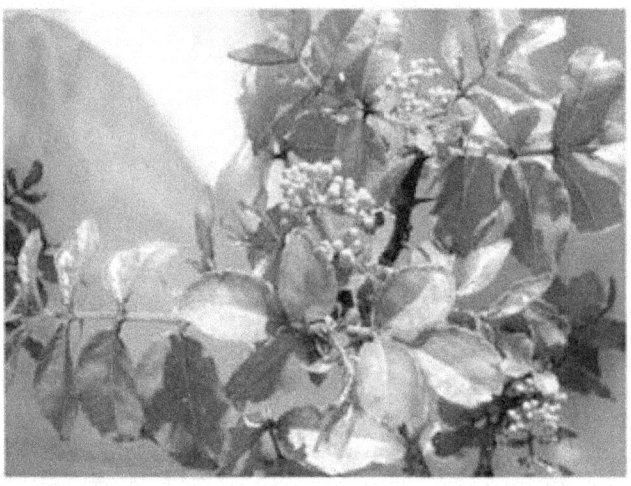
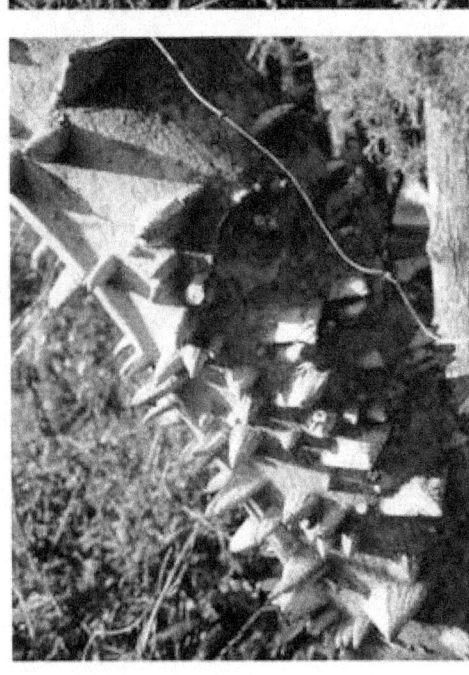
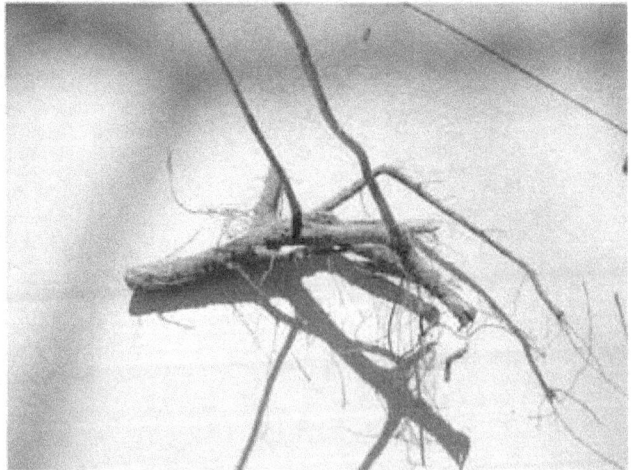

PRICKLY ASH
Zanthoxylum americanum [formerly seen *Xanthoxylum*]
[Northern Prickly Ash,
Or
Zanthoxylum [formerly seen *Xanthoxylum*] *Clava-Herculis*
[Southern Prickly Ash]
Fam. Rutaceae

Common and Regional Names
Zanthoxylum americanum: Toothache bark, Angelica Tree, Yellow-wood

Zanthoxylum Clava-Herculis: Sea Ash, Hercules Club, Pepperwood, Toothache Bark

History and Common Usage
Indigenous to the Eastern United States and Canada the northern prickly ash is found from Quebec to Minnesota and southward to Virginia and Missouri. The southern occurs from southern Virginia to Florida and west to Kansas and Texas. Prickly ash is not related to the true ash and there is often confusion between various species due to common names being used for several different trees or shrubs. *Zanthoxylum*, or *Xanthoxylum*, as both spellings are still in common use, is a Greek word meaning "yellow wood" and *americanum* refers to North America. *Clava-Herculis* means the "club of Hercules" possibly as a reference to the damage the spines could inflict if used as a weapon.

The southern prickly ash is often confused with *Aralia spinosa*, the angelica tree, which is also called by the common name, "prickly ash." The bark of the angelica is smooth externally with slender prickles in transverse rows. The spines of the prickly ash are irregular.

Known among the Native Americans as a medicinal plant, especially efficacious in the care of the teeth and gums, *Zanthoxylum* was introduced to the early American settlers. It entered cultivation records in the United States around 1740 and transitioned from an indigenous folk remedy to official pharmacopeias some time around 1826 to 1829 when alkaloidal substances were first identified. The use of prickly ash as an effective masticatory as used in folk medicine for the treatment of teeth and gums has yet to be scientifically researched.

It is recommended in traditional herbal medicine as a tonic to stimulate circulation in cases of chronic rheumatism, in the treatment of ulcers, as a stimulant to the cardio-vascular or lymph system, as a gastro-intestinal tonic to treat some cases of low blood pressure and as a flavoring agent in beverages and foods. The 21st Edition of the United States Dispensatory lists prickly ash as an official drug plant but states the volatile oils *"probably have no therapeutic effect except…of a mild aromatic."*

Description
Prickly ash occurs as a shrub or small tree that can attain heights of 25 to 45 feet with a trunk diameter of 18 to 30 inches. There are minor differences between the northern and the southern in appearance and growth habits but there is no distinction between the two for medicinal use. While the bark is considered the most valued medicinal part all parts of the tree can be used therapeutically.

The northern is usually found as a 10 to 12 foot high shrub rarely seen over 25 feet. Its leaflets are from 5 to 11 in number and from 1 1/2 to 2 inches long. The greenish-yellow flowers appear before the leaves, usually in April or May. The branches are covered in brown, cone-shaped strong prickles. The northern does not always develop spines on the trunk although in older specimens they may be present.

The southern is taller but seldom attains a height greater than 45 feet. Its leaves consist of 5 to 17 leaflets from 1 1/2 to 3 inches long, and its small, greenish flowers appear in June after the leaves are out, borne in large clusters at the ends of the branches. The trunk bark turns a handsome light grey in older trees. The entire tree is covered with sharp, irregular spines or thorns.

As the twigs or stems mature into branches the thorns lose their juvenile reddish coloration becoming gray or brown. As the tree matures the spines develop into individual raised bumps with spines or thorns at the top which are extremely hard and sharp and which increase in size year after year as the tree grows.

Growing Conditions and Propagation
Prickly ash is pollinated by insects, wind and bird borne seeding and propagates from its underground rooting system. It is easily, albeit slowly, propagated from seeds. A young tree or sucker can also be cut from the parent root system during the winter dormant period and trees can also be easily ordered from nurseries. Because of their thorns, eventual size and vigorous growth habits, some careful thought should be given to where they are planted.

Seeds are collected in the late fall when they are dry and wrinkled and planted in their permanent location. They will winter over before germination. Due to the low germination rate it is necessary to plant more seeds than are needed. Leave them for a year or two and then thin out the weakest leaving only the healthiest 4 or 5. Of these all but one should eventually be sacrificed in favor of the most vigorous. This final thinning is done when they have attained between 2 to 3 feet in height.

To contain the tree within the available space cut away any suckers that will readily grow from the roots. Keep the lower branches trimmed as the tree grows so that eventually the lowest branches on the tree will be above head height – at least 7 feet from the ground - and it is wise to enclose the trunk in a wire cage to help prevent accidental injuries. The cage should be of a sufficient diameter to never touch the trunk and of a sufficient size to allow for growth, made of a sturdy material [strong wire is a good choice] and securely fixed in the ground with metal stakes.

Harvesting
In the wild prickly ash is sometimes found in thickets which are impossible to penetrate without injury. In order to collect branches or handle them in order to harvest the ripe seeds, gloves and long handled pruning shears are necessary. To avoid accidental injury take a cardboard box to the site and cut all the small twigs and branches on location trimming them to the size of the box for transportation home.

Both the bark and ripe berries are used in folk medicine. If the berries are desired their medicinal properties are higher in the fresh fully ripened fruit before they show signs of drying. They are picked by hand and used fresh or placed on trays to dry in the sun until they are withered and dried to a leather-like state. They are then stored in the usual manner.

When harvesting the bark stout gloves and a very sharp knife are necessary to peel or scrape away the outer bark and thorny spines. The inner bark is then cut into small pieces and dried, or can be dried whole, and after drying cut or ground into smaller pieces.

In an emergency a leaf or a young and tender twig of the tree can be cut and chewed to bring relief from a toothache or sore gum as the following suggests has been done for centuries: *26. [Q] What is the reaction of the Prickly Ash Bark on the gums? [A] It is nature's preservative for STRENGTHENING the tissue about the teeth themselves. The very NATURE of it, from its name as given by the aborigines - that toothache bark indicates its very nature! 1800-26*

Use in the Edgar Cayce Readings

Prickly ash is a companion plant. Perhaps its most frequent use is in a very effective remedy for the treatment of Pyorrhea originally named IPSAB[88] after the letters of the primary ingredients. The formula was first developed in 1925 and in 1934 in transcript 1800-20 instructions were given on how to advertise and label this new product. Note the reference to the *"Indian herb"* described as the *"basis of the thing"* which must have been in the original Sunker Bisey[89] "Atomic Iodine."

1800-20 Special

13. [Q] To meet all requirements of the pure food and drug laws, what printed material should appear on the label for Ipsab?
[A] Give the formula; NOT the quantities. As this:

> **Calcium Chloride**
> **Atomic Iodine**
> **Water [or Aqua Pura, if it's desired in the correct way]**
> **Essence of Peppermint**

These, of course, will make for the analysis; and when they attempt to analyze the compound they DON'T FIND the basis of the thing - which is an Indian herb - when it is powdered with the others!

14. [Q] What should appear on the carton for Ipsab?
[A] I-P-S-A-B. Recommended in the treatment of Pyorrhea, Rigg's Disease, Gumboils and other Mouth ailments.
15. [Q] What directions should appear on the label as to the proper use of same?
[A] Massage gums, boils or ulcers in mouth at least once each day, rinsing the mouth after its use.

The following describes how and why this formula works:

1800-21 BUSINESS

11. Then, this is what happens when Ipsab is used where…there is the bleeding or the receding *[Author's note: receding gums]*… **First: The properties in same act upon the defective conditions to produce a cleansing, and an attacking of the influences that make for the conditions that are destructive to enamel and to the tissue itself. Also there is a stimulation to the glands, that make for an activity in the system itself to produce a greater activity in the direction that will overcome those conditions in the system. So, if these properties are used in a consistent way and manner, we will bring to such a body a normal, HEALTHY condition in the mouth; PROVIDED, to be sure, that the condition does not arise from some more subtle cause in other portions of the body, or that there is not taken such**

---

88   The Heritage Store, P.O. Box 444 WWW, 314 Laskin Road, Virginia Beach, Virginia 23451. 757-428-0100, 1-800-862-2923. http://www.heritagestore.com
89   See 1734-2 Reports

properties as iron in certain states, or lead, or copper, to make for destructive forces to the enamel itself, or of the glands in the system.

It is difficult in these modern times to grasp what a dreaded disease Pyorrhea was before the wide spread recognition of the need for good oral hygiene, the advent of present standards of dental care and antibiotics. Pyorrhea alveolaris, an anaerobic bacterial infection, is a serious inflammatory disease in which the gums are swollen in the early stages, and then develop a bright red or reddish-purple coloration. At this stage the gums begin to bleed easily and they may be tender to the touch but painless otherwise. Breath odor from the infection becomes evident and the infection causes the tissues that surround the teeth to atrophy resulting in the teeth loosening in their sockets. At this point the disease becomes very painful as abscesses may form in addition to the infection. In the later stages of the disease the jaw bone itself becomes infected leading to bone re-absorption, more loss of teeth and receding gums. Most common in persons over 40 the primary cause is poor oral hygiene [lack of brushing and flossing] combined with irritation of the gum tissues by dental tartar.

Cayce described the cause of gum disease and the mechanism of IPSAB in 1934 as follows:

1800-21 BUSINESS
6. As to that which may be given respecting the effect of this solution upon disorders that arise in the gums and in the enamel of the teeth themselves: It is known by scientific research [or so called scientific research] that the accumulations of the film [or you may use, of course, if so desired, the technical name of same - if you desire to be impressive or appear to be verbose in thine own expression of thine knowledge; but better use it in the plain words and let ALL understand] upon the teeth and gums are through the use of cooked and soft food, more by the very fact or act of using very hot and very cold foods or properties in the mouth of an individual. For nature attempts to protect the enamel and the gums themselves from such sudden changes. And this accumulation of foods makes the acids in the system. For we know by the proper tests that the secretions of the salivary glands are of an alkalin nature, and these are turned by the accumulations of decaying or changing food values - or the film's accumulations upon the gums and teeth. Thus there is made place for the germ of what is called Pyorrhea, Rigg's Disease, or such conditions that gradually arise in the mouth. First there is produced an irritation that makes for the loosening of the gum from the enamel. Then there is the accumulation of these same particles of film, and of those secretions that arise in the mouth, just below the edge of the gums; as the heat and cold that arise from the mastication of that taken - or that drunk by a body - makes for the accumulation of these under the edge of the gum itself, where the enamel is not protected so much as that which is in active use by the mastication of foods.

7. Now, in the very nature of the teeth, the enamel of same is a secretion of the body itself; as also are the toe nails, the finger nails, the hair of the head, the hair of the body, and the cuticle itself; that ability of the body through any portion where irritation may come - as we find in the hands of those who toil with tools, these are those things that must be created by the body itself. And it should be considered by all: There is no greater factory in the universe than that in a human body in its natural, normal reacting state. For there are those machines or glands within the body capable of producing, from the very air or water and the food values taken into the body, to take from or to reproduce ANY element AT ALL that is KNOWN in the material world!

8. What happens when there are those excesses of heat and cold, by the use of hot foods or cold foods; cold drinks more especially, or hot drinks? There is the attack first upon the thin edges of the film of the tissue of the gums themselves.

One of the oldest known cases of evidence of Pyorrhea has been discovered in skeletal remains found in an elaborate tomb in the ancient Phoenician seaport city of Sidon, now Saida, Lebanon. The burial site dates back some 2500 years. A crude dental appliance was found still intact holding the teeth of a middle-aged man securely in place in the mandible. An X-ray of the jawbone revealed the typical atrophy of Pyorrhea – the disease still progressing at the time of his death.[90]

The following simple home made formula for IPSAB was given on April 1, 1925

760-3 F 50
2. EC: …we find there are indications of the bacilli of in the lower back teeth, especially the second one from rear, one of molars. This we find produces the inflammation and irritation that affects the third and fourth nerve of the face, and this tooth would be better removed. This, however, could be saved, were the care and attention given same to destroy the nerve that is exposed and relieve the pressure as produced by pus being formed through the creating of the streptococci in the blood in the eliminating from this distressed condition. …

3. On the gum, near where the tooth was removed in the lower jaw, we find there the sore abrasion produced by inflammation from sympathetic condition in the teeth. These may be treated by the solution as prepared from this:

4. To 6 drams of Wild Prickly Ash Bark, [Simple formula for what later came to be known as Ipsab.] add 6 ounces of distilled water. Reduce to 1 ounce by simmering, and strain. Wash the barks before putting in for this reduction. Then, when strained and reduced, add common table salt until the solution takes up all that it will in producing saturated solution, adding to this 2 minims Tincture Iodine, with 1 minim Essence of Peppermint. Use this solution by rubbing the gums with finger, not with cloth or brush, getting in the sore or abrasion places, treating locally the condition in the teeth where the air breaks in to exposed nerves. This we find will reduce the condition….

In this formula, easily made at home, prickly ash bark is reduced by gentle simmering in distilled water and iodized salt is added together with a small amount of oil of peppermint:

1800-1 BUSINESS
4. As to how this , or Gum-ese, would be prepared: [It was later [from 1925 on] referred to as Ipsab*.]

5. To six ounces toothache bark, or Prickly Ash Bark, add 16 ounces rain, or snow, water.

6. Reduce by simmering [not boiling too severely] to one-half the quantity. Then add iodized, or salt treated with iodine, to the amount of 8 ounces; this stirred well in while the solution is very warm, adding at the same time to these properties 2 minims of Oil of Peppermint.

---

90   *Surgery in Lebanon* by Antoine Ghossain, MD., FACS: Fuad Freiha, MD, FACS; Nagib Geahchan, MD. JAMA. Archives of Surgery. Vol. 138. February 2003

7. Use or place in container wherein the solution may be used by rubbing on gum with the finger, and the mouth rinsed with plain water after rubbing for two to three minutes. This solution should be used where has begun at least twice each week, until the gums and soreness is relieved.

Then once each month. Should solution become hard from exposure, and from evaporation, add small quantity of water and the solution will be ready for use. Best that these properties, then, be put in small containers.

* [10/17/72 GD's note: The name was suggested by Gertrude Cayce, combining the first letters of the main ingredients: iodine, prickly ash bark [or peppermint], salt. Soon the readings started using the name.]

A formula for commercial production is shown below:

1800-34
7. As to the formula for Ipsab...This is the formula:

8. With the bark that has been indicated, - the Toothache Bark, - use Sea Water. Boil these together until the solution tests hydrometer four [4], see?

9. Then to this, after it has been strained off and allowed to cool, add to each pint the following - and then reheat it, not to the boiling point but just until it begins to simmer; adding these in the order named:

>   Atomidine.....................1/4 ounce,
>   Salt............................2 ounces,
>   Calcium [ground, or in such
>   nature as the crystal].......2 grains,
>   Essence of Peppermint.........1/2 ounce.

10. This will keep, - it is a preservative, it is a cleanser.

3211-1 M 55 Dentist BUSINESS
9. [Q] As I have patented dimethyl cellulose for use in a dentifrice, what is the best chemical combination to use same in a liquid form?
[A] This depends upon what it is used for, whether it is to be for the gums or merely for the protection of the teeth themselves. If it is to be as a protection, then the use of those properties found in what is known as toothache bark [Prickly Ash Bark] will supply sufficient elements not only to protect gums but to form a resistance against many of those forms of diseases that attack teeth and gums.

Internal Use

Prickly ash is recommended over 60 times as an ingredient in compound formulas or tonics taken internally describing it as an "activative force" in the liver, the gall duct, and that it works as a stimulant to the pancreas and "spleen's activity." In other transcripts it states it acts on the lacteal ducts.

13. We would begin, then, with first preparing a compound to be taken internally, in this manner:

14. To 1 gallon of Distilled Water, add:

      Wild Cherry Bark.........................1/2 ounce,
      Sarsaparilla Root........................1/2 ounce,
      Yellow Dock Root.........................1/2 ounce,
      Burdock Root............................1/2 ounce,
      Prickly ash Bark........................1/4 ounce,
      Elder Flower............................2 ounces.

15. Reduce this by slow boiling [not in an aluminum container, but enamel - not cracked or broken, and NOT with a tin top; an enamel or glass top] to 1 pint. Strain and while it is still warm, add 1 ounce of PURE grain alcohol [195 proof; NOT 90], with 1/2 dram of Balsam of Tolu cut in same. [10/52 Note by Francis deSales Woidich, M.D.: "100% equals 200 proof. % and proof not used together."]

16. Shake well the solution before the dose is taken, which would be 1/2 teaspoonful 3 times each day, after meals.

Immediately after the meal take 1/2 teaspoonful, 3 times each day. Don't take it unless you eat! for it will act with the GASTRIC juices of the stomach; they each having their effect upon the various portions of the organisms that supply for blood forces. That is:

17. The first ingredient, the Wild Cherry Bark, is a direct activative force upon the pneumogastrics and the pulmonary system.

18. The Sarsaparilla works with the gastric juices of the stomach, and the eliminations in the peristaltic movement through the intestinal tract.

19. The Yellow Dock acts with the DIGESTIVE fluids themselves.

20. The Burdock is an activative force with or in the juices through the hydrochloric area, or in the pylorus.

21. The Prickly Ash Bark acts directly with the activative forces in the liver itself, in the gall duct, and as a stimulant to the pancreas and spleen's activity.

22. The Elder Flower acts with the increasing flow for the NATURAL eliminations through the system to the organic activities of the system in its relation to the sex activities of the body.

23. Then the preservative, with the activative forces in the gum, makes for an effectual activity without producing a disagreeable effect in the activity of the others.

5. To relieve the condition for this body we would keep those forces for the system much as we have at the present time. We would only take those of a stimulation to the body to give the correct vibration through the system with the air and water as is being shown or given in the body, as in this:

6. To one gallon of rain water we would add:

Wild Cherry Bark...............4 ounces,
 preferably from the North side of the tree,
Yellow Root....................2 ounces,
Red Root.......................2 ounces,
Prickly Ash Bark...............1 ounce,
Elder Flower...................1 ounce.

7. Reduce this by simmering, not boiling, to one quart, strain, while warm add:

Balm of Gilead.................2 drams,
Grain Alcohol..................6 ounces.

8. The dose with this would be teaspoonful four times each day before meals. The effect with this on the system is to give the stimulation to the organs and to the eliminating forces in the system, as in this:

9. The active principle from the Wild Cherry Bark with the other ingredients is a stimulation to the lungs, throat and bronchials and those organs above the diaphragm.

10. The Yellow Root is for the pneumogastric forces and gastric juices of the pyloric end of the stomach itself.

11. The Red Root is a stimulus for the secretions given by the pancrean forces and the spleen in its functioning from the blood cell forces as destroyed there.

12. The Prickly Ash Bark is for the blood supply as acted upon in the emunctory forces of the liver itself proper.

13. The Elder Flower is as that in the functioning of the organs of the pelvis with the action of the kidneys, with the stimulation from the alcohol and Balm of Gilead in these organs.

The following is included to illustrate the action of prickly ash bark in a compound formula:

457-3 F 26
8. ...The Wild Cherry Bark is for cleansing the blood supply. The Sarsaparilla Root is an active force in the lactic fluids of activity in the digestive area. The Elder Flower is to be effective with the organs of eliminations as related to the generative organs. The Prickly Ash Bark is for the lacteal ducts and their activity in dissemination throughout the system.

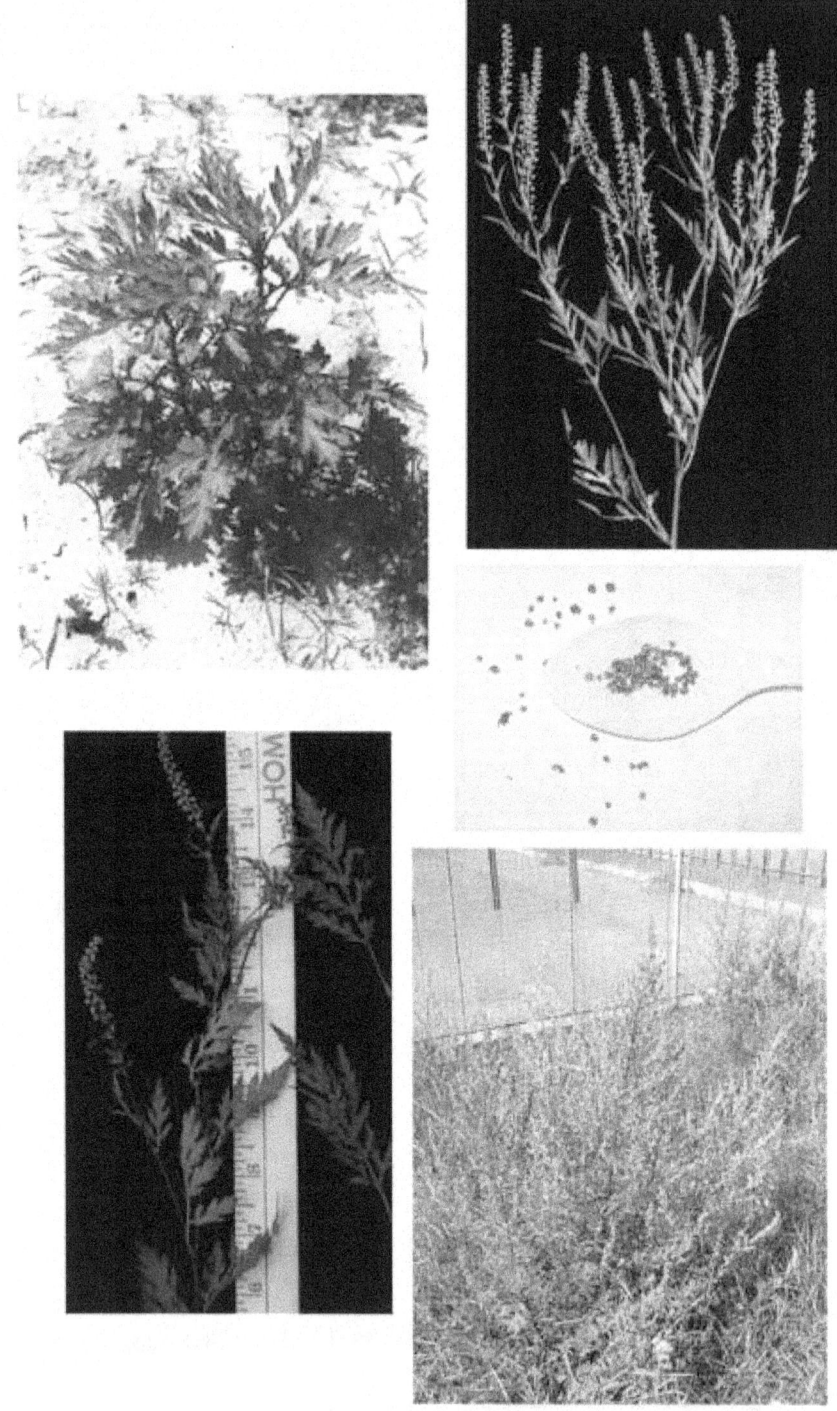

RAGWEED/AMBROSIA
Ambrosia artemisiifolia, Ambrosia trifida, Fam. Asteraceae

Common and Regional Names
Hayfever Plant, Roman Wormwood, Hog-weed, Bitter-weed, Pigweed, Bitter Weed, Blood Weed

History and Common Usage
Ragweed is thought to have originated in what is today Canada, North America and Central America. It is also found throughout Europe, Africa, Central and South America, Australia and New Zealand and in many places is considered an invasive. It is especially abundant from British Columbia in Canada to Mexico. The two most prevalent species of Ragweed are *Ambrosia artemisiifolia* and *Ambrosia trifida*.

Ragweed is famous for making some people miserable. Ragweed pollen is the cause of hay fever in sensitive individuals and a small percentage of the population even experiences a contact rash when touching the plant. It yields prodigious amounts of pollen beginning as early as June in some areas until as late as October.

Ragweed does not claim a significant presence in traditional herbal lore nor is a distinction made between *A. artemisiifolia* and *A. trifida*. According to the 21st US Dispensatory either plant can be used. Ragweed is described for use as an astringent and stimulant and as an insufflation or gargle in nose and throat infections.

Description
Ragweed is a coarse, weedy herb characterized by small, greenish, unisexual flower heads. Each plant produces thousands of seeds which turn brown to near black as they mature. The upper leaves are small, thin and alternating, the lower leaves are larger with a lacy appearance. *A. Trifida* can grow to 6 feet but *A. artemisiifolia* is usually found between 2 and 3 feet in height. It is classified as a noxious and pernicious weed.

Growing Conditions and Propagation
Ragweed is a vigorous and most prolific self-seeder. It likes sunny locations and well-drained soils but will do well under any conditions. It is an opportunistic weed, favoring feed-lots and pastures, the edges of fields and gardens and can be found thriving in ditches.

The tiny greenish flowers develop on upright stem tips at the top of the plant. Both male and female flowers appear on the same plant. The male flowers release billions of grains of pollen beginning in August and ending in October. Most pollen is released in midmorning when the dew evaporates and is most prolific on warm, windy, dry days.

The small seeds mature on the plant and dry in place. It a simple matter to strip the stem tips by hand storing the small seeds in plastic or paper bags. They can be scattered on prepared ground in the spring in the same manner as flower seeds. The seeds are viable for up to five years and will often spring up seemingly out of nowhere. Weed control is exercised through pulling and discarding the unwanted plants. Young plants are also easily transplanted. Once one plant is established nature will take care of the rest.

Harvesting

Only the leaves are used in the Cayce system. The active principles are highest if they are picked in the early morning for immediate use. For drying they are washed under cool, clean water and spread out in a warm area protected from direct sunlight. Ideal drying temperatures are between 70° and 80°F. Depending on humidity the leaves should be dry enough to store in three to five days. Dried leaves are powdered by rolling them inside a brown paper bag or plastic food storage bags with a rolling pin until they are pulverized, or small amounts at a time may be processed in a food processor or blender. The dried leaves, whole or powdered, are then stored in plastic freezer bags or sealed in glass jars stored out of the light. The bags or jars can also be stored in the freezer.

Use in the Edgar Cayce Readings

Ragweed is used alone and as a companion plant. Mentioned nearly one hundred times in the Cayce system ragweed is used in a variety of tonics for intestinal and digestive disorders ranging from appendicitis, uricacidemia, constipation, debilitation, diabetes, and ulcerative colitis.

The green leaves are to be chewed, ignoring their bitter taste, or used as a tea to stimulate the liver, act as an eliminant or as an intestinal purifier. Although fresh is always better either fresh or dried leaves can be used.

The question must be raised that if this plant, classified as a noxious weed, is the cause of so much suffering, why would anyone want to deliberately cultivate it?

The answer is that the plant, according to Cayce, if properly used, is a natural antigen. By using ragweed internally BEFORE it begins producing pollen the plant may relieve or even prevent the allergic reaction. Transcript 903-35 states that by choosing a young plant and chewing the leaves it will relieve the allergy or eliminate the cause of the hay fever – _**for this body,**_ the last sentence indicates that hay fever _**"is not caused by the same in all:"**_

903-35 F 41 HAY FEVER

16. (Q) Where would be the best place to go to aid the condition of her hay fever, and what will relieve her now?
(A) A higher altitude would be better, and where it is somewhat drier. These are the conditions that are conducive to hay fever.

If remaining in the lower altitude, (Authors note: she lived in New York City) the use of an inhalant such as we have indicated for hay fever would be very well. [see directions [which were enclosed] [261-8] for preparing inhalant.]

17. (Q) What particular weed or flower is causing it?
(A) Ragweed!

18. (Q) Since hay fever is usually caused by an allergy, can the Forces describe the particular allergy which is causing this condition to this body, so that the body can stay away from it?
(A) As just indicated, smell one of the weeds, try it on self and see! But if you chew it as it is growing, you may relieve yourself from it! It's a good eliminant, too! It is one of the best eliminants with a vegetable base. But it must be chosen very young, and the leaves alone chewed - but don't spit it out because it is bitter! It's not poisonous, and it is a good eliminant, and it will relieve the allergy - or

eliminate that causing the hay fever FOR THIS PARTICULAR BODY! For it is not caused by the same in all.

Another hay fever sufferer was given similar advice but to make a tea of the ragweed or ambrosia leaves instead of chewing the young leaves. The information then goes on to give directions for the compounding of a simple home tonic to be taken throughout the season as a preventive:

5347-1 M 35 HAY FEVER

4. These reactions come from what may be called or set up as vibrations in certain centers between sympathetic and cerebro-spinal system, and thus the body in such periods is subject to conditions which manifest in irritation to mucous membranes of the nasal passage and throat, bronchi and larynx or, as sometimes called, rose fever or such natures. These, for this body, are particularly from the ragweed.

5. Thus, we would find in this particular season, before there is the blossoming of same, the body should take quantities of this weed. Brew same, prepare, take internally and thus war or ward against the activity of this upon the body itself.

6. Then, through the period, also take that as an antiseptic reaction upon the nerves of the nasal passages, or the olfactory nerves of the body.

7. These will prevent, then, the recurrent conditions which have been and are a part of the experience of the body. This will enable the body to become immune because of the very action of this weed upon the digestive system, and the manner it will act with the assimilating body, too. Well, just don't get too heavy, for it will make for an increase in the amount of assimilation and distribution of food values for the body.

8. Thus we would prepare the compound in this manner: Take a pint cup, gather the tender leaves of the weed, don't cram in but just fill level. Put this in an enamel or a glass container and then the same amount (after cleansing of course, don't put dirt and all in but put in same amount by measure) of distilled water, see? Reduce this to half the quantity by very slow boiling, not hard but slow boiling, strain and add sufficient grain alcohol as a preservative.

9. Begin and take it through the fifteen days of July and the whole of August, daily, half a teaspoonsful each day.

This kind of information naturally gives rise to the question: does this work? The following letter speaks to the efficacy of this simple, and more importantly - cost free - remedy.

September 12, 1971

Gentlemen:

Words will never be able to express my appreciation for the July issue of the A.R.E. Journal[91] I am 40 years old and have suffered from a lifetime affliction of ragweed allergy. I have never bothered taking the troublesome*

---

91   [*] *Blessed Ragweed-The Most Hated of Weeds*
by Robert O. Clapp ARE Journal – Vol. 6, No. 4 – July 1971

shots preferring to suffer through the 6 to 8 week ragweed season. Neither had I seen a doctor for quite some time having concluded years ago that the prescription antihistamine pills and allergic pills were no more superior than those sold over the counter.

So the hay fever season for me was one of staying in where the air conditioning did some filtering of pollen from the air and taking endless antihistamine pills and nose sprays and generally suffering thru the agonizing symptoms of hay fever. Some antihistamine pills seem to help, some don't, some seem to wear out on their effectiveness, and anyway they can only be taken for short lengths of time because extreme drowsiness sets in after two or three days straight on the pills. I always had to curtail swimming during August because the chlorinated water was too abrasive on the red, swollen and sensitive nostrils and eyes. But thanks to the Cayce readings printed in the July A.R.E. Journal, this year was quite different.

I began eating the leaves of the ragweed plant immediately upon reading the article July 7, 1971 and continued thru September 11, 1971. True to the Cayce readings I found the ragweed leaves to be quite bitter in taste on the first occasion but I didn't mind it after that. Also true to the Cayce readings a little over indulgence caused some marked differences in assimilation and elimination. But the beautiful thing about it was that throughout August no hay fever symptoms ever developed. This year I rode my bicycle up and down roads which were lined with ragweed and also walked thru woods and pastures which were thick with ragweed. (Iowa has the highest ragweed pollen counts of any location in the nation.) This was one of the worst seasons for hay fever sufferers and all of my ragweed allergic friends suffered terribly even though some had been taking the year round shots. I went swimming throughout August with no discomfort at all and forgot about pills.

The fact that I was not suffering from hay fever this year caused quite some consternation among my hay fever suffering friends. I frankly told them all what I was doing and the source of the information, but nobody believed a word of it. Some called their doctors and demanded to know why they couldn't be cured of hay fever, but their doctors told them there was nothing they could do but take shots the year around or the pills. All the experiences I had with friends who are sufferers would fill up a letter in itself. I would be glad to give many more details about this whole subject if you are interested.

Looking back over this past hay fever season it now seems about unbelievable to me; a cure for hay fever is miraculous.

Many thanks again for publishing that article on ragweed.

Yours truly, H

*Harold D. Armentrout
6801 Devonshire Drive,*
Cedar Rapids, IA 52402

Certainly the most unusual of all the uses of ragweed in the Cayce system is described in the following in which having ragweed as a portion of the diet deters appendicitis:

644-1

21. (Q) What are the influences brought to bear that seem to cause appendicitis to come in epidemics?

(A) These are both mental attitudes of individuals and the astrological influences, combined with the very nature of the elements that people take under certain seasons; or the lack of vitamins in that which grows in the products used as food. Hence are the combination of all of these. Some families, some groups, being more sympathetic than others are more easily affected by the conditions, both from the mental attitudes and the diets in that particular family or vicinity; for - as it will be seen in such epidemics - the diets of those individuals in certain territories or surroundings are lacking in the necessary vitamins; for with the making of many things used in the seasoning of foods, or in the applications for those things where synthetic conditions have brought about the making of things, they leave OUT the vitamins that NATURE has prepared - and does prepare - in all food values.

22. (Q) Is there any correction for this, generally?
(A) If the most hated of the weeds were used as a portion of the diet, it would never occur - Ragweed.

23. (Q) How should this be prepared or taken?
(A) Either taken as a medicine or as a portion of the diet

The following two excerpts are examples of how ragweed is used in the Cayce system:

369-12 F 29 LIVER KIDNEY INCOORDINATION
15. (Q) Is the Simmons Laxative which I took, the same as Simmons Liver Regulator recommended in reading [369-11 on 8/4/34]?
(A) Not exactly the same; this was made to take the place of the Liver Regulator and to meet some requirements that were necessary. Where this is given for anyone, the better preparation would be to make it out of the Ragweed, which is the basis of same - either the green (but dry same) or the dry, which may be preserved or bought in bulk, and made in the form of a tea - in this manner (this isn't for this body in the present - may be necessary later; but we have given those things necessary for this particular body in the present), and in this proportion:

To 8 ounces distilled water add 3 drams dried Ragweed. Reduce to 6 ounces, or reduce to the quantity then it is necessary to add even more water to make 6 ounces. Then add a preservative, which would be 1 ounce of grain alcohol.

And you have better than Simmons Liver Regulator for activity on the liver! This for anyone! This is the BEST of the vegetable compounds for activities of the liver. Of course, if made commercially we would add some few other things to it. [See 562-1 on 5/29/34.] [5/11/39 See 1880-1 not recommending Simmons, but Ragweed. See also 1880-1 Reports in re Simmons and Ragweed or Ambrosia. Some years later the Simmons Liver Regulator went off the market, but not during Edgar Cayce's lifetime.]

389-3 M 55 INTESTINES:COLON:PLETHORA
26. (Q) What causes intense pain in side? Is it the appendix, or just a natural result?
(A) A natural result from removing the fecal forces that have caused the pressure in the system. Necessary, then, that there be kept the removal of the pressures in the colon, and that there be the proper reaction in the digestive area.

189

It would be well for the body to at least once a week to take ragweed; and plenty of it grows around the place! Strip the leaves and dry into a powder; or take the ragweed green and chew a good mouthful of it, swallowing the juice. Or, take that known as Simmons Liver Regulator, the dry; a quarter teaspoonful in water once a week. This will clear out all the disturbance.

This does not mean that the enemas should not be taken. They need not be taken so often, but - as indicated - they are necessary to keep down the irritation.

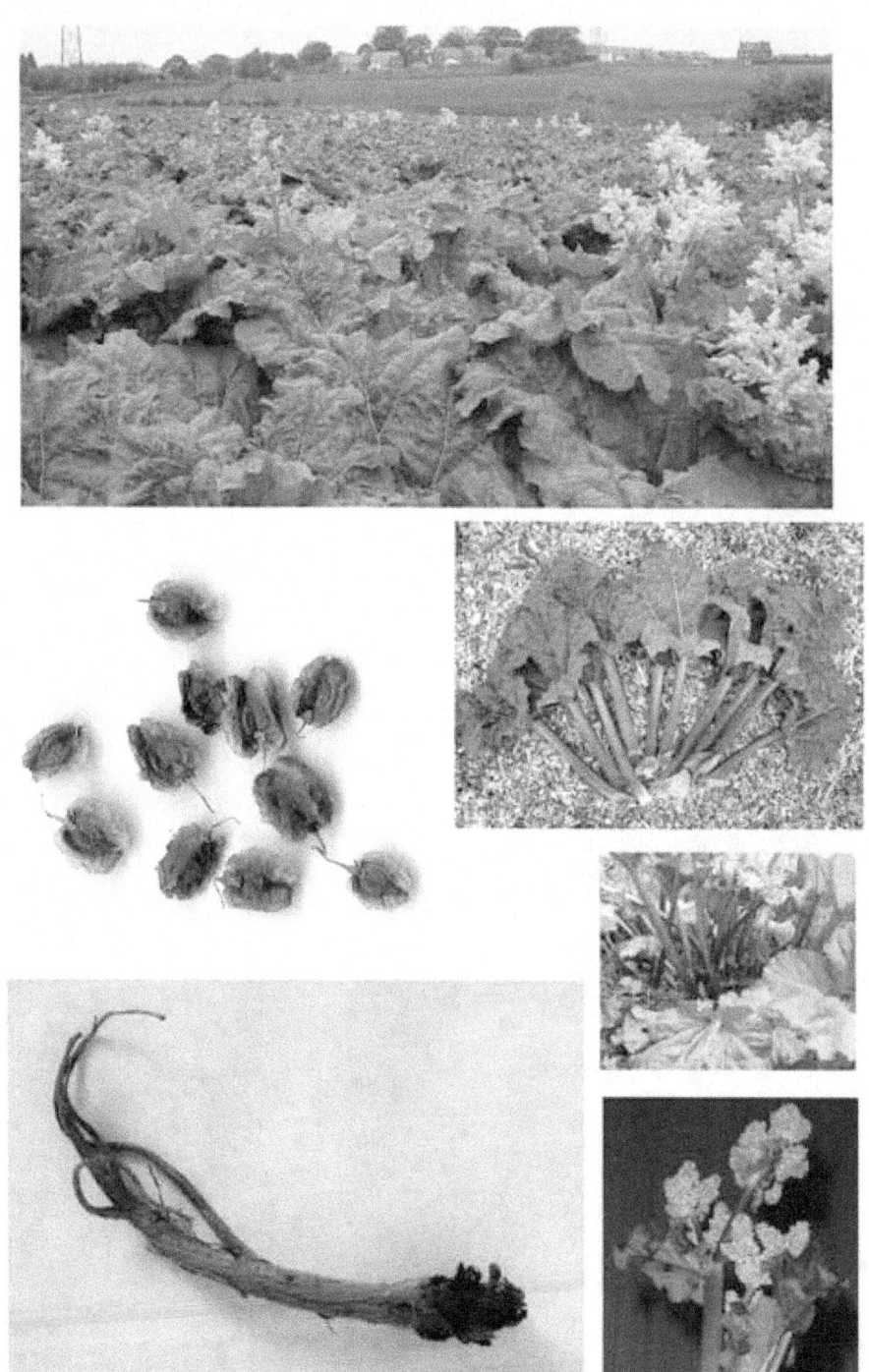

Rhubarb/Pie Plant
Rheum officinal or Rheum palmatum, Fam. Polygonaceeae

Common and Regional Names
Pie plant, garden rhubarb, Russian Rhubarb, Turkey Rhubarb, Chinese Rhubarb

History and Common Usage
Rhubarb root was officially recognized as a medicinal plant 3,000 years before the birth of Christ. It is cited in the Chinese herbal *Shen Nong's Ben Cao Jing*, which as previously stated is thought by most scholars to be a re-compilation of even earlier works dating back possibly 5,000 years B.C.

There are now about 25 identified species all believed to have evolved over eons from one original species that originated in Asia; a region today which includes Tibet and Western China. Other distinct varieties are found in the area of the Black Sea. Rhubarb is thought to have been the plant referred to in the first century A.D. by Pedanius Dioscorides as "Rha." Scholars disagree whether Rha is taken from the Greek rheo 'to flow' alluding to the purgative properties of the root, or from the ancient name of the River Volga.

As early humans migrated around the globe identification of the different varieties of rhubarb became confused and one variety came to be known by many names. Because it was an important commodity for commercial export rhubarb would be sometimes named after the country of origin. As confusing as this is it sheds some light on the routes by which it traveled to European markets and into European record keeping.

Rhubarb is recorded as having entered cultivation in Italy in 1608 and around 20 or 30 years later had made its way throughout most of Europe. In 1653 Nicholas Culpepper mentions the use of a plant by the name of rhubarb [or Raphontick] in his <u>Complete Herbal</u> but this is not the rhubarb root used in medicine. Records are found in 1764 of its cultivation in the Botanical Gardens in Edinburgh, Scotland. In 1777 an apothecary in Banbury, Oxfordshire by the name of Hayward is recorded as successfully raising rhubarb from seeds sent from Russia in 1762. Rhubarb root was used only in medicine as far as western record keeping is concerned until around 1790 or 1800 when the plant began to be used as a potherb throughout all of Europe. French chefs began using the leaves in soups finding its flavor superior to the leaves of sorrel. Sometime around 1846 deaths began to be attributed to the plant. Several historical sources published in 1846 to as late as 1910 cite death by oxalic poisoning by means of ingesting rhubarb leaves.

Rhubarb has the unique ability to combine within itself the properties of a relaxant, stimulant and astringent. It is a dietetic, an eliminant and a purgative. It has also been used in some medical traditions as a topical dressing or poultice in the treatment of thermal burns, sores and ulcers. Rhubarb was official for use as a laxative in both the United States and British pharmacopeias during the time the Cayce information was being given.

Description
Rhubarb is a handsome plant characterized by emerald green leaves with beautiful red, pink or green stalks which are tart but edible. The leaves should never be eaten as they contain oxalic acid which is poisonous.

The roots are long lived and it is not unusual for a single plant to live for 12 to 15 years. The size of the plant depends upon the variety grown some reaching 4 feet in height with leaves 2 feet in length while others can be 12 to 18 inches in height with leaves 6 to 8 inches in length. The root, which is the medicinal part, is dark brown and branches from a crown, which grows just above the level of the soil. Leaves develop from buds on top of the crown in the early spring, folded and wrinkled, and of a dark reddish brown color. Warmed by the sun they spread taking on a beautiful dark, emerald green color. The stems of the leaves, called petioles, form the edible portion of the plant. The stalks grow quite large, sometimes an inch in diameter and 1 ½ feet in length.

After the leaves have reached their prime the plant sends up a stem topped by small, greenish-white clusters of flowers. The small dark brown seeds develop from the loose clusters of flowers as the season turns to autumn.

Rhubarb varieties are classified as red or green. The green types are again differentiated as green and speckled [pink]. In the United States commercial production of rhubarb is concentrated in Washington, Oregon and Michigan. Victoria is a popular red variety well suited for home gardens.

Growing Conditions and Propagation
Rhubarb is a cool season perennial. It is pollinated by wind and insects and propagates by seeds and through root division. Rhubarb tolerates winter temperatures to –20°F but does not thrive in sustained summer temperatures exceeding 85°F. When the summers are too warm the plant will appear dormant, and as the temperatures decline the foliage growth will resume. It can be grown as an annual in some southern climates but if summer temperatures reach 90°F the plant soon wilts and if these temperatures continue the plant dies. It requires sustained temperatures below 40° F to break dormancy. Rhubarb does best in the northern United States from Maine to Illinois and west to Washington State. Canada is also well suited to rhubarb as is its close southern neighbor, Michigan.

Rhubarb can be grown from seeds but it takes a long time for the plants to become established. It is easier to propagate from roots, which are readily available through local nurseries, mail order catalogues and often by way of a neighbor with a plant ready to be divided.

The plant needs well-drained soil and full sun. Rhubarb can thrive in most soils but prefers rich, well-drained soil high in organic matter. It does best at a soil pH of 6.0 to 6.8. It is one plant that needs fertilizer so each plant should be fed one cup of 10-10-10 each spring, applied in a circle around the plant just as growth starts. Rhubarb can also be composted with well-rotted manure in the fall but do not bury the crowns.

When planting dig extra large holes for the roots and mix the soil with composted manure, or work fertilizer well into the soil. Spread the roots out as much as possible without damage, firming the soil around the root. Keep them watered – but not wet - while they establish. If planted in rows in the garden allow 4 feet each way around the plant to allow room for both the leaves and for garden maintenance. Some varieties will spread 4 feet in diameter attaining heights of 3 feet.

In areas where there is an occurrence of standing water for any length of time, or sustained and excessive rainfall, the crowns will rot and the plant will die. Roots live for many years but due to inroads by insects or disease it is common practice for serious gardeners to rest a bed every 4 to 5 years. This is done when the stalks begin to be spindly or small or the crown of the plant can be seen to be too crowded with buds and stalks. It is time to dig them up, divide the roots and trim them back to only 4 or 5 buds before planting them in a new area. Discard any crowns that show rot or damage from excessive water. Plan on letting them grow for 2 full years before harvesting the stalks.

Harvesting

The root is harvested from plants that are 4 year old or older. They are usually dug in October, washed under cool, clean running water, and all rootlets and fibers are removed. The covering or "bark" of the root is scraped or rasped to remove the bark or outer skin and the root is then cut in transverse pieces for drying. If the root is very large it should be cut in half before slicing transversely. Smaller roots can be dried whole. Pieces can be sun dried if drying conditions are favorable and in some cultures the pieces of root are hung on cords and dried in the sun. Where high humidity is present the roots can also be dried in a home oven on its lowest setting. The dried pieces can be stored in plastic food bags or sealed in sterile jars. The dried pieces are also chopped and pulverized into powder for use in syrups and tinctures.

When cutting the stalks it is good to get into the habit of first cutting the leaves from the stalks and then cutting or breaking the stalks from the crowns. This helps keep the oxalic acid levels lower in the stalks. Wash them well under running water for a few minutes before cooking.

If rhubarb is damaged by a freeze or frost the stalks can still be eaten provided they are still firm to the touch and upright. If they are even the least soft or mushy they should be discarded as the oxalic acid crystals in the leaves may have migrated to the stalks. The damaged stalks and all leaves can be safely used for compost.

Use in the Edgar Cayce Readings

Rhubarb is used as a companion plant combined with other herbs in mixtures and tonics variously described as tonics, eliminants, laxatives, and as remedies for coughs and expectorants in cases of cold and congestion.

It is recommended over 140 times, 70 of those citations calling for syrup of rhubarb which contains cinnamon, rhubarb, potassium carbonate, distilled water and syrup which is usually simple syrup made with cane or beet sugar. In only 5 cases is rhubarb to be taken alone. It is recommended as a dietary item in 30 cases and always where increased eliminations are necessary. Often other "laxative" foods are mentioned as well, such as prunes or figs.

In 10 cases CRC tablets were recommended. No longer available these tablets were made of calomel, colocynth and rhubarb.[92]

As a dietary item rhubarb is often seen recommended as follows:

1206-16 F 18 June 10, 1944
5. We would add more raw vegetables, more fruits, more which are laxative; as prunes, pieplant, such things. The rhubarb stewed, rhubarb pie in various manners is excellent, especially at this period of the year. Especially fruits and vegetables, change about, and we will have bettered conditions for the eliminations.

92   Calomel – called also mercurous chloride – a purgative. Colocynth. From Citrullus colocynthus, related to the watermelon. A Mediterranean and African herbaceous vine, the spongy fruit of which yields a cathartic.

The following are excellent examples of expectorants made with syrup of rhubarb that can easily be made at home. Often Cayce describes more than one benefit from a given formula:

772-6 F 49
10. As a cough syrup compound or solution, we would prepare this:

11. To 2 ounces of Syrup of Horehound, add - in the order named:

> Tincture of Valerian............1/4 ounce,
> Syrup of Rhubarb................1/2 ounce.

Shake the solution, and take a teaspoonful whenever there is that tickling in the throat or tendency for a cough.

12. In the diet, keep away from too much starches or fats.

13. Be mindful that there are good eliminations kept, using as a laxative the vegetable compounds preferably, or those that are of the senna base [Castoria, Syrup of Figs, Elixir of Senna, Tam, etc.] These would be the better for this present condition.

This formula doubles as an expectorant and a tonic to assist in assimilation:

1278-7 F Adult
8. We would prepare rather than a cough syrup or an expectorant, those properties where there would be these combined in same, that will not only make for the relief of the mucous membranes but assist in assimilation and give to the gastric flow of the digestive system activities and principles from which the assimilating system may gain strength; relieving this tendency for soreness and nausea through the alimentary canal, as well as through portions of the stomach itself - that is, if all of these are combined together - all of the treatments, see?

9. To 2 ounces of Strained Honey add 2 ounces of Distilled Water. Let this come to a boil. Skim off the refuse. Set aside to cool, and then add to this 2 ounces of Grain Alcohol [85% pure]. Then to this as the carrier, add - in the order named:

> Essence of Wild Ginseng............1/2 ounce,
> Syrup of Rhubarb..................1/2 ounce,
> Syrup of Senna....................1/4 ounce.

Have this shaken together before the dose is taken, which may be taken every two hours - unless there is too great a coughing or too great a strain upon the nervous systems of the body. Every two hours give half to a teaspoonful, unless there is too great amount of coughing - when a little or a small quantity may be sipped.

The following case of a lady recovering from pneumonia is given a formula that Cayce states will act as an aid to eliminations, an expectorant and a tonic AND can be made at home:

464-22 F 62

2. These properties may be so combined or compounded as to act as an eliminant, an expectorant and a strengthener also; and preferably would be combined by self, in this manner:

3. To 2 ounces of Strained Pure Honey, add 4 ounces of water. Let this come to a boil. Strain or skim off the refuse forces or drosses that rise to the top. Then put this in about an 8 ounce bottle container, and add to same - in the ORDER NAMED: [Obtain each of the ingredients separately, you see, and add in the order and proportion indicated]:

> Apple Brandy.......................4 ounces,
> Syrup of Wild Cherry Bark.........1/2 ounce,
> Syrup of Rhubarb..................1/2 ounce,
> Syrup of Horehound................1/2 ounce,
> Glycerine.........................1 teaspoonful.

Shake the solution well before each dose is taken, which would be a teaspoonful about every three or four hours. This as we find will not only aid in eliminations, clear the cough and the hoarseness but make for a general stimulation for the body.

481-3 M 31

10. Then, as an expectorant - and for a healing with same - we would prepare this:

11. Put 2 ounces of Strained Pure Honey in 2 ounces of Distilled Water. Let come to a boil. Skin off the refuse. Then add, in the order named:

> Syrup of Wild Cherry Bark...............1 ounce,
> Glycerine............................1 1/4 ounces,
> Syrup of Rhubarb......................1/4 ounce,
> Syrup of Horehound....................1/2 ounce,
> Gordon Gin.............................2 ounces.

Shake the solution, not too hard but shake it before the dose is taken; which would be a teaspoonful three to four times each day.

In this formula the alcohol called for would be pure grain alcohol:

5683-1 F Adult NEURASTHENIA

8. First we would prepare as this: We would take Wild Ginseng 1 ounce, to 8 ounces of distilled water. We would reduce this body slow boiling to 6 ounces. Then, to this we would add [when this is strained, we would then add] as this:

> Tincture of Stillingia...............20 minims,
> Syrup of Rhubarb.....................20 minims,
> Tincture, or Essence, of Indian
>   Turnip............................2 minims,
> Alcohol...........................1 ½ ounces.

The dose of this would be half teaspoonful 3 times each day.

9. Now, the pathological effect of this upon the system is to react through the assimilating system to both the eliminating and assimilating ducts and glands of the body. These [save the Stillingia] are for a stimuli to the active forces of the ducts of the body. The Stillingia is as a sedentary action for the glands of digestion, or the lacteals, WITH those that will make for a better coordination of the mucomembranes in the intestines, that will clarify poisons from the body. [That's in the Syrup of Rhubarb, see?]

One of Cayce's "smart formulas," its intended multiple purpose function is to create equilibrium between the liver and the kidneys, while assisting in eliminations through the alimentary canal:

5508-1 M 29 Eliminations
9. First, we would prepare THIS as MEDICINAL properties for the system, to create an equilibrium in the activity of the liver with that of the kidneys; also of the cleansing of the system throughout the alimentary canal:

10. To 6 ounces of distilled water we would add the dried Ambrosia weed 3 ounces. Reduce this by simmering, not boiling, to 1/2 the quantity. Strain while warm and add:

> Tincture of Stillingia...........1/4 ounce,
> Simple Syrup......................2 ounces,
> Syrup of Rhubarb.................1/4 ounce,
> Tincture of Capsici...............3 minims,
> Pure Grain Alcohol................1 ounce.

Shake the solution together before the dosage is taken, and this should be at least TWICE each day until there is the thorough reaction through the alimentary canal. Then it may be taken only once each day, the dosage being half a teaspoonful at a dose.

Dietary Examples

367-1 M 14
19. Mornings - citrus fruit juices or stewed fruits; preferably prunes and the pie plant [rhubarb, you see], and when this is stewed the sugar added should preferably be the heavy brown sugar or saccharin or beet sugar.

433-4 F 45
6. [Q] What would be the proper diet for me?
[A] As we would find, it would be well that the juices of fruits be taken, or the citrous fruit diet; preferably, however, those of grape juices and grapefruit juices, and those of lemon, than too much of the orange, though these may be mixed at times WITH the grapefruit juices or with the grape juice FOR the palatability of this as a beverage, or as a drink. These of mornings. Alternate these occasionally with stewed rhubarb, prunes and prune juices, figs - that are stewed, not in sugar, but dry figs stewed.

633-6 M 26
13. [Q] What particular diet at this time?
[A] A general diet that includes those active forces that have a tendency for laxative reaction; as prunes, figs, stewed raisins - all of those activities that include such. The pie plant or rhubarb, those of such natures that tend to make for not merely weight but an activity to the mucous membranes to the LOWER intestinal system.

This last excerpt is included only as an interesting example of Edgar Cayce's clairvoyant abilities:

5421-1 F Adult
1. EC: Now, we have here the body of [5421], ..., Texas. They have been and are giving properties, medicinal properties to this body that have not been compounded in the way as was given here.

The senna and rhubarb and other properties as were given to this body, part were compounded from old stocks that have carried with them another resistive force. Through their rebuilding and channels they produce microbes in this so that their action and reaction in the system, instead of producing an active principle to carry out the action of the digestive tract and carry from the system the feces were trying or producing more of a condition.

The saffron that should have been given to this body, they are using a substitute. Those powders that act as a sedative to the duodenum are overcharged from fumes thrown out by other properties when this is set near it.

All of these combined produce a bad condition in the system. Let them have this prepared again and follow the channels if we would reduce the fear and condition that we have in this system.

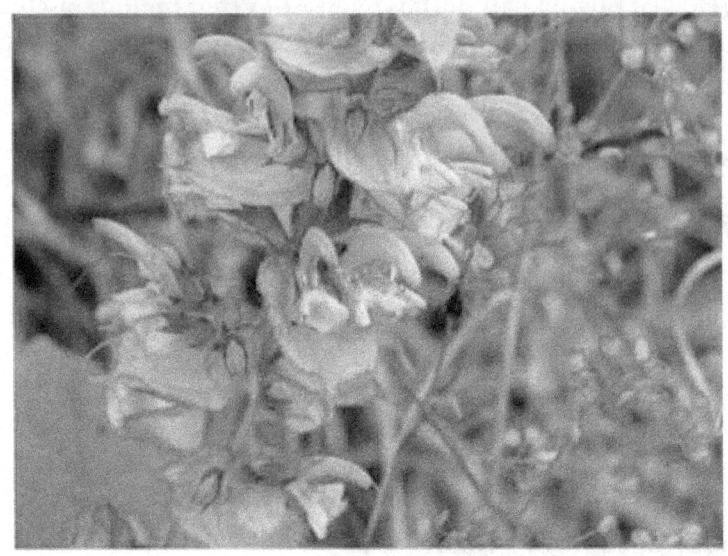

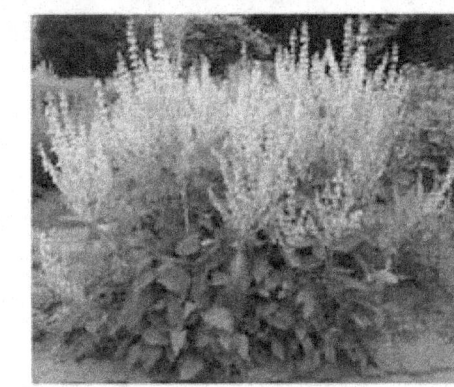

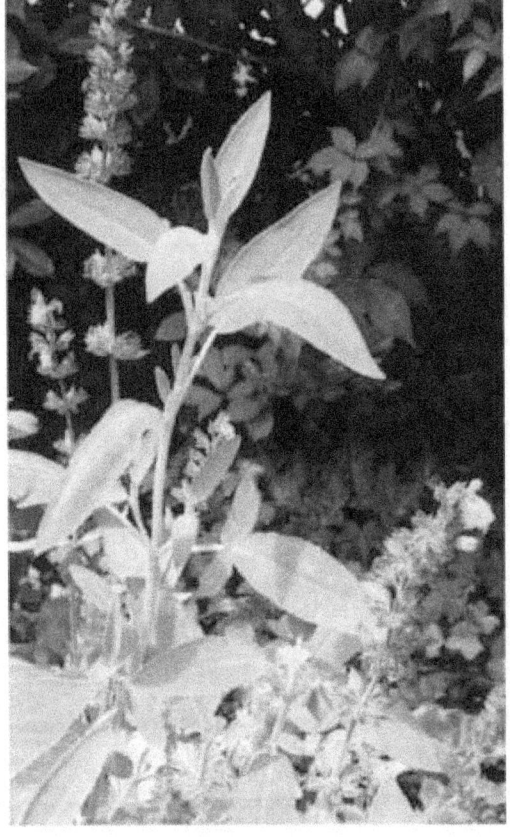

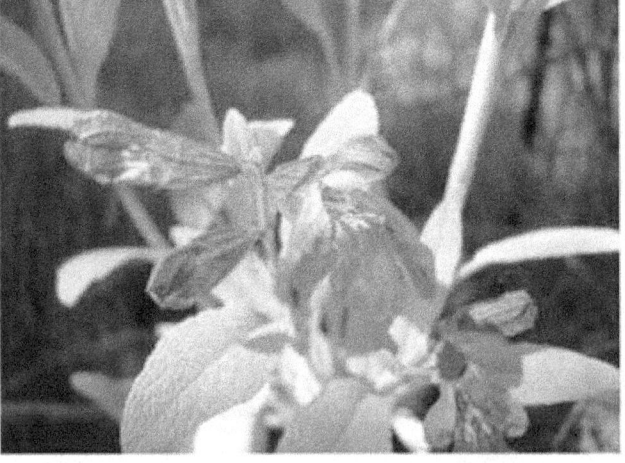

SAGE-CLARY WATER
Salvia officinalis and *Salvia sclarea, Fam. Lamiaceae [formerly Labiatae]*

Common and Regional Names:
Salvia officinalis: Sage, Garden sage, common sage, white sage

Salvia sclarea: Sage, Clary sage, clarey sage, Clara Sage, clarywort, musoatel sage, Eyebright, See Bright

History and Common Usage

Sage is the common name of a very large genus of about 900 flowering plants in wide distribution throughout the world. The name is from the original Latin "salvere" in reference to the curative properties of the plant meaning "to be saved." The word devolved to Sauja and Sauge [from the French] into the old English "Sawge" which further changed over time into the present word sage. The sages were formerly classified as members of the *Labiatae* family but are now officially listed as *Lamiaceae*.

Sage is related to the mint family and is said to have originated in the Mediterranean and in areas from Southern Europe to Asia Minor. It has long been used as a flavoring agent for food, cheese, beer and wine and as a medicinal plant. Through archeological evidence it is known that sage was grown in home gardens by the ancient Egyptians but it does not appear in their pharonic pharmacopeias. Pliny refers to many kinds of sages in his time and cites their varied uses. In AETHIOPIS:FOUR REMEDIES he says: *"Taken in white wine they are curative of affections of the uterus, and a decoction of them is administered for sciatica, pleurisy, and eruptions of the throat. The kind, however, which comes from AEthiopia is by far the best, and gives instantaneous relief."*

The Book of Medicines lists only one remedy used by the Syrians calling for clary sage given for, among other complaints: *"cold of the stomach, and for the kidneys…and it beautifieth the complexion."* Administered in extract of leeks the formula contains 25 other ingredients and is said to be *"well tried."*

Sage has been used as a hair rinse and hair tonic, a flavoring for tobacco, as a tea or poultice in the treatment of eye infections, insect bites and stings, and as an antibacterial agent on cuts and scrapes. As a tea it is used to ease the symptoms of menopause and to soothe and heal stomach and mouth ulcers. It is recommended as a stimulant, tonic, carminative, digestive aid and as a gargle for sore throats. Sage is probably most famous for its use in various kinds of stuffing for roast turkey and chicken and as a spice in sausage and other prepared meats. Lactating mothers are advised not to drink sage tea as it has the action of drying the mammary glands thereby reducing or inhibiting the production of milk.

Clary sage, or *Salvia sclarea*, is officially recorded as being introduced into the British Isles from Syria in 1562 where it quickly gained a place as a medicinal. It is cited in many pharmacopeias for its effectiveness in drawing out foreign bodies from the eyes. The seeds are soaked in water to release their mucilaginous properties and then placed over the closed eyelid as a poultice for inflammation of the eyes and lids giving rise to the common name of eyebright.

Clary Water is a formula found in the Cayce information made with sage as the base but it is not original to Cayce. The original "Clary Water" formula was in widespread use throughout Europe as a tonic and digestive aid as far back as at least the Middle Ages. It contained clary-flowers, brandy, sugar, cinnamon, and a little ambergris. Clary Water was at first individually compounded from a "folk recipe," then later it was prepared commercially and sold for a number of years throughout Europe. In 1900, just as Cayce began his career, Clary Water had fallen out of fashion, commercial production declined and both the time-tested old formula and knowledge of its efficacy faded into obscurity.

Around 1903 Mr. Cayce attempted to obtain information to help Mr. 5676. No copy of that transcript survives but the following from his diary mentions the discovery of Clary Water being made in Paris fifty to seventy five years earlier:

B5676-1 M Adult
"About that time I received a request from a Mr. [5676] in New York City for a reading on himself. This was my first experience in trying to give information for one at a distance. Mr. L. [Al C. Layne] conducted the experiment in the presence of several physicians, for I made a trip to Hopkinsville for that purpose. In this there was clary water suggested for him. We did not know whether this was a preparatory medicine, or whether there was any such thing or not, but the information written at that time was sent to Mr. [5676]

"Some weeks later, as he had been unable to obtain the preparation, he asked that we try to give the formula for making it. This reading was conducted by Dr. B. [Blackburn] in Bowling Green, with quite a number of prominent persons present – business men, professors and doctors. A formula was given [See GD's note below]. Something like a month later I received word from Mr. [5676] that he had received a letter from a man in Paris, France who informed him that his father fifty or seventy-five years before had made and marketed a preparation under the name of clary water, and the formula was identical with that which had been given in the reading to Dr. B. Mr. [5676] reported receiving a great deal of benefit from the taking of the clary water."

[GD's note: We do not have a copy of the check-up Physical Rdg. conducted by Dr. Blackburn. However, in a letter 10/12/31 Edgar Cayce wrote out the formula for Mrs. [5480], [a diabetic] from memory - 5480-1, Reports:]

Put 6 ounces of the clary flower [or garden sage, dried] in 32 ounces of distilled water. Reduce by slow boiling, or steaming, to one-half the quantity. Strain while warm and add:

> *Simple Syrup..........................1 ounce,*
> *Ambergris.............................15 grains,*
> *dissolved in Grain Alcohol.......1 ounce,*
> *Gordon Gin...........................8 ounces,*
> *Cinnamon [preferably in the stick]...1 dram.*

Shake solution together before dose is taken. [Dose: 1/2 teaspoonful 4 times each day, after each meal and before retiring.] You will be able to obtain ambergris from either Lehn & Fink or Eimer & Amend, N.Y.C.]

The 21st Edition of the United States Dispensatory lists sage among the unofficial drug plans but does not attribute any therapeutic value. It is described as only a tonic and a condiment.

Description

Both *S. officinalis* and *S. sclarea* have the square stems characteristic of the mint family. *Salvia officinalis* grows to a foot or more in height and has gray to whitish-gray green thin leaves set in pairs on square, wiry stems. The leaves are smooth underneath and covered with short whitish fuzz on top, giving rise to one of the common names of white sage. The purplish-blue flowers appear at the tips of the stems in July or August.

Salvia sclarea is a much larger plant. It is a biennial which grows 3 to 4 feet tall on a square, brownish stem with large, broad-ovate green leaves that are fleshy and distinctively veined. The tap root can penetrate 20 inches and plants have been known to grow to 6 feet in height. The white or lilac to blue flowers appear on spikes at the top of the plant as early as June and as late as July or August. The whole plant is covered with tiny hairs tipped with glands with a pronounced and somewhat disagreeable odor. *Salvia sclarea*, or clary sage, can naturalize very quickly becoming an invasive if growing conditions are favorable.

Growing Conditions and Propagation
Both *S. officinalis* and *S. sclarea* are pollinated by insects and reproduce by seeds.

S. Officinalis is a shrubby perennial which, if ignored in the garden, degenerates in two to six years [depending upon the quality of the soil and growing conditions] so that new plantings have to be made every three or four years. To keep sage healthy and long lived, harvest frequently, and prune the plant every autumn. It can be grown from seed or seedlings are easily available from local nurseries and will do well in ordinary soil. They prefer full sun although they will tolerate some shade. Once a plant is well established, a simple method for propagation is through layering as sage will readily produce new plants from the adult stems. In the early spring cover a length of the stem with an inch or two of soil and anchor it so that it will not be disturbed, leaving the tip supported above the ground. By May or June new plants will develop and can be either left to grow from the old stalk or cut from the mother plant and replanting in a new location.

S. Sclarea is a biennial propagated by seeds. In its first year it appears as a multi-leaved rosette low to the ground, and in the second year it sends up a tall spike, flowers, produces seeds and dies. Seeds are sown in the garden in the early spring or late fall where they can winter over. When the seedlings appear they should be thinned to at least 18 to 24 inches apart because they become rather large plants.

Harvesting
The leaves and flowers are used both fresh and dried. The leaves are collected in the early morning or late evening when the plants are mature but before they have begun to bloom. They can be washed under cool running water, patted with paper or linen toweling to remove excess moisture, and spread out to dry in a warm, dark place. They should be stirred occasionally to encourage even drying and dried to the brittle stage.

Pick the flowers in the early morning or in the late evening, preferably on the first day of bloom when the active principles are at their highest. Used them fresh or spread in a warm, dark area until completely dry, stirring occasionally to ensure even evaporation.

Clary seeds are collected when the plant dies back in the fall. The flowers develop seed pods that turn black as they mature. They separate easily from the plant and should be spread to dry for a day or two before breaking them open to collect seeds.

As long as the leaves are kept free from moisture, they will retain their aromatic properties for years, but for medicinal use they should be collected fresh each year and stored out of direct sunlight in sterile containers.

Use in the Edgar Cayce Readings

Sage is both used alone and as a companion plant. It is mentioned over 130 times as a tea often combined with yellow american saffron or catnip to soothe the stomach and aid digestion. The formulas are quite precise in calling for either fresh or dried sage. Cayce frequently refers to sage as common garden sage which is also called white sage, however either *Salvia officinalis* or *Salvia sclarea* can be used.

Clary Water is used to address a variety of assimilation and elimination problems the most serious of which is diabetes or diabetic tendencies, but unfortunately this original formula can no longer be compounded in the United States as it calls for ambergris. It is illegal to obtain or even to possess any whale products or whale by-products in the US or in the British Isles. Cayce describes the action of ambergris, always dissolved in a small amount of grain alcohol, on the pancreas as follows: *"and with the sediments from the Ambergris as stimulated by the alcohol and beet sugar, will give the action necessary to the pancreas and duodenum to receive the incentive for their functioning."* 4156-2.

And more specifically in 953-26: *"The ambergris acts in the human system as that necessary for the juices or the excretions from the pancreas to not turn so much sugar in the system – acting, then, in a way and manner as do those properties are as secreted by the pancreas proper, OR the pancrean fluid concentrated and reacted in the system through that of the hypodermic [insulin], see?"*

Ambergris is a solid, fatty, inflammable, waxy exudate of a gray or blackish color, sometimes variegated like marble, which is a natural by-product of the intestines of the spermaceti whale, *Physeter catodon*. Cayce prefers ambergris from the Gray Sperm Whale.[93] [see 13-1; 953-15; 2192-1 and 3932-1]. A note by Gladys Davis Turner states that Mr. Cayce always pronounced ambergris as "ambergray" when giving a reading.

Ambergris can sometimes be seen floating on the surface of the ocean and is frequently washed up on beaches. In earlier times it was collected from shallow waters and used in trade as a perfume fixative. The exudate in its raw state, harvested from the ocean, has a sweet, earthy odor. When harvested from the intestines of the whale it has a foul odor and must be cured before it can be used. The raw material is sealed in an airtight container where it is left to ripen for up to twelve months. At the end of this time the ambergris is cured, all traces of the foul odor are gone, a sweet odor characteristic of the fresh product is present and it is ready for use.

As demand grew the world market could not be satisfied with harvesting the natural product from the ocean where it occurs "in nature" and whales were hunted to near extinction in order to harvest ambergris and other by-products such as oil for various commercial markets. This eventually resulted in a ban against all whaling by the United States and England in 1977 putting an end to the availability of legal ambergris with which to compound the Cayce formula for diabetes, however naturally harvested ambergris is still legal to possess in some countries of the world.

---

93   Rhachianectes glaucus of the northern Pacific. Also locally called devil-fish; grayback; hardhead; mussel-differ and ripsack.

Three Sample Formulas with Clary Sage and Ambergris

480-39 F 25 Diabetes:Tendencies

13. To 6 ounces of Garden Sage [dried], add 12 ounces of Distilled Water. Let this simmer until it has reduced to at least, when drained off, 6 1/2 ounces. Keep this warm and set aside.

14. Then prepare: To 1 ounce of Strained PURE Honey, add 2 ounces of Distilled Water. Let this come to a boil. Skim off the refuse. While warm add this to the other solution, or the Sage or Clary Water solution, see?

15. Dissolve 15 grains of Ambergris in 1 ounce of Pure Grain Alcohol. Have this thoroughly dissolved. Add this then to the other solution while warm, and stir.

16. Then, put 2 sticks of Cinnamon [good size Cinnamon sticks] in 6 ounces of Gordon's RE-DISTILLED Gin. Let this set for at least an hour.

17. Then add the other solution to the Gin, not the Gin to the other. That is, add the solution of the Sage, the Honey and the Ambergris, TO the Gin solution.

18. Shake this together and the dose will be a teaspoonful before each meal, and half a teaspoonful at bedtime.

730-1 M 51 DIABETES

17. Before the meals we would take the clary water compound, which would be to those activities of the gastric flow of the stomach itself and to the activity of the pancreas and the system, aiding the assimilations, with the proper balanced elements for the whole system. This would be taken at least twice or three times each day, before the meals - not more than a teaspoonful at the time; and would be prepared in this way and manner:

18. To 16 ounces of distilled water add the 6 ounces of Dry Garden Sage. Boil slowly [not in aluminum, but preferably in an enamel container - with an enamel or glass cover; NOT tin], until the quantity has been reduced to 8 ounces. Strain, and while it is warm, add:

    Simple Syrup............................1 ounce,
    [but not made with cane sugar;
    preferably beet sugar]
    Cinnamon, preferably in stick...........1 ounce,
    Ambergris [dissolved in 1 ounce
     of grain alcohol]...................15 grains,
    Gin.....................................4 ounces.

Shake this well together each time before the dose is taken.

19. The active principles of each of these ingredients will act upon the digestive system in these manners:

20. The Cinnamon with the carriers are as laxatives for the system that make for active forces with the upper portion of the digestion of the body.

21. Ambergris in its actions is not for the sedimentations but the active forces to allay the tendencies for the glands that secrete or make for accumulations of sugar to be reduced in its quantity.

22. The Gin acts upon the flow for the kidneys, if used in the manner indicated.

911-1 F 24 DIABETES

In this line, as we will find, those properties found in the clary water will - WITH the manipulations - CLARIFY the hepatic circulation and make for the activities in the glands that are in sympathy with the lachrymal circulation toward an even balance. This would be prepared in this manner, which will affect also the diet - so that this may be outlined as a diet that would make for general BUILDING of the system:

To 1/2 gallon of distilled water, add 3 ounces of clary flower or dried garden sage. Reduce this by slow boiling to 1 quart. Strain, and while warm add 15 grains of ambergris dissolved in 1 ounce of grain alcohol. Then add 2 ounces of simple syrup made with beet sugar only, or 2 ounces of the sugar to 2 ounces of the distilled water heated and made into the syrup. Then add Gordon Gin 4 ounces, with 10 minims Oil of Juniper, and 1 dram of cinnamon.

Shake the solution together before the dose is taken, which would be a teaspoonful four times each day - before the morning meal, before the lunch, before the evening meal, and at retiring.

Other sage based formulas similar to Clary Water but not requiring ambergris were also given as stimulants, eliminants [as differentiated from cathartics or laxatives] and tonics. This suggests that *"sage is an active principle with the digestive forces of the INTESTINAL tract themselves, acting PARTICULARLY WITH those of the circulation in the duodenum, pancreas and liver area, giving for the jejunum a better activity with that of the coating as is necessary to prevent seepages in the intestinal tract..."* 2352-1.

The following three excerpts are examples of Clary formulas without ambergris which are easily made at home:

2352-1 F 50 PSORIASIS TOXEMIA

12. First, WE would prepare as this to be taken for the change in the organs of the digestion, as well as to make for a better lymph circulation in the whole of the digestive system:

13. Take 3 ounces of clary flower to 16 ounces of distilled water. Reduce by simmering to 1/2 the quantity. Strain while warm and add 15 grains of ambergris, dissolved in 1 ounce of alcohol. Then add:

> Simple Syrup..............................1 ounce,
> Oil of Juniper.............................1 dram,
> Alcohol [grain - 90%].....................2 ounces,
> Cinnamon [preferably in the stick]........1 dram.

Shake the solution together before the dosage is taken. The dose would be teaspoonful 4 times each day, half an hour before the meals and before retiring.

4094-1 F Adult Urethritis
13. Do that. The clary water is prepared for this individual in this manner: Sage or Claraflower, eight ounces into half a gallon of rainwater or distilled water, simmered, not boiled, until reduced to one quart. Add six ounces of Cane Sugar, four ounces of Grain Alcohol, three drams Sweetgum dissolved, five drops Oil of Juniper. This must be shaken well before a dose is taken. We are through. - No operation at all; no operation.

25-3 M 18 RHEUMATISM TUBERCULOSIS:TENDENCIES
5. To the mixture of the 6 ounces of dried Garden Sage, added to 16 ounces of distilled water, simmered, NOT BOILED, but reduced to 8 ounces, and strain. This as the base, see?

Add:

> Tincture Valerian.............1 ounce,
> Extract Stillingia............1 ounce,
> Tincture Polk Root...........20 minims,
> Fluid Extract Wild Cherry.....2 ounces,
> Syrup of Sarsaparilla.........1 ounce,
> Extract Calisaya Bark.........1 ounce.

6. Shake the solution well to-gether, see. Then add 4 ounces grain alcohol, with 2 drams Balsam of Tolu cut in it. Then add this to the solution. Shake this well to-gether each time before dose is taken, which would be two teaspoonful four times each day, and this we find will bring about the condition necessary to relieve this body, [25].

Other interesting uses for sage follow in the tradition of some of the earliest historical citations for its use on the hair. When asked what effect sage tea has the answer was given: *"That's the coloration, see, that strikes through, see – as does that of the COMBINED action of the acid that makes same pliable, soft, and easy for the coloration as carried in same to be helpful – see?"* [658-5]

In another case a 48 year old lady asked about an application to cover gray hair and was told that a commercially product named Colorbak was acceptable, however a *"preferable compound may be made… which…in connection and conjunction with such a diet as indicated…"* 920-2 and went on to suggest a formula utilizing Essence of Walnut, sage and coffee:

920-2 F 48 Physiotherapy:Applications:Coffee:Hair:Color Restorer
13. However, as we find, a much preferable compound may be made in this way and manner which, in connection and conjunction with such a diet as indicated, will make for the proper relationships to the scalp:

> To 1 ounce Essence of Walnut, add:
> Essence [or reduced properly] of Sage...2 ounces,
> Coffee, made from coffee grounds........2 ounces.

BOIL these together. Then add sufficient alcohol for a preservative. Use this to comb into the hair. Of course, this should be strained and filtered.

14. [Q] Will this bring back the natural color to one's hair?
[A] It will bring back the natural color, whether red, dark or light; although it will make the light hair somewhat darker.

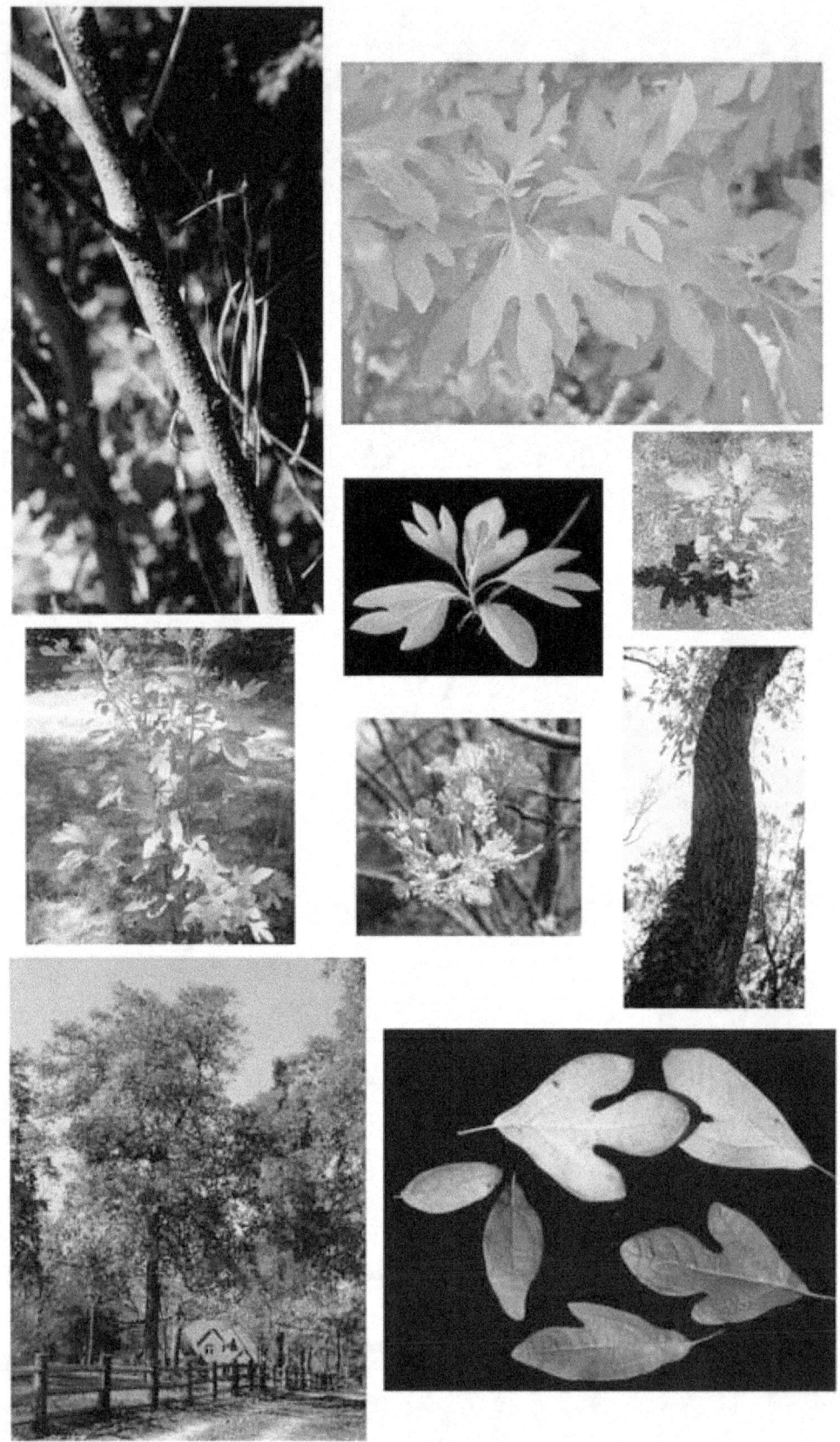

SASSAFRAS
Sassafras albidum [Nuttal, Sassafras officinale [L], Fam. Lauraceae

Common and Regional Names
Ague tree, Mitten plant, Saxifrax, Saloop, Cinnamonwood, Tea tree

History and Common Usage
Sassafras is a long lived tree indigenous to the United States most commonly found throughout the east, extending west to Kansas and south into Mexico. It was imported to Europe during the early American settlement period where it entered into cultivation and is now naturalized.

Sassafras was used by the Native Americans for its volatile oil in liniments, the pulverized leaves as a thickening agent in soups and stews, and the pith of the dried stems for its mucilaginous properties for burns, abrasions and eye infections.

The leaves of the sassafras are very high in mucilage. They can be dried and pulverized for use as a thickening agent in soups, gravy or stews. In the southern United States this is sometimes referred to as "gumbo filet." It is easily made at home by rubbing the dried leaves until they are very finely powdered after which the material is sifted to remove large pieces, stems and veins. The resulting powder can be stored and used in the same manner as cornstarch. "Filet" is commercially available in the United States on most supermarket shelves in the spices and condiment section.

Soon after the importation of sassafras to England a beverage containing powdered sassafras called "Saloop" began to be sold on the streets much in the way coffee and tea is available to early morning commuters today. Saloop is a mixture of sassafras tea, salep, [a starchy meal ground from the dried roots of old world orchids such as Orchis and Eulophia] milk, sugar and sometimes cinnamon. It remained a popular beverage until it fell out of fashion in the mid 1800's when coffee became less expensive, but is still commercially available in powder form sold as Salep and Dondurma. The drink is also seen marketed variously as Salepi, Sahlab, Sahlep and Saloop.

Sassafras is used as a demulcent, stimulant, diaphoretic, diuretic and there have been many anecdotal claims for its healing properties in cases of rheumatism, and in poultices for ulcers and eye infections. Many early settlers in the United States used sassafras tea as a spring tonic to cleanse the blood, to bring relief from cold and congestion, or simply as a pleasant tasting beverage.

Sassafras oil has been used in perfume and as a flavoring agent to mask the unpleasant taste of some medications. It is especially used in cough syrups and in the manufacture of root beer.

The production of sassafras oil through distillation of the root and root bark constitutes a small industry in the southeastern area of the United States. In 2002 the American Food and Drug Administration renewed a ban on sassafras oil for use as a flavoring and as a food additive. This is because sassafras root contains safrole, which is considered a carcinogenic.[94] A safrole free extract of sassafras oil is now in use.

The 21st United States Dispensatory lists the official preparation of sassafras as the dried bark of the root, however all parts of the plant yield both medicinal and flavoring properties and can be used. The

---

94   http://www.cfsan.fda.gov/~lrd/FCF189.html See Title 21 Sec. 189.180 Safrole

volatile oil of sassafras is lost if the fresh plant materials are heated to too high a temperature for too long a period making cold percolation and extraction methods desirable. Tea from the fresh twigs and leaves should never be boiled but gently steeped in simmering water and taken while warm.

Description

Sassafras is generally found as a small tree – usually about 35 to 60 feet in height. The largest tree on record in the United States is in Kentucky,[95] roughly 97 miles from Edgar Cayce's birth place. It measures over 100 feet tall and the trunk of the tree is 21 feet in circumference. This rare giant is thought to be between 250 or 300 years old and is a dramatic example of the magnificence of the original forests discovered by the early American settlers.

The mature trunk bark of sassafras is grey and furrowed while the bark of the young sapling is a mottled green and grey. The twigs are bright green and the tree has the peculiar distinction of producing three different shapes of leaves which are often found growing on the same twig making it easy to identify the sassafras. One leaf is shaped like a mitten, one is three-lobed and the third is oval.

The flowers appear before the leaves, usually in the latter part of April or early May. The flowers are used as a tea or decoction. They are small and greenish-yellow, the male flowers having 9 stamens; the female flowers 6. The resulting fruit is a bright-blue oval somewhat larger than an English pea, born on small red stems called peduncles. The fall foliage varies from yellow, orange to a dull red.

Growing Conditions and Propagation

In northern climates sassafras appears as a shrub or small tree and in less severe climates it grows as a tree. It propagates from its underground rooting system as well as by seeds. The underground rooting system sends up young saplings a few feet from the parent trunk in all directions creating colonies of small shrubs.

If the tree is grown from seeds they should be planted in the fall and the area watched for seedlings in the spring. Plant the seeds 1 inch deep in rich, well worked soil in an area that receives full sunlight for at least half of the day, preferably in the early morning. Plant more seeds than are wanted and thin the young trees when they have reached 8 to 12 inches in height.

The easiest propagation method is to dig or pull a young sapling from a well established colony and transplant it where it will receive sufficient light and moisture. By allowing the underground system to produce young shoots provides the homeowner with a constantly renewing supply for home use.

Harvesting

The flowers can be picked from the tree in the early spring for use as a tea or decoction. They are best picked on the first day of bloom. Their delicate fragrance is refreshing and makes a pleasant tasting drink. The leaves and small twigs can be used fresh at any time. Small twigs can be dried and chopped or pulverized without removing the bark and stored in airtight containers away from the light. Leaves can be dried and pulverized for use as a thickening agent as mentioned above.

Branches and smaller trunks can be cut and dried to extract the pith. The pith of sassafras contains mucilaginous properties used for eye inflammations and in the treatment of dysentery. The branches are split and the dried pith extracted. It is then soaked for several hours in cool, distilled water which is

---

95   http://www.roadsideamerica.com/tip/7879

later filtered through a purified piece of cotton cloth such as a good quality cotton sterile handkerchief to remove the tiniest pieces of pith.

The root is gathered either in the very early spring or late in the autumn. It is white when first taken from the ground and almost immediately discolors turning dark brown, brownish gray or black. The root bark is easier cleaned of its outer bark when fresh. The outer layer is peeled away with a sharp knife revealing the inner bark which is then, depending upon the size of the rootstock, chopped or sliced transversely for drying. The root can be air dried out of direct light but if humidity is a problem it can be dried in a very gentle heat source such as a convection oven with the temperature kept as close to 100° F as possible. The root can also be used fresh.

Use in the Edgar Cayce Readings
Sassafras is both used alone and as a companion plant in the Cayce system. Sassafras is recommended in over 390 cases, oil of sassafras being recommended in 286 of those. During the time the Cayce information was being given natural sassafras oil was used.

Cayce departs somewhat from the historical and traditional use of sassafras as there are only three recommendations for its use as a tea. In other applications it is not used alone but always in combination with other ingredients. The root bark is often called for and in a few cases Cayce stipulates it should be fresh, or "green." It is recommended in two cases as an ingredient in steam cabinets and vapor baths, once as the sole additive and once in combination with witch hazel. By far the most frequent use of sassafras is as an ingredient in compound massage oils.

Steam Cabinet and Fume Bath Additive
3254-1 F 36 INJURIES:SPINE:COCCYX:AFTER EFFECTS
11. Poisons then have made for conditions through the lymph body. These cause the organs of the sensory system to suffer at times, as the eyes, ears, nose and the like.

12. As we find there should be taken a series of hydrotherapy treatments, of this type or nature, however: Begin with not a dry heat bath but a Fume Bath using an equal combination of Witchhazel and Oil of Sassafras Root in the water boiling in the cabinet to produce the fumes.

13. In the rubdown following this, unless grain alcohol is used rather than wood or denatured alcohol, it will cause a rash. But we need to stimulate the superficial circulation.

14. Follow each Fume Bath with the needle shower, and then a thorough rubdown - after the body has had at least ten minutes of the Ultra-Violet Light with the green glass projected between this and the body; so as to stimulate not only the structural portions of body, - but with the relaxing, do use those periods for dedicating self for a real service.

15. Follow same with the Pine Oil rubs rather than other characters of oils for this body.

16. Have such a hydrotherapy treatment once each week for five to six weeks. Then rest from these for three weeks. Then have another series, and so on.

4557-1 F 35 DERMATITIS OBESITY

2. As to the physical forces as may be assisted in this body here, to rid same of those conditions wherein the humor at times shows in the effect as is created in the eliminations, and in the manner in which the distribution of same is carried on in the body - this, then, is the cause of these conditions physical that arouse in the system that of the rash, or the conditions as seen in exterior portions of system: To cleanse these we would use first, every third day, take the vapor baths, and in the vapor as is created for same let there be that of the oil of sassafras applied in same. To the half pint of water [this as proportion] add ten minims, or drops of the oil of sassafras. After this is taken there should be the thorough rub down over the whole system of the body with the coarse towel, or cloth, to get a stimulation to the capillary circulation.

Compound Massage Oils

265-10 F 71 ELIMINATIONS:INCOORDINATION

4. Twice each week massage the whole cerebro-spinal system for two to five minutes with a saturated solution of Epsom Salts; as warm as may be applied to the body; that is, with cloths wrung out of this saturated solution. This will naturally make for the accumulation of the circulation, both as to nerve and blood supply, to the various ganglia along the cerebro-spinal system. Of course, the hot applications will tend to open the pores of the skin.

5. To prevent any cold arising from such applications, compound a solution to massage into the spine following [immediately] such a rubdown, see? in this manner:

6. To 4 ounces of rub alcohol, add:

>   Russian White Oil[96*]..............2 ounces,
>   Witchhazel.....................1 ounce,
>   Oil of Sassafras.........5 to 10 drops.

7. Pour a little of this in a saucer, dip the fingers into it and massage over those portions that have been massaged with the saturated solution of Epsom Salts. This will leave a pleasant, tingling sensation, and - for the first time or two - leave a little burning [as from the Oil of Sassafras], but will restore more and more the normal equilibrium and coordination throughout the whole system, overcoming the tendencies for the active forces in the lymph and the circulation that make for the disturbances.

5525-1 F 59 ARTHRITIS TENDENCIES

After such a treatment is given, massage thoroughly into the cerebro-spinal system - from the base of the brain to the coccyx - those of equal parts of the Tincture of Myrrh, Olive Oil, and Sassafras Oil. Heat the olive oil, adding the myrrh and sassafras oil; using only sufficient to give a thorough massage, see? that is, only prepare sufficient at the time. After the fourth to fifth treatment, leave out the Sassafras Oil, for we will have created then an irritation to the exterior portion of the body, along the cerebro-spinal region, especially in the lower portion of body. This will disappear with the leaving off of the Sassafras Oil, but this we desire to create in the system to be assimilated by the system through the action of the cuticle, or the skin itself, and we will find with the keeping up of these conditions that within six to eight weeks the conditions will disappear.

---

96   * Russian White Oil is light weight mineral oil

421-8 F 23 ANEMIA Cold:Congestion:Feet

7. We would also apply MOST consistently these conditions for the feet and lower limbs, that will aid the most in the circulation to the feet, to the lower extremities, preventing tired feet, preventing taking cold, preventing the decrease in weight:

8. At least once each week do ALL of this:

9. First, before retiring in the evening, bathe the feet in a warm salt solution. To a gallon and a half of water put a level teaspoonful of table salt, see? Keep the feet in this and rub them during the time, for at least twenty minutes.

10. Wipe the feet dry and then use a solution of tanic acid, which - as we find - may be best made from coffee grounds that are ready to be thrown away. To a gallon and a half of water put two cups full of coffee grounds that are refuse. Let this come to a stiff boil, boiling for two to two and a half minutes. Set aside, and have this WARM when the feet are put in this, for five to ten minutes. Be sure the feet are rubbed with this; not hot, not just tepid but WARM.

11. While, the salt water ought to be as hot as the feet can stand, see?

12. Bathe from the knees to the bottoms of the feet, especially massaging thoroughly the heels, the toes, and the arches of the feet.

13. EACH day [including the day on which the above would be used] bathe the feet and massage thoroughly into them and the lower limbs, including the knees, a preparation made in this manner:

14. To 4 ounces of Russian White Oil, add:

      Witchhazel......................4 ounces,
      Oil of Sassafras...............10 minims,
      Rub Alcohol.....................2 ounces,
      Spirits of Camphor............1/2 ounce.

Massage this into the feet and limbs, only what the body absorbs.

15. And then the diet: Don't eat so picayunishly! Yes, it's a very good word for the body's eating; scimping over!

456-1 F Child POLIOMYELITIS:AFTER EFFECTS

10. Then, in meeting the needs of the conditions for this body in the present, to be sure these will require patience and persistence; but this may be done by those about the body. Prayer, meditation, sincere desire, and the APPLICATION not as rote - that it is told thee to do - but with the expectancy in the heart as the applications are made, that there will come to this body the opportunity, the privilege, of its being more and more capable, more and more able to function the nearer normal in its physical activities.

11. Then, prepare as this - only when these are to be used: Olive oil, Tincture of Myrrh, and Sassafras Oil. Heat a tablespoonful of Olive Oil, not to boiling but just heat until warm. Then mix with same a tablespoonful of Tincture of Myrrh. Stir together. Then add five minims of the Sassafras Oil. Pour a

small portion in a saucer or open basin, and - just dipping the finger tips in same massage the lumbar and sacral area, following along the lines of the greater nerve centers along the limbs; particularly the left limb. This should be done each day.

628-4 F 7 COLITIS CURED
8. We will find that the rubs will be well also for this body; preferably with a compound prepared in this manner:

9. To 2 ounces of Olive Oil as the base, add:

> Witchhazel.................1 ounce,
> Russian White Oil.........1 ounce,
> Sassafras Oil............20 minims.

10. All of these will tend to separate. Shake together before these are massaged into the body. This should preferably be done in the evenings as the body is ready for retirement. Well that the body be cleansed afterwards with the use of rub alcohol.

386-3 F 20 Feet:Arches:Weak
25. [Q] Why have my arches always been weak? Can I ever go without wearing arch supports in my shoes?
[A] To be sure, especially if the limbs and feet especially the bursa in the heel, or the Achilles bursa are stimulated. For such stimulation [besides the massage to the sacral and lumbar plexuses that stimulates impulses to the lower limbs], we would advise using a compound prepared in this manner [which will give the body a good deal to do for itself!]:

Each evening before retiring, bathe the feet and limbs to the knees in a very mild tannic acid; which may best be made [for such conditions] from coffee grounds. When they are ready to be thrown out, put on a cupful to a gallon and a half of water. Let boil for ten minutes, pour off and allow to cool sufficiently so that the lower limbs may be bathed in it. Massage the limbs and the feet, especially the heels and the arches and toes, all the time they are in the solution, see? The whole quantity being used, of course; drain the dregs off, or the grounds; and keep the limbs and feet in same for twenty minutes.

After taking them out of the solution, massage them with THIS compound for five to ten minutes; putting the ingredients together in the order named:

> Russian White Oil................1/2 pint,
> Witchhazel........................2 ounces,
> Rub Alcohol.......................4 ounces,
> Oil of Sassafras...................3 minims,
> Tincture of Capsici................2 minims.

That would make it hot enough! Massage only the amount the skin will absorb. Shake the solution together, for the tendency will be for the Oil of Sassafras to rise to the top - see? Pour a small quantity in a saucer, and only massage into the feet and to the limbs to the knees, including the knees. And do it yourself! And we'll be rid of all this trouble, and it'll help the body in many different ways. It'll walk ten miles instead of five!

Sassafras Tea

556-16 M 59 ASSIMILATIONS:ELIMINATIONS:INCOORDINATION
4. Especially through this spring period it would be MOST helpful for the body to use Sassafras Tea about three times a week. Make it as ordinary tea, with strength as to taste. Do not use cream, though, in this.

1739-6 M 36 NEURASTHENIA
1. EC: Yes, we have the body here, [1739] - this we have had before. Very good are the conditions in the physical forces of the body. There should be those clarifications in the blood supply. See that with the food values, or with those properties taken, there is a clarification of the blood stream - especially as related to the capillary circulation. Quantities of the sassafras bark, or tea - or as medicinal properties - or sulphur and soda or cream of tartar - THESE will clarify the better. Keep the physical forces and mental forces active and well balanced. Keep the manipulations as will keep a normal balance, but not over-active as to same as to OVERDO the conditions for the physical forces. Ready for questions.

4436-1 F Adult BACILLOSIS CANCER:LUNGS
16. Direct the mind forces as this acts in the system. Keep those properties for the diet as will give the reviving forces through the nerve tissue. That of vegetable matter that grows above the ground. That of broth, or of meats of wild game. Little of other kinds of meat. Keep the water that is taken in the system carrying at all times a very small quantity of elm, and of sassafras root tea.

Used Internally

125-1 F Adult Abrasions CANCER
3. The continuation of those treatments as have been and are being applied would be well to keep. We would not change much from these. There may be added as another stimulant, taken occasionally, those properties as would be in this:

> Tincture Valerian.....................1/2 ounce,
> Elixir Calisaya........................1/2 ounce,
> Tincture of Capsici.....................2 minims,
> Oil of Sassafras.......................10 minims,
> Peptotol, or lacted Pepsin
>   sufficient to make...................4 ounces.

Shake solution well to-gether, and the dose would be teaspoonful in water or plain, as would be needed. These may be taken every two hours - these will act better than bromides for the system - may be used with that as being administered as the sedative, but will not act against that being administered. The conditions are serious and need close attention, yet we find these may bring bettered conditions.

129-3 F Adult Skin:Abrasions

2. We would take those properties in the system that will give the healing forces and produce coagulation in the blood supply, and these would be found in these, for this body at the present time.

Ragweed 6 ounces, added to 8 ounces of water, and reduce to 4 ounces by simmering. Strain. While warm, add: [when it is dissolved and cut in alcohol]

> Balsam of Tolu................3 drams,
> Oil of Sassafras ....20 minims,
> with
> Extract of Cayenne...........2 minims.

3. The dose would be half teaspoonful in half glass of water taken 3 times each day.

207-2 F 35 ULCERS:STOMACH

5. Take 3 ounces of ragweed [green]. Add this to 8 ounces of water. Reduce this by simmering [not boiling] to about 4 ounces - that is, half the quantity. Strain this off - set it aside, see? Then take 16 ounces of water, with Wild Cherry Bark 8 ounces, and reduce to 8 ounces, see? of water. Strain this off. Add these two to-gether - that is, that of the ragweed, that of the Wild Cherry Bark, and then to this add 4 ounces of sugar, first dissolved in 1 to 2 ounces of hot water, see? Then add to this 2 ounces pure grain alcohol, with 2 drams Balsam of Tolu cut in it. As this is cut, add 3 to 5 minims of Oil of Sassafras. The dose of this will be teaspoonful 3 times each day.

244-3 M 71 Digestion TOXEMIA

8. For the condition as is seen in the mesenteric system, and the trouble as experienced with the body in this manner, well that that of the salve [Tim for hemorrhoids] be used, as the rectum shows irritation from the system showing congestion or laxness. This would remove irritation by the use of this, being injected in the rectum after each stool, see? a small quantity on finger or swab may be applied to these protruding parts, or in the mouth or end of rectum, see?

9. Also we would take OCCASIONALLY - once a day, or once every other day - a good swallow of a preparation of this:

10. Take six [6] ounces of horehound. To this add eight [8] ounces distilled water. Reduce by simmering [not boiling] to one-half the quantity. Then dissolve one [1] ounce of rock candy in two [2] ounces of eighty-five percent [85%] alcohol, see? adding solutions to-gether. Then add to this - after this has been compounded to-gether -

> Oil of Sassafras......................5 minims,
> Oil of Peppermint......................5 minims,
> Senna.................................1 grain.

11. Shake this Solution to-gether, and let the dose be taken of a teaspoonful, see, once a day or once every other day, whenever necessary for the system to complete digestion throughout the whole of the mesenteric system.

8. We would also ADD, though, this - as the properties to aid in digestion and in the proper vibrations as will be set up in the system: We would prepare first as the carrier, this: Take 4 ounces of wild cherry bark, put in 8 ounces distilled water. Reduce by simmering, or very slow boiling, to at least 6 ounces.

Then add:

        Simple Syrup......................2 ounces,
        Compound Syrup of Sarsaparilla....1 ounce,
        Tincture Stillingia.............1/2 ounce,
        Syrup of Rhubarb.................60 minims,
        Oil of Sassafras.................20 minims,
        Elixir Calisaya.................1/2 ounce,
        Essence of Elixir, or
        Tincture of Elder Flower.....1/4 ounce,
        Tincture Capsici..................2 minims.

Cut 1 dram Balsam of Tolu in 1 and 1/2 ounces grain alcohol and add to solution.

9. Shake solution together before the dose is taken. The dose should be half teaspoonful every 4 hours. When the body rests we would not disturb same for medicinal properties.

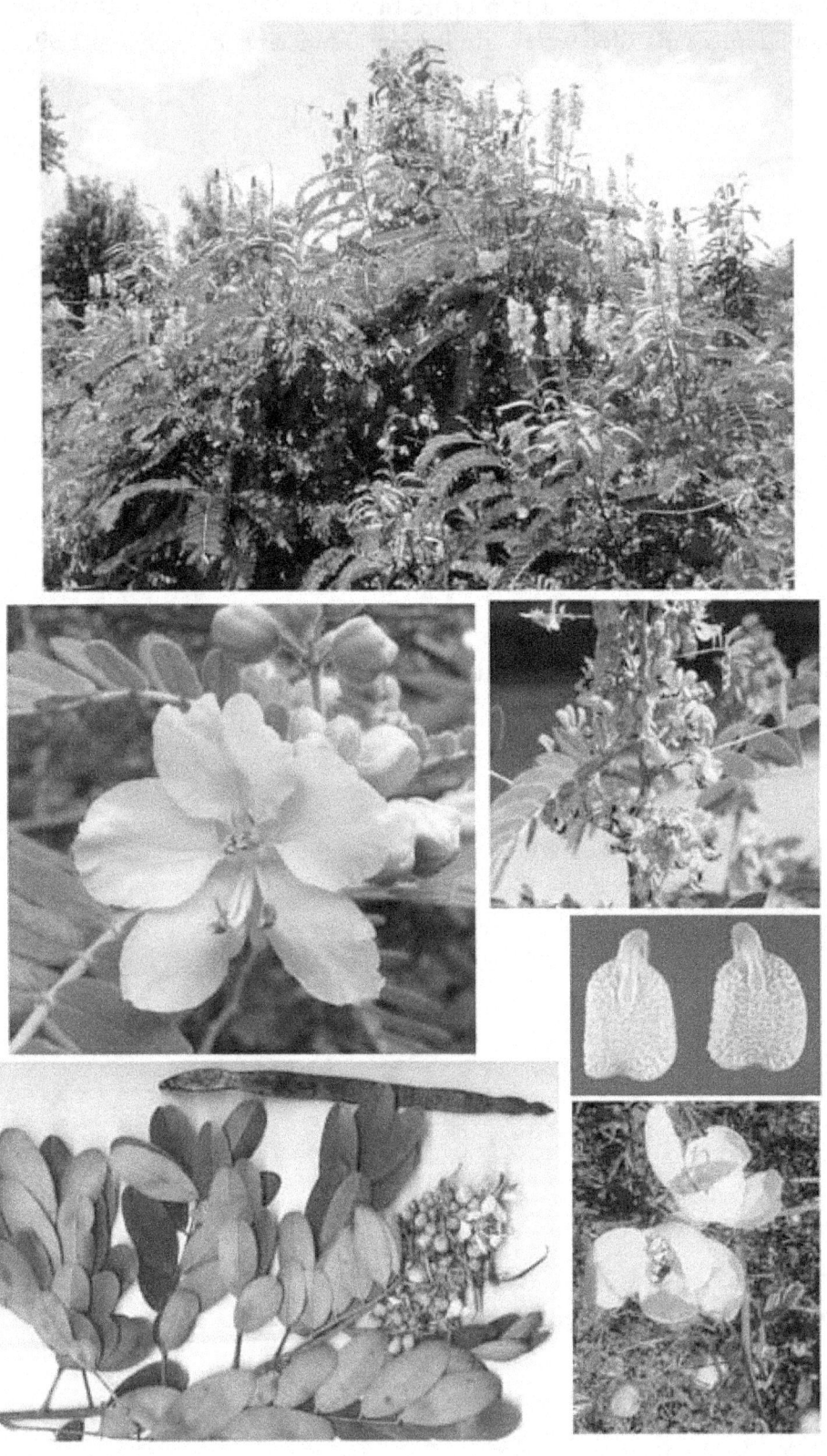

Senna

Cassia acutifolia and *Cassia angustifolia, Fam. Leguminosae (now Fabaceae)*

Common and Regional Names

Alexandria Senna, Tinnevelly Senna, Casse, Black Draught, Indian Senna, Khartoum Senna, Sena Alejandrina, Sene d'Egypte, Sennae folium, Sennae fructus, Sennae fructus acutifoliae, Senna fructus angustifolia, True Senna

History and Common Usage

Senna is thought to be indigenous to the Anglo-Egyptian Sudan region. It now grows in southern Asia, Egypt, Nubia, Sennar, Africa, and India. Senna is produced commercially in India, with a large commercial concentration in Rajasthan, a state in Northwest India. There are about 600 species known within the genus Cassia, most of which are native to the tropics, including trees, shrubs and herbs. The senna of the Cayce era comes from the two best known medicinal varieties: *C. acutifolia* and *C. angustifolia*, both of which are grown only in the tropics.

Senna superseded castor oil as a laxative or cathartic about 800 years ago. Senna is an Arabian name and it is first cited, within the time of present recorded history, in Arabian medical texts. It is believed senna was first brought to use by Arabian physicians Serapion[97] and Mesue.[98]

Senna was cultivated in England around 1620 forced in hot-bed plantings but without success. The plants could be brought to flower but they would rarely produce seeds leaving English physicians to rely on imports from Nubia, India and Cairo. Senna consistently appears in British Pharmaceutical works from this time as a cathartic and is also listed officially in the United States Pharmacopeia of the Cayce era.

Description

Cassia acutifolia is a perennial shrub which grows from 2 to 10 feet high with a stem that is erect and smooth. It has alternating narrow leaves which grow in pairs of 4 to 8 on each stem. The flowers are bright yellow, which in turn produce slightly curved pods. The seeds of the *C. acutifolia* are ash-colored. The *C. angustifolia* is considered an annual even in the tropics and is replanted each year from seeds. The seeds of the *C. angustifolia* are deep brown.

Growing Conditions and Propagation

Senna can only be grown in the tropical regions of the world. It is a perennial and some varieties self-seed. Some small experimental plantings have been made in the extreme southern regions of Florida, Texas and New Mexico but without great success. *Senna alexandrina* or *Alexandrian senna* is cultivated in the Virgin Islands. The only source of *Acutifolia senna* and *Angustifolia senna* at this time in the U.S., Canada and the British Isles is through import.

Harvesting

When the plant dies back at the end of the growing season the whole plant is cut and stacked to dry in the sun. The cheapest form of senna is made from using the whole plant, pods, stems and all.

---

97   Yuhanna Ibn Sarabiyun, known as Serapion in Europe, a Syriac physician of the 9th century.
98   Ibn Masawaih, son of a pharmacist in Jundishapur, studied under Jibrll ibn Bakhtyashu, died in Samarra in 857. Known in Euroope as Mesue, sometimes seen as Msue Major or Mesue the Elder.

Some growers pick the pods and leaves separately. The pods can be bought separately either whole or ground. The leaves can also be found on the market either whole or ground. The consumer will also find combinations of pods and leaves whole or ground together. Tea can be purchased in bulk or in ready to use tea bags.

Use in the Edgar Cayce Readings

Mentioned in over 250 cases senna is used alone and as a companion plant in the form of syrup of senna. It is frequently recommended to be taken as a tea in an alternating fashion with another type of laxative. The Cayce system advocates not using just one type of laxative but alternating a vegetable with a mineral.

Senna is not always used as a laxative. The following is a case in which it is used in a compound formula recommended as an expectorant for the relief of a cough in a case of cold and congestion:

538-43 F 57 Cold:Congestion:Flu
4. Then, as an allaying for this irritation to the mucous membranes, as the congestion will be somewhat relieved by a released circulation and better conditions from the manipulations, make not so much an expectorant as a cough syrup - in this manner:

5. To 1 ounce Compound Simple Syrup, add:

> **Syrup of Horehound................1/2 ounce,**
> **Syrup of Senna....................1/4 ounce,**
> **Chloroform.........................5 minims,**
> **Syrup of Squill...................1/4 ounce,**
> **Grain Alcohol.....................1/2 ounce.**

6. Shake well before the dosage is taken, which would be about three-quarters to a teaspoonful, and this only when there are the irritations or the coughs.

Cayce often combines syrup of senna with syrup of figs:

935-2 F Adult Hemorrhoids Eliminations
11. For the eliminations we would use a vegetable compound, - not so much as to cause irritation or bleeding, but such as a compound carrying Senna, or Syrup of Senna, as combined with Syrup of Figs. These would react as an eliminant, as well as act upon the liver.

Often a number of ingredients are combined with senna to tailor an eliminant to the needs of the individual. In a number of cases syrup of senna is used as an additive to commercially prepared laxatives such as Fletcher's Castoria for Children. Syrup of senna appears in the United States Dispensatory during the time the Cayce information was being given. It contained a fluid extract of senna, oil of coriander, sucrose and water.

Senna Tea

585-7 F 45 TUMORS:LYMPH Hair Loss
13. (Q) What is the best laxative for me to take?
(A) Senna Leaf Tea.

641-5 M 27 PSORIASIS:TENDENCIES
7. Be sure there are the full eliminations through the alimentary canal each day; preferably use enemas instead of too great a quantity of cathartics or laxatives. But when laxatives are used, alternate with the various properties that have the senna base. These are better for the body.

1553-27 F 75 DROPSY Eliminations
THEN the high enemas or colonics, with Senna tea as the best eliminant, might be combined with these applications; though the senna tea may be necessary to take twice instead of once a day. The Senna tea is better than the Syrup of Senna, for the syrup would become hard upon the kidney reaction, while the regular senna tea - made from the senna pods or leaves - will set better drainage and better activity in the association with the drying effect upon the lymph. Just the regular senna tea, you see, made rather strong, to be sure, for the body, but at least a good teacup full.

543-28 F 30 EPILEPSY Assimilations:Eliminations:Incoordination
6. (Q) Would the senna pod tea be beneficial at this time?
(A) Senna pod tea or syrup of senna would be beneficial. The senna pod tea would be the more effective to be taken a long period, and about an ounce - not too strong, but this taken as a laxative and an addition to the activity of the gastric flow, will be helpful.

2941-1 F 23 ANEMIA:TENDENCIES Headaches
13. And with these keep a good elimination through alimentary canal. As we find, for this body, this may be done preferably by taking the Senna Tea; this taken regularly - when treatments are begun - for at least a period of five to six days. Then leave it off for five days, and then take another series of same. This would be about an ounce and a half to two ounces of the Tea taken each evening when ready to retire.

5319-1 F 55 CANCER:TENDENCIES:PELVIC CELLULITIS
9. Increase the eliminations by the use first of a senna base eliminant and then the next time with the mineral salts eliminant, or we would use senna leaves. Take the senna leaves each evening that these are to be taken, and about twice a week we would take the senna pod. Put about three pods in a teacup. Pour boiling water over this and let it stand for thirty minutes and then cool and drink. The mineral salts when these are used, about once or twice a week, take Sal Hepatica a heaping teaspoonful, not other than to keep the eliminations bettered.

Compound Formula Laxatives

903-4 F 25 INTESTINES:COLON:IMPACTION
4. For relief for these conditions we would use the packs of saturated solution Epsom Salts, as hot as the body may well stand, see? These, with a cathartic in the form of this, will relieve this condition and set the system aright. Use six (6) ounces of Ambrosia or Ragweed in sixteen (16) ounces distilled water. Reduce by simmering (not boiling) to eight (8) ounces. Strain. Then add simple syrup two (2) ounces, alcohol two (2) ounces, with two drams Balsam of Tolu cut in same. We would also add one-

half (1/2) grain of Senna, if the dried weed is used. If the green weed is used do not use the Senna. The dose would be half teaspoonful three (3) times each day until there is the full evacuation of the intestinal tract, see?

388-1 M Adult MALARIA Eliminations:Poor

20. After the second enema is taken, begin with capsules prepared or compounded in this manner and take three at each period, letting one day elapse between each capsule, see? This proportion would be in each capsule:

> Podophyllum...................1/4 grain,
> Leptandrin....................1/2 grain,
> Sanguinaria...................1/2 grain,
> Senna........................1/4 grain.

21. After the third dose is taken, rest another day and then begin with Fletcher's Castoria - taking a whole bottle (or 900 drops), half a teaspoonful every hour.

760-9 F 53 ACIDITY LIVER:SLUGGISH

1. EC: We have the body here - this we have had before. Now, we find there are still those aggravating conditions as produce gas and the acidity, or super-acidity, throughout the system; caused most at present from conditions of the liver in ITS activity in the system. Worry and the action of the system towards KEEPING the system in that condition where the acidity is reduced, brings the greater distresses to the system. We would use that as would AROUSE the liver to activity at present. PREFERABLY, as we find, would be in this: At least TWO doses, and this in each dose:

> Podophyllum...................1/2 grain,
> Leptandrin.....................1 grain,
> Senna.........................1/2 grain,
> Sanguinaria...................1/2 grain.

2. This should be taken preferably one day apart; that is, one day elapsing between each dose. Then continue with those properties that will reduce acidity in the body, being careful of the diet. ALSO giving plenty of the oil, that, that as is begun by the action of Podophyllum and Senna may be kept in the activity of the liver.

Syrup of Senna

1112-5 M 63 COLD:CONGESTION ELIMINATIONS

8. As a laxative we would on the morrow also give equal portions of Syrup of Rhubarb and Syrup of Senna; not more than a teaspoonful of the combination, though this may be combined with other properties if most desirable.

303-11 F 49 CYSTS

18. (Q) Is there anything the body may do that will bring about normal eliminations?
(A). Do those activities that have been indicated as to the diets; these are the more preferable way. When cathartics are needed for the eliminations, use an alteration between such as the Syrup of Figs and Castoria, or a combination of Syrup of Senna and the Syrup of Figs - as Caldwell's Syrup of Figs

- mixed equal portions. Take a teaspoonful at a dose of the mixture; while the other two when taken would be two to three teaspoonsful, not at once but half an hour apart. Do not take any one for a long period of time, but alternate - see?

326-13 F 74 COLD:CONGESTION

6. Then, begin with this first, - take a small size bottle of Fletcher's Castoria. Take out a teaspoonful and add in its place a half teaspoonful of Syrup of Senna, (which is the basic force of Castoria, you see) - shaking it thoroughly then. Shake for five to six minutes, very, VERY thoroughly mixing it together. Then begin taking it about twenty drops every half hour, until there is full elimination through the alimentary canal.

361-7 M 14 PARALYSIS POLIOMYELITIS

2. We have a return of some of those conditions arising from the localization again of poisons that have been as accumulations in the system, by indiscretions in eating and indiscretions in the activities of the body.

3. As we find, the more preferable manner would be first to start the general eliminations of the system, by the use of the Fletcher's Castoria; but prepare and take it in this way:

4. With the small-sized bottle of the Castoria, take off a teaspoonful. Add in its place one-half teaspoonful Syrup of Senna, and one-half teaspoonful Syrup of Cascara. Shake this thoroughly. Take in broken doses; that is, one-half teaspoonful every half hour.

379-6 F 56 Bronchitis

4. But on the morrow we would take the Castoria. However, to the small-sized bottle, add half a teaspoonful of the Syrup of Senna (pouring out half a teaspoonful from the bottle, taking it if so desired). Then shake it WELL together. We need more Senna as an active force for this body in the present. This we would take in about four to five doses through the day, see? that is, the small-sized bottle of Castoria with the Senna added as indicated.

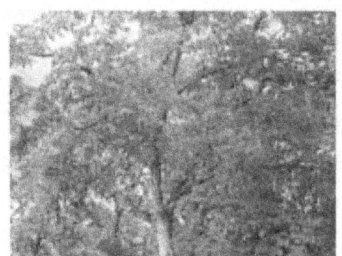

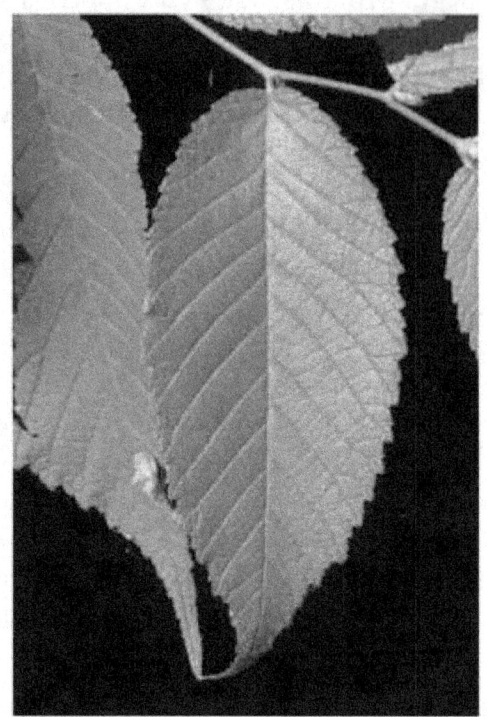

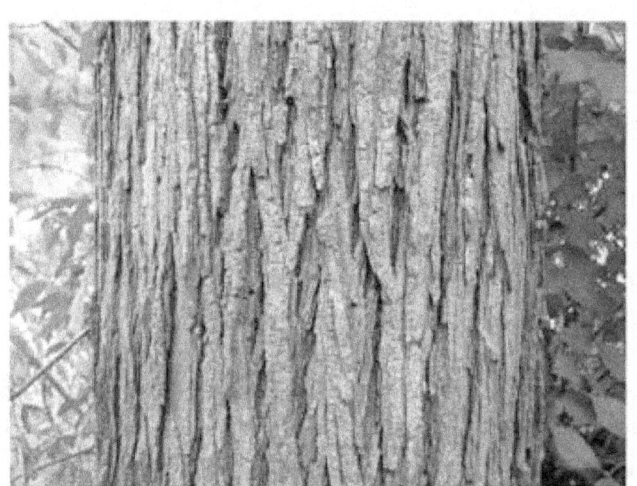

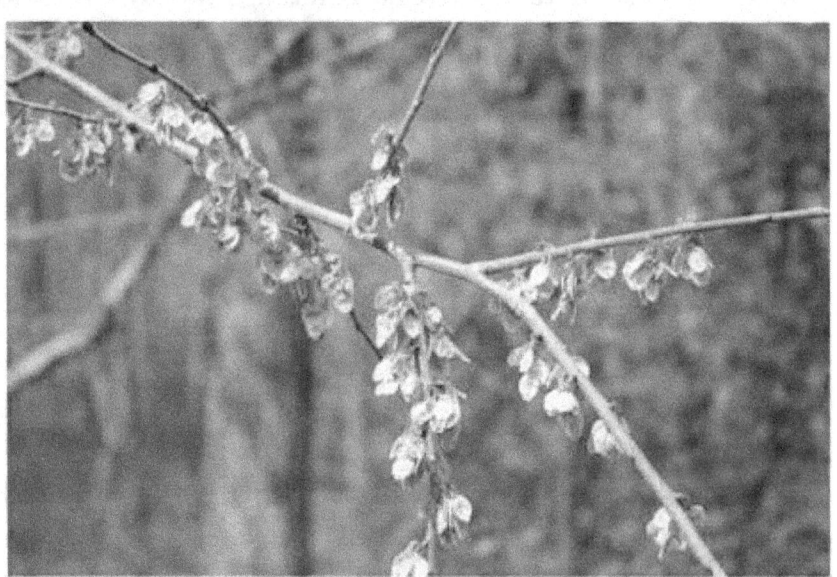

SLIPPERY ELM
Ulmus fulva, Fam. Ulmaceae

Common and Regional Names
Red Elm, Moose-elm, Indian Elm, American Karaagaci, Sweet Elm, Rock Elm, Winged Elm, Gray Elm, Soft Elm, Slippery Elm

History and Common Usage
Slippery elm is indigenous to the Northern Hemisphere, native to the eastern half of the United States and adjacent regions of southern Canada. Originally found in only the eastern half of the United States its range now extends westward to the Dakotas and northward to western Quebec in Canada although it remains most abundant west of the Allegheny Mountains. It is found in Virginia except in the high mountains but is not abundantly represented. Slippery elm was introduced to the early settlers by the Native Americans.

The Native Americans used the inner bark in all cases of inflammatory irritation of mucous membranes treating sore throats, coughs, duodenal ulcers, acute gastritis, enteritis, urinary problems, dysentery and diarrhea. It was also used as a topical application in the form of a poultice, plaster or dressing in the treatment of wounds, burns and infected skin areas and to relieve poison ivy.

The early people in what is today the United States and Canada discovered that slippery elm bark has the property of preserving fatty substances, preventing them from turning rancid. Bears fat was melted with the bark in proportions of one drachm[99] of the powdered bark to a pound of the fat, heating them together for a few minutes, and then straining off the fat.

Slippery elm is usually grown as a landscape ornamental and is not grown for commercial use to any great extent. Since the wood is moderately durable it is used for coarse construction purposes as ribs for small boats, crossties, agricultural implements and fence-posts.

The 21st edition of the United States Dispensatory lists slippery elm as an official drug plant used as an *"excellent demulcent"* and recommending powdered slippery elm bark in water to treat diarrhea and coughs.

Description
The slippery elm family boasts 15 genera and 200 species. Mature specimens of slippery elm attain heights of 50 or 60 feet with a trunk between 15 to 40 inches in diameter. The alternating leaves, a medium to dark green, closely resemble those of the familiar American elm and are often from 2 to 3 inches wide, reaching lengths of 4 to 7 to 8 inches. The edges of the leaves are doubly serrated and the undersides are slightly hairy. The bark of the tree is dark grayish-brown, broken by shallow fissures into flat ridges. The slippery elm shares the elm family vulnerability for the Dutch elm disease which is carried by beetles.

---

99   Dram = A unit of weight in the apothecaries' system. Sixty grains, or 1/8 oz apothecary weight or 1/16 oz. Avoidupois. "A small amount."

Growing Conditions and Propagation
Slippery elm is pollinated by wind and insects and propagated by winged seeds with thin, tan colored, papery margins which assist their dispersion by the wind. Seeds appear from April to June depending on weather and location. They are large, usually about ¾ to 1 inch across. They develop from bell-shaped reddish flowers covered by a dense russet down, which appear before the leaves develop in the spring, usually April to June in most areas of its habitat.

Slippery elm also sprouts readily from viable stumps and from roots that form during the seedling stage. Roots can also be developed in 12 months by the layering method and the rootstock of slippery elm is often used to propagate hybrids. Young slippery elm grows rapidly in the open sun light and does well in open shade but takes many years to attain any girth. The largest known specimen of record in the United States is located in Perry County, Pennsylvania and is 90 feet tall and 76 inches in diameter.

Slippery elm prefers moist, rich soils of the lower slopes of stream banks, river terraces and bottom land. It will tolerate occasional flooding for periods of 2 to 3 months but will not reproduce or grow well if flooding is too frequent or too prolonged. It will thrive in drier soil if limestone is present. The life zone for slippery elm requires an average annual temperature range from 40° F to 70°F. The lowest temperature range it can tolerate is 5° F to 54°F and the highest sustained temperature from 60°F to 95°F. The frost-free period required for best performance ranges from 90 to 280 days.

Harvesting
The best product comes from inner bark which has been harvested before the sap begins to flow. Bark can also be collected during the dormant season. Only bark from 10 year old or older trees should be harvested.

At 10 years of age most slippery elm will have attained at least 1 inch in diameter under the worst of growing conditions and manually stripping the outer bark is not too difficult. If larger specimens are harvested the outer bark does not peel easily, as it is thick and difficult to separate from the inner layer. The thin inner bark, called the bast, is the desirable product. These thin pieces, 1/8th to 1/16th of an inch in thickness, are cut into manageable lengths and bound together with wire to hold the pieces flat as they dry. The fresh bast is very pliable and has a slippery feel and a mucilaginous and insipid taste. The bark is placed in a warm, dry, dark area and kept from the sun until it has cured. Small amounts can also be dried in a home oven, heat never to exceed 105°F.

Dried bark can be manually cut into smaller and smaller pieces, which, when very dry, can successfully be put through a home meat grinder. Subsequent grinding with smaller and smaller screens result in a finer product, which can then be more easily pulverized in small amounts in a home blender or food processor.

Small pieces of the bark can also be chewed. Chewing a piece of the dried bark and swallowing the saliva delivers the same medicinal benefit as the powdered product. Small pieces can also be soaked in water, strained and drunk as a decoction or tea. The powder can be saved for drinking and the coarser material for use as poultices.

For commercial harvesting the tree is fully stripped and the tree dies. At the present time there is no re-forestation plan in place in the United States for the slippery elm and its numbers are in decline. As the trees are best harvested at 10 years of age, harvesters are taking younger and younger trees further reducing the population. Commercial powdered slippery elm is frequently adulterated with bark from other varieties of elm, which have lesser amounts of the mucilaginous properties of the true slippery elm reducing its effectiveness. The powder should be grayish or fawn colored and if it is dark or reddish it is a sign of adulteration.

The homeowner can sacrifice a sizeable branch of an elm without killing the entire tree leaving it to continue seed production for the future. Since only a pinch of the powdered bark is used at a time small branches will produce enough slippery elm for a year or more.

Use in the Edgar Cayce Readings

Slippery elm is used alone and as a companion plant. It is recommended alone or in an alternating fashion with yellow american saffron, sometimes chamomile, Knox Gelatine or Glyco-Thymoline.[100]

The gum of elm is sometimes used in compound formulas. In transcript 133-5 given January 15, 1935 for a 55 year old woman living in West Virginia rare instructions are found for the collection of elm bark:
… In the surroundings there may be obtained the elm; the slippery elm bark, not the exterior but that next to the root itself (and it's a good season to gather same).

Slippery elm is recommended in over 160 cases for conditions ranging from allergies to baby care, from cancer to colitis, and from ulcers to pinworms. The use follows closely both folk medicine and official practices. It soothes and coats mucous membranes and acts as an intestinal antiseptic. It absorbs acids in the stomach and intestines, produces better lymph flow and improves the secretion of lactic fluids in the stomach and supplies nutriments. Case 4841-2, indexed as gastritis, calls for using powdered slippery elm as follows: "*…water produced from the bark of the elm, to act as a rebuilding force to the mucus coat of the intestine and lower duodenum itself.*"

In the following excerpt precise instructions are given as to how to prepare the bark and how to take it:

2884-5 F 23 11. In practically ALL of the water that is taken, or especially that taken at home and at meals, have the gum from the slippery elm; that is, put a pinch of the Powdered Elm in a glass of water - or in each glass of water. Do not let it stand too long before drinking, and yet do not drink it before it has formed an activity in the water; for if this forms in the system it would work to a disadvantage. Yet if the powdered elm becomes too old or stale in the water, this would be harmful also. Just let it set a bit, not to become so thickened as to be obnoxious to the body, but stir and let set for fifteen to twenty minutes - then drink - a pinch of the powdered elm in each glass of water taken.

The following four excerpts are only a few of the many ways slippery elm is used:

3373-1 F 74 PSORIASIS
11. In at least two or three glasses of the water taken each day, a few minutes before it is taken, put a pinch of ground elm bark in the glass of water and stir it. Let it begin to become active, not wholly dissolved, and drink it. Don't drink it just dry and have it in patches through the stomach, but prepare it properly and drink at least three glasses of this elm water every day.

---

100   An alkaline reacting mouth wash frequently recommended by Cayce. See The Heritage Store at http://www. heritagestore.com/.

480-34 F 25 PREGNANCY

9. [Q] My mouth has seemed quite dry - what can be done for same?
[A] Rinse same with a little elm water occasionally; this is helpful; or a little sweet gum [this better fresh]. Any of these as a rinse for the mouth, you see, and then if any of it is swallowed it is all the better for the general condition of the body.

257-214 M 46 HEMORRHAGE:INTESTINES

10. Each morning, before any meal is taken, stir a pinch of elm [slippery elm bark, you see, ground very fine] in a glass of water and let it stand for about ten to fifteen minutes before it is taken. Only fix this each time as it is to be taken, see? Now, a pinch means between the thumb and forefinger; do not take more or less than that! Take it AS indicated!

A slightly more complex formula calling for the gum of elm is shown below:

3125-1 F 40 ALLERGIES

11. As the suggestions are made, begin taking internally those properties to change the whole chemical reaction that forms the basis of this breaking between the sympathetic and cerebrospinal systems. Prepare a compound very carefully, in this manner:

12. To 2 gallons of Distilled or Rain Water, add - in the order named:

> Yellow Dock Root......................2 ounces,
> Burdock Root..........................1 ounce,
> Calamus Root.........................1/2 ounce,
> Black Snake Root, or Snake Root.......1 ounce,
> Red Root.............................1 ounce,
> Buchu Leaves.........................1 dram,
> Cincho Bark..........................2 grains,
> Podophyllin [dry]....................1 grain,
> Elder Flower.........................4 ounces.

Reduce by slow boiling, in an enamel container with an enamel or glass top [not tin or metal], to 1 gallon. When partly cooled, cut 4 drams of Gum of Elm in the alcohol - that is, cut 4 drams of the Tolu elm, or Balsam of Tolu, in 6 ounces of Grain Alcohol, and add to the solution.

13. The dose will be a teaspoonful four times each day, before each meal and at retiring.

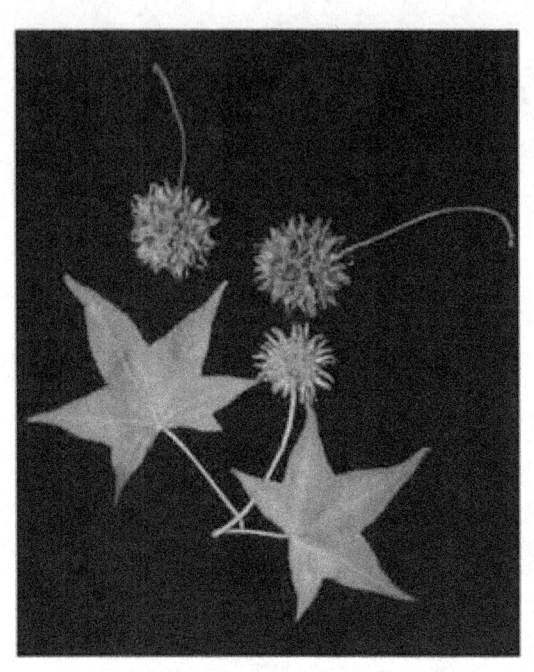

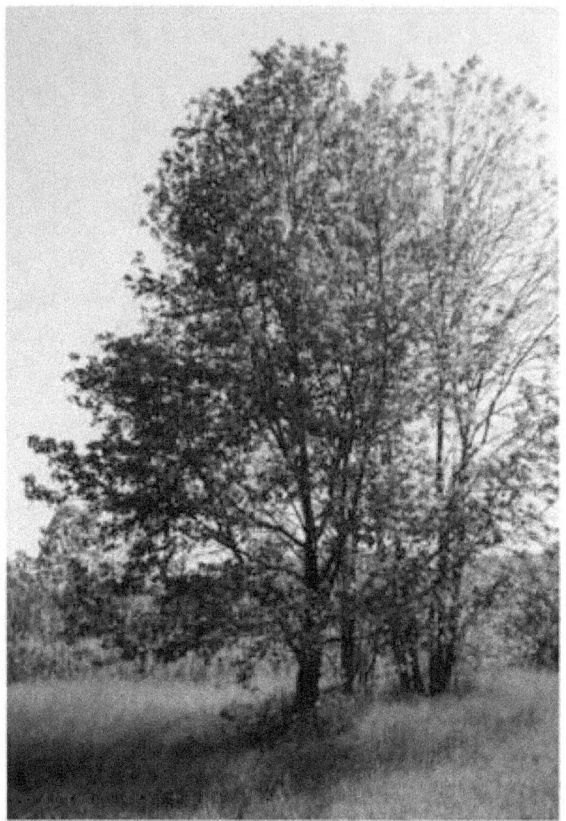

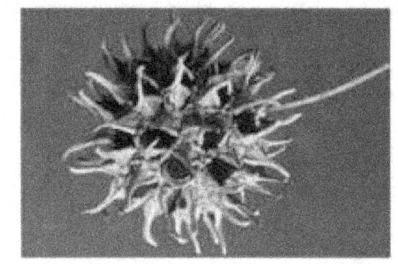

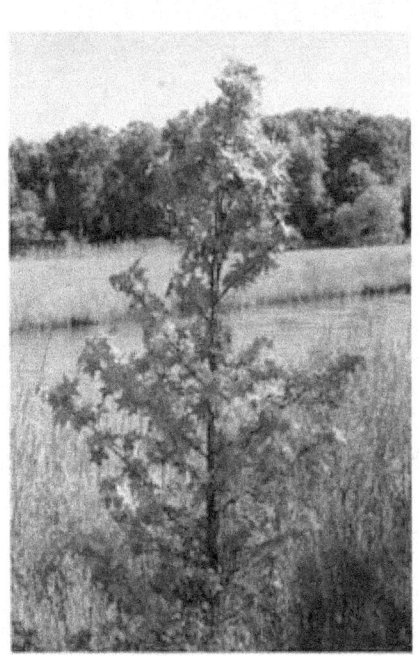

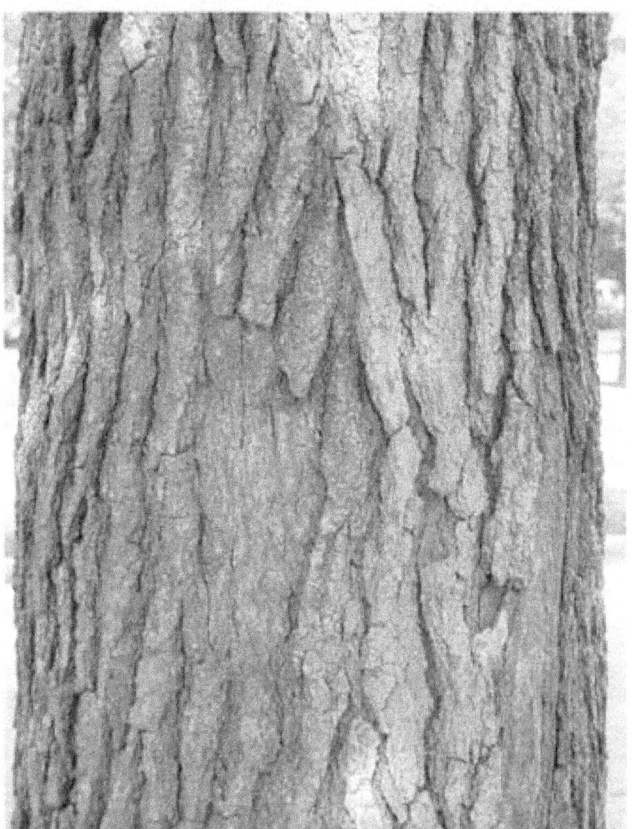

SWEET GUM
Liquidambar styraciflua, Fam. Hamamelidaceae

Common and Regional Names
Sweetgum, gum ball, southern gum ball, American sweetgum, redgum, sapgum, star-leaf gum, bilsted, satin-walnut, white gum, Alligator-Tree, opossum-tree, gum-wood, copalm balsam

History and Common Usage
Sweet gum, also called a gum ball tree, can be considered a living fossil. Twenty extinct species are known, the oldest found in the Upper Eocene rocks of Greenland during a time when that continent had a sub-tropical climate some 55 million years ago. Today there are three existing species of *Liquidambar*. One is found in Formosa, one in Turkey and one is native to the United States. Sweet gum resin has been used since pre-historic times as a chewing gum, an expectorant, and occasionally as an antiseptic ointment in cases of scabies and dermatitis. Medicinally known as "copalm balsam" the resin has been used in ointments, cough syrups [obtained by boiling the young branches] and in cases of dysentery and diarrhea. It is also used as a perfuming agent in soap.

The currently accepted scientific name for sweet gum is *Liquidambar styraciflua*. An important derivative of the tree resin is storax, [also seen as styrax] a constituent of compound tincture of benzoin. Storax from sweet gum can be used as a substitute for the official storax or styrax which is obtained from a close cousin *Liquidambar orientalis*. [101]

Styrax was used medicinally by the ancient Egyptians although not extensively. They may have used *L. orientalis* and not *L. styraciflua* although the latter probably would have grown in nearby Turkey. One typical Egyptian formula found on page 44 of the Ebers is referred to as a "Remedy to cool" and calls for:

Styrax ½ ro[102]
brain of a fat ox 16 ro
sdr-drink 15 ro [un-translated word]
honey
Mixed and injected into the anus.

The Book of Medicines makes far more extensive use of styrax than the Egyptians, citing its use in over 20 formulas. One of the most complicated [and time consuming] remedies is named *Antidote Ariston*. This prescription is said to be for a bad condition of the liver, phthisis, protracted pains of the liver and *"every kind of disease"* provided *"that a man useth it with the skill and understanding which are meet."* Thirty-three ingredients are listed among them dry Styrax, opium, safflower and dried roses. All the dry ingredients are to be mixed and steeped in wine for three days. All the soluble ingredients are mixed in wine with honey, oil of balsam was added and the mixture was boiled and then set aside for six months before it is ready to be dispensed. The standard dose is one drachm *"for every ailment."*

---

101   Liquidambar orientalis was not known botanically until the 18th century when it was grown in England having been imported from the Middle East.

102   The Egyptians used measurements of capacity not weight for both dry ingredients and liquid. A ro is generally accepted to be roughly 15 cubic centimeters, or a spoonful.

L. styraciflua was first described in English literature by Nicholas Monardes when new plant materials were brought back to Europe from early expeditions to the New World. Nicholas Monardes named the sweet gum resin *Liquidambar*. He obtained his first sample through his trading operations in what is now Mexico.

Sweet gum is an important commercial lumber source used primarily for veneers and plywood. The lumber is used to make boxes, crates, furniture, interior trim and millwork. The veneer is used for crates, baskets and interior woodwork. Sweet gum is also used for crossties and fuel, and small amounts are used in fencing, excelsior and pulpwood.

The 21st Edition of the United States Dispensatory lists sweet gum as an official drug plant citing its derivative storax, or balsam, as a "stimulating expectorant." Mixed with olive oil it was an effective remedy in the treatment of scabies and taken in the form of syrup it was said to be effective in cases of diarrhea and dysentery, especially in young children.

Description
Sweet gum is a handsome long-lived tree often confused with maple because the leaves are similar, but the branches of sweet gum are alternating and not opposite as in the maple. The bark is a uniform grey in color and deeply corrugated in a flat top diamond pattern. Sweet gum leaves are lustrous and bright green above and paler green underneath. When bruised, the leaves give off a pleasant resinous scent.

They are large trees, sometimes reaching heights of 100 to 200 feet, and at this height will be 3 to 4 feet in diameter. They are a long-lived species with older specimens reaching 200 or more years of age. The largest and oldest trees in the United States are located along the well-drained ridges in the Mississippi River bottomlands. They are also found from Connecticut to Florida to Texas and in northwestern and central Mexico, Guatemala, Belize, Salvador, Honduras and in Nicaragua. It is one of the most adaptable of the hardwoods in its tolerance to different soil, water and site conditions.

The leaves of the sweet gum produce beautiful fall colors ranging from bright yellows, reds and purples on through bright oranges and browns. All the leaves do not turn at once providing a constantly changing panorama of fall color.

Growing Conditions and Propagation
Sweet gum is pollinated by wind and insects and readily sprouts from seeds and from cuttings. Young trees are a source of winter browsing for deer and other animals. Under ideal conditions the young trees can put on as much as 2 feet of height in a growing season. They begin to produce seeds at between 20 and 30 years of age and if undisturbed they continue seed production for at least 150 more years.

The seeds are contained in a 1 to 1-1/2 inch spiky ball known as a gum ball. Each gum ball can produce as many as 50 seeds to as few as 7 or 8 in poor growing conditions. The seeds are small, usually 2/10 of an inch in length. Ripe gum balls are brown to brownish black in color and their appearance on the tree instantly distinguishes the tree from the maple. Each tree produces a great abundance of seed balls and as the tree reaches between 30 to 60 years of age these can become a great nuisance to the homeowner. Gum balls are shed throughout the year with last year's seed balls often seen on the tree with the young green seed balls of the current season. When fully mature they are very hard with strong, sharp spikes making walking barefoot a risky business. They do not burn easily and often remain in the soil for years without decomposing. They make poor mulch although some sources claim slugs are somewhat deterred by their sharp spines. Gum balls collect in rain gutters and downspouts requiring constant cleaning and removing them from driveways and sidewalks is an on-going chore. A few are collected and used in various arts and crafts applications, spray painted various colors and used to adorn or construct center pieces and wreaths, but they have not made a significant place for themselves in arts and crafts.

Harvesting

The sap or resin of the sweet gum is sometimes produced naturally by an injury or limb breakage due to wind, fire, ice, lightning or other accidents. The sap is yellowish and slightly viscous with a not unpleasant, faintly turpentine like after-taste. It runs freely at first but slows as the site of injury seals over. The resin or balsam can also be extracted by boiling the twigs and young branches in a similar fashion to that of witch hazel.

The resin can also be obtained in the very early spring by making a small V-shaped cut with a sharp axe in a limb or trunk. Over a few days time the resin bleeds or oozes from the cut and through natural evaporation becomes a soft residue, which can be collected by hand and rolled into balls. Sap collection is possible throughout the year but collects more slowly as summer progresses.

Sealing the resin pieces in plastic bags or small glass jars to halt further evaporation is the best storage method. The resin will keep for years if sealed in an air tight container.

Use in the Cayce Readings

Sweet gum is used alone and as a companion plant. It is mentioned in 15 cases as an ingredient in compound tonics, as a mouth wash and an inhalant. A unique use is in a steam sitz bath, akin to the "fumigation" technique of ancient Egypt, in the treatment of female sterility.

As A Steam Sitz Bath Ingredient

2428-1 F 29 Sterility Cured
44. [Q] Why do I not become pregnant, and what can I do to correct the condition of sterility?

…To be sure, from the experiences, there has been a hindrance by the very position of the organs.

Not as a charm, but once a week at least use this:

Put a pellet of sweet gum, the size of a buckshot, in hot water and sit over same, with the vagina exposed to same.

This, - with the mental attitude, - will have an activity upon the body. We refer to the sweet gum from the sweet gum tree, you see.

45. [Q] Will we have any more children, or should we adopt a child?
[A] This depends upon the application of self in those directions indicated; and this is not self alone, but in unison of purpose - as indicated - ye must learn.

Like so many people who were helped by Edgar Cayce Mrs. [2428] did not send any announcement of her pregnancy for their second child. The only notification of the results of this unusual recommendation are found in this exchange of correspondence where Mr. Cayce is helping her to find the recommended gum followed by a note mentioning the birth date of the second child, a son, born recorded as July 4, 1942.

4. 2/26/41 EC's ltr. to [2428]:

Virginia Beach, Va.

Dear Mrs. [2428]

Have yours of the 24th – sorry you are having trouble obtaining the gum. Felt sure you would find it at the place in N.Y. – would suggest you write S. B. Penick & Co. – Crude Drugs, Ashville, N.C. as they gather much of their products from the mountain side. Am sure they will get it for you. May be that you can best get attention through your own local druggist, as wholesalers, usually wish to have requests come through such.

Do hope you will find it. If you don't have ready response let me hear and will see what can be done further, but feel sure you will obtain this here.

Thanking you and hoping you are feeling much better.

Sincerely [signed] Edgar Cayce

R5. 7/24/43 Letter: "I would like to have a joint reading for our two children, [...] [baby son], born 7/4/42 in ..., N.J., and [5043] born 10/1/37 in ..., N.J.

5090-1 F 40 CONCEPTION STERILITY
5. There have been, of course, physical defects in the associations of the companion of the body. But if there is the care and the attention this may be accomplished.

6. When there are those preparations for such, do this to insure conception, if this is desired at a special period [and those periods just before the menstrual period are the preferable for conception]: Put into a hot basin of water a sweet gum ball about the size of a small agate, or say the end of the thumb, in hot boiling water.

7. Sit over this for some ten minutes, and you needn't fear, there will be conception.

Samples of the other ways sweet gum is used are shown below:

Internal Use
59-1 F Adult Toxemia
To give this balance to this body we would take this into the system: To one gallon of rain water - we wish the nitrates in this - we would add:

Wild Cherry Bark	**4 ounces,**
Sweet Gum	**2 ounces,**
Balsam of Tolu	**1 ounce,**

```
Calisaya Bark......................1 ounce,
Sassafras Root.....................2 ounces,
Mandrake Root....................15 grains,
Buchu Leaves.....................30 grains.
```

This would be reduced by simmering, not boiling, to one quart.

To this we would add 4 ounces of sugar, dissolved in sufficient warm water to dissolve same, and 4 ounces of grain alcohol.

The dose of this would be tablespoonful three times each day, half an hour before meals. Do that.

1010-1 F 51 Eliminations:Incoordination
6. Correct these conditions and we will find this body will be able to pass the century mark on this plane if it so desires. These we would accomplish by keeping the ever rebuilding thought in the mind and spiritual entity of the individual and have as physical forces to give the correct incentives to the functioning of the hepatic circulation, this of course including the whole digestive tract.

7. Take this in the system only when the body feels it is needed to give the balance, so should be kept on hand and only taken occasionally: Take two ounces of the rag weed in its green state gathered as we would find at the present; this we would put into six ounces of water and steep until reduced to four ounces; to this we would add the same quantity made from the green plant known as horehound; add to this four ounces of grain alcohol with two drams of sweet gum dissolved in it. Do that. Take teaspoonful when necessary for the correction of the condition through the intestinal tract.

8. Let the diet be only vegetable forces. Do not lower the plane of development by animal vibrations.

As An Inhalant
1866-2 F 34 DEBILITATION:GENERAL TUBERCULOSIS
3. Then, to bring the better condition for the body at the present time, we would give those inhalations as would be found in this:

4. To 4 ounces pure grain alcohol, add:

```
Eucalyptol...............20 minims,
Tincture of Sweet Gum
   [in solution]........30 minims,
Canadian Balsam..........10 minims,
Rectified Oil of Turp.....5 minims,
Benzosol.................10 minims.
```

Shake solution well together. Inhale both through the nostrils and into the lungs through the mouth, see? Not taken internally; inhaled only. That is, once or twice inhale through nostrils, for the inflammation as is seen in this portion of the body; into the lungs, that the respiratory system may be lightened from the burden as is seen from the conditions as existent there.

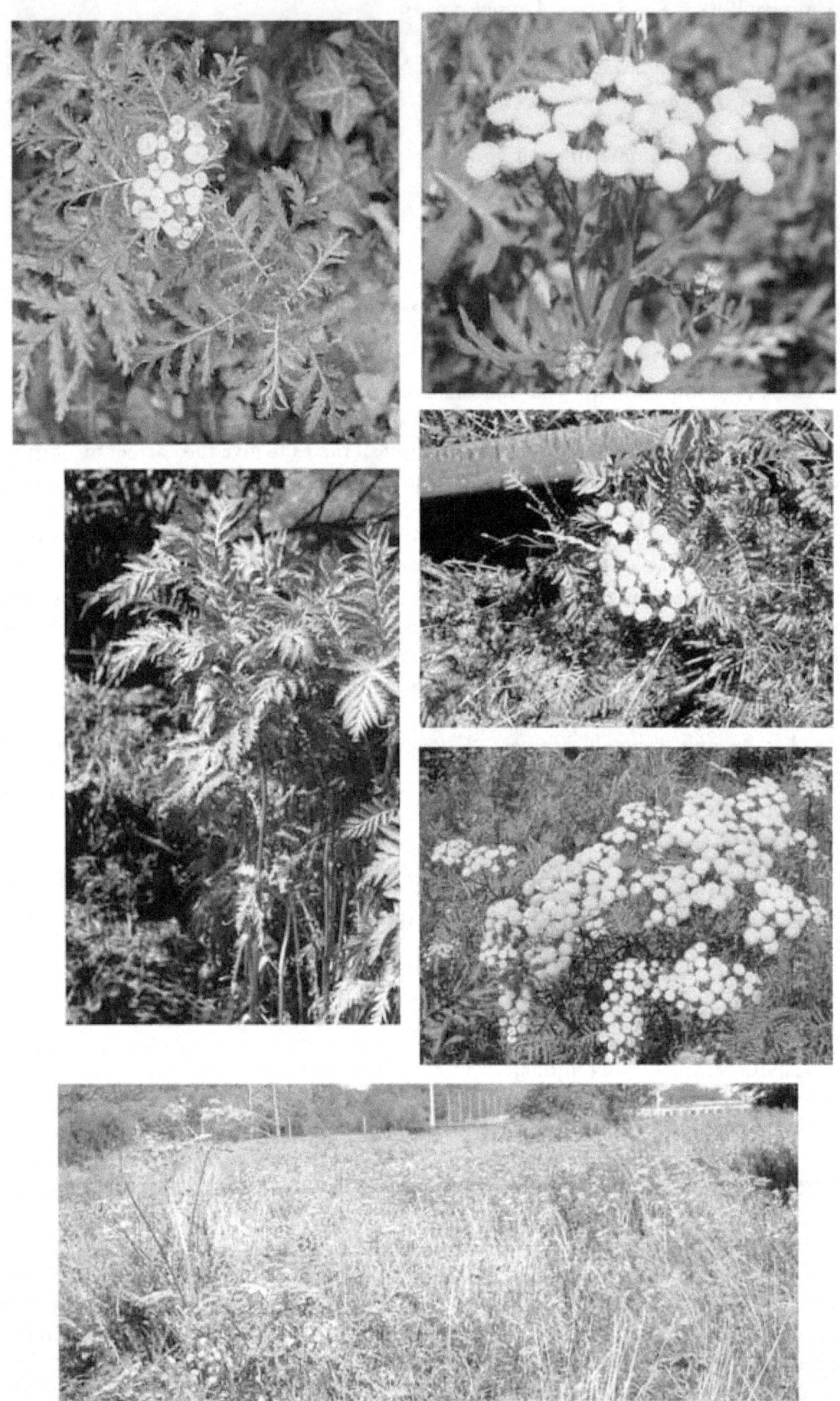

TANSY

Tanacetum vulgare, Fam. Compositae

Common and Regional Names
None

History and Common Usage

Tansy has been found in archeological deposits in Norfolk, England that pre-date the Devonian era of 416 to 359.2 million years ago. It is indigenous throughout Europe and was brought to the New World by early settlers being carried first to Nova Scotia, then south to Georgia and west to Nevada and Oregon. It occurs now throughout the United States and Canada. There are 30 species in this genus world wide, 2 are established in the United States. The plant has been used as a vegetable, in folk medicine and as an insect repellant.

Tansy has been cited in herbal lore and indigenous medical traditions for centuries. British physician and herbalist Nicholas Culpepper mentions the efficacy of the common garden tansy in the treatment of worms, especially in children, and recommended the application of crushed leaves placed on the stomach as a means of prevention of miscarriage. It was also planted in fruit orchards to keep insects from the trees, an early pesticide method which seems to have worked. Tansy has found very limited use throughout history as a condiment. The dried flowers of some varieties, such as Crispum, are used in present day arts and crafts.

Early medical practices made use of tansy as a tea to stimulate menstrual function and to medicate sitz baths in the treatment of female pelvic disorders and local [tub baths] baths in the treatment of rheumatism. Tansy should never be taken by pregnant women, those hoping to become pregnant or nursing mothers. The oil, greenish-yellow and very pungent is expressed from the seeds and leaves. It is considered an excellent rubefacient.

After long winters the people of Medieval Europe were hungry for fresh greens and the early shoots of tansy were among the plants eagerly picked and boiled, sometimes eaten raw and very often scrambled with eggs. The use of tansy actually came under regulation by the early Catholic Church and for a time in some parts of Europe it could only be eaten on Palm and Easter Sundays, *"and their neighbor daies."*[103] This may be attributed to tansy being one of the native plants originally dedicated to the Virgin Mary, perhaps the Church leaders of the time may have felt tansy was deserving of greater respect. Tansy is also identified as one of the original "strewing plants" as cited by British physician Thomas Tusser in 1557.

Strewing herbs were much in use during medieval times when insect infestations and odor control were constant household concerns. Plants were chosen for their aromatic and pest repellant properties. They were especially cultivated for this purpose and were strewn on floors for the purpose of keeping down fleas, a daily chore for household servants.

In a time when structures were closed for months at a time against cold weather and the lack of hot and cold running water made both personal hygiene and household cleaning difficult, the aromatics contributed a great deal to a more tolerable environment. Contrary to modern thinking the householder of this time, whether of a hovel or castle, was not insensitive to a clean and pleasant smelling personage

---

103   Thomas Tusser, A Hundred Points of Good Husbandrie, London 1557, expanded as Five Hundred Points of Good Husbandrie. London 1571, 1573

and surroundings. A great deal of time and resources were spent in developing aromatic products such as pomanders to be worn around the neck and the mixing of various plant products, both fresh and dried for use on floors and in chests where textiles were stored.

Description
Tansy is a handsome ornamental with a somewhat fern-like appearance. It can attain heights of 3 to 4 feet and the branching, plume like stalks are covered with dark, rich green leaves which grow directly from the root and from spreading rhizomes in the same manner as asafoetida and licorice.

Beginning in June or July in most areas flowers begin to develop. They are small bright yellow flower heads with tightly curled petals causing the flowers to be referred to as "buttons." Their tiny seeds develop from these bright yellow buttons which are used to express oil.

Growing Conditions and Propagation
Tansy is pollinated by wind and insects and propagates from seeds. It also spreads vigorously through its root system. Fernleaf is a very decorative variety which does not spread as quickly as some others. It retains a more compact form and if grown in the home garden Fernleaf is a good choice.

Tansy will thrive in almost any growing conditions. In some areas it has done so well it is classified as a noxious weed. The shoots are eaten by cows and horses in the very early spring but as it matures into the summer season they will avoid the plant. Sheep and goats, however, will eat the mature plants without any ill side effects. These animals are often used by farmers and ranchers as "walking weed control agents." They eagerly eat the plants down to the soil level, frequently including the roots.

Harvesting
Tansy leaves should only be harvested in the early spring and dried out of the sunlight in a warm, dry area. The root is not used. Mature tansy leaves contain large amounts of a bitter principle called tanacetin which in large amounts is poisonous. The symptoms begin with abdominal pain, vomiting, violent convulsions, respiratory distress and death through paralytic asphyxia. Again, pregnant and nursing mothers should not drink tansy tea.

Use in the Edgar Cayce Readings
The Cayce system departs from traditional herbal traditions by only using tansy once out of the 9603 physical transcripts, and then as a companion plant in combination with horehound in an expectorant which calls for several other ingredients to be added.

337-18 F 43 LUNGS:EXPECTORANT ECZEMA
Well, also, for such as THIS to be prepared, and this would be well for most every condition in its beginning, or termination. Prepare first as this: This as a carrier: Take 16 ounces distilled water, and Wild Cherry Bark 8 ounces. This should be boiled, or steamed together, and reduced to 8 ounces when strained off. Also prepare Horehound and Tansy, 3 ounces of each in 12 ounces of water. Reduce THIS to half the quantity. Put the 2 solutions, then, together. Add to this 4 ounces of simple syrup, reducing again until there is 8 ounces, see? Then, to this add:

Oil of Sassafras...........................1/4 ounce,
Syrup of Rhubarb..........................1/4 ounce,
Spirits Frumenti [at least 90% pure].........4 ounces,
Tincture of Capsici................................3 minims.

Shake it together before the dose is taken, which would be a teaspoonful at a dose, and it may be taken WHENEVER necessary, preferably just before retiring and on arising of morning.

This is an excellent expectorant.

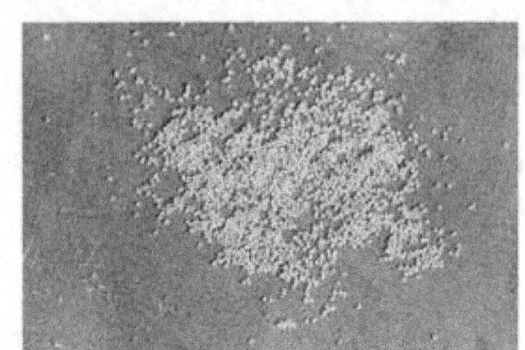

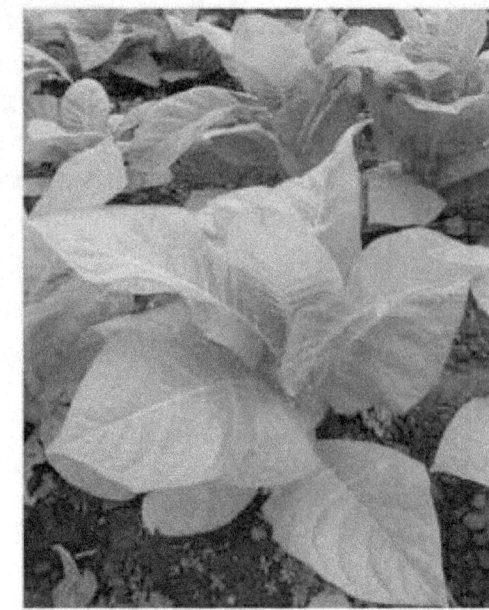

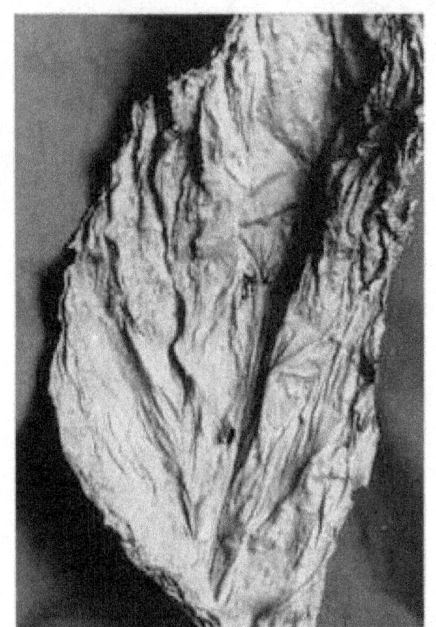

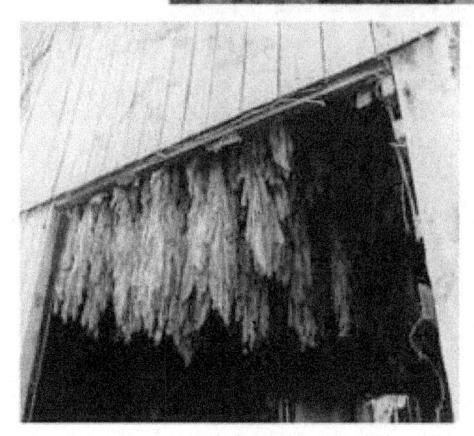

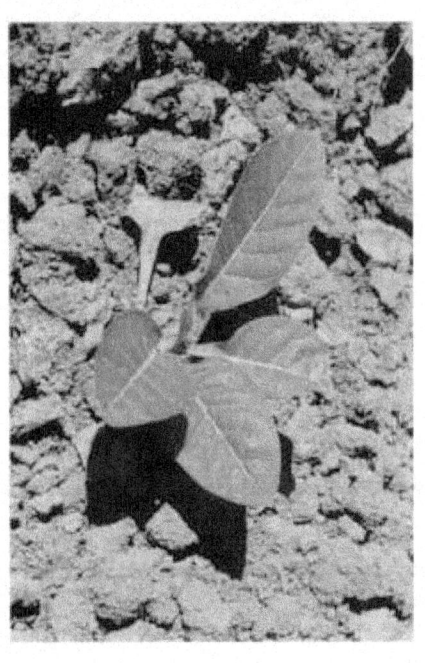

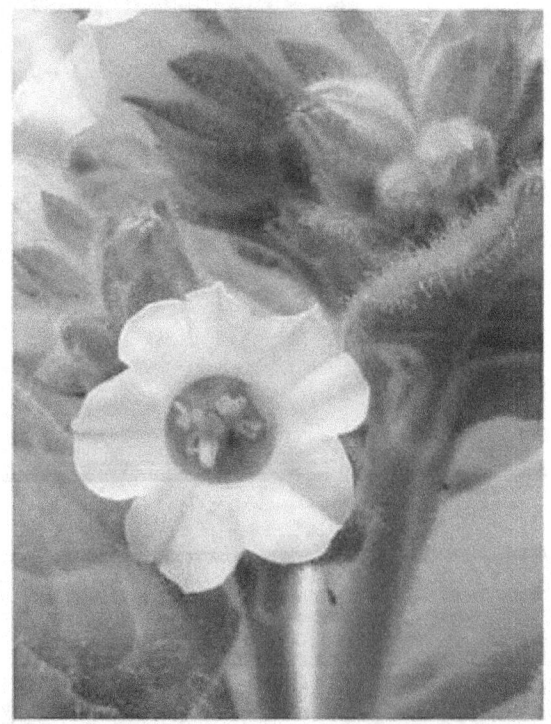

Tobacco
Nicotiana Tabacum, Fam. Solonaceae

Common and Regional Names
Smokes, Snuff, Chew, Dip, 'Baccy

History and Common Usage
There are 67 recognized species recorded to date in the *Nicotiana* family. *Tabacum* is believed to have originated with the other members of the *Solonaceae* family in what is today South and Central America. It can be safely conjectured that the inhalation of smoke from different kinds of plants began very early in the history of mankind; however documentation of the use of *Nicotinia tabacum* is relatively new and very controversial.

Analysis of a smoking pipe dating to approximately 300 B.C. from the Boucher Site, a Middlesex-complex from Vermont in the Northern United States, has yielded evidence of nicotine decay products.[104] At a somewhat later period, between 470 and 630 AD, the Mayans and Toltecs are known to have begun to immigrate to other areas taking the plants and seeds with them. Another early record of its use is found on a piece of pottery from Uaxactun, Guatemala dated between 600 and 1000 AD. A Mayan male is depicted smoking a roll of tobacco leaves tied with string.

The Mayan word for smoking was *sik'ar* or sicar which transitioned into the European word for cigar. The leaves, frequently mixed with other substances such as coca, have long been chewed or smoked by Mayans and Toltecs. Some researchers posit that smoking, especially on the part of the upper classes, was part of a religious ritual, and indeed smudging, smoke and the burning of incense form a part of certain religion practices even today. This does not, however, adequately address the addictive nature of the habit of smoking tobacco.

At present there are no known pre-historic records of the use of tobacco and it is not until the late 1500's that plants and seeds were brought to Spain, Portugal and England by early explorers. Italian explorer Christopher Columbus is credited with first introducing tobacco to the Europeans. The Island of Tobago in the Republic of Trinidad was named by Columbus for the native tobacco pipe he found in such widespread use there. The European cultivation of tobacco began in roughly 1556 and the first tobacco plantations in the United States were established in 1612. This single crop is largely responsible for the initial colonization of the New World.

The various uses of tobacco by indigenous peoples of Central and North America were first adopted by European explorers and soon thereafter the use of snuff, chewing tobacco and the smoking of rolled leaves became a widespread social practice.

Tobacco contains a poisonous substance called nicotine, named after French ambassador Jean Nicot.[105] Nicot was on assignment in Portugal in 1559 where he was first introduced to the new plant. He sent tobacco products back to France and upon his return home he brought with him both tobacco plants and seeds. He is credited with introducing the use of snuff to the French court and in 1753 Carolus Linnaeus named the genus *Nicotina* in his honor. Linnaeus described two species at this time, *nicotiana rustica* and *nicotiana tabacum*. The origin of the word tobacco is in question. Some sources believe it comes from the

---

104   Rafferty, Sean M. Journal of Archeological Sciences. Volume 33. Issue 4. Pages 453-458. April, 2006.
105   1530-1600

Arabic word tabbaq or tabco dating from around 1410 AD while others believe it originally comes from one of the Caribbean languages called Arawaken encountered by Christopher Columbus in his original travels to what is today Trinidad.

Whatever the origin of the common name may be there is no escaping the present medical and legal controversy over the use of tobacco, the admittedly dangerous adulteration of cigarettes and other tobacco products, and the ban against smoking in public places which is slowly becoming a world wide standard.

Tobacco does not have a presence in folk medicine despite the fact that Nicholas Monardes originally hailed the plant as a cure for toothache, falling fingernails, worms, halitosis, lockjaw and cancer. Tobacco is listed as an unofficial drug plant in 21st Edition of the United States Dispensatory citing the practice of smoking as both a stimulant and a relaxant but further warning of the danger of fatal poisoning if pure nicotine is absorbed through the skin.

Description
Tobacco plants often grow to over six feet in height and 3 or 4 feet wide. The leaves are dark to medium green becoming yellow as they mature. In the United States they are grown as annuals although in more tropical regions the plant appears as a biennial, or in some cases even a triennial. They have large, pointed heavy leaves that have a distinct narcotic odor. The root is fibrous and the stem or stalk of the plant is round and slightly hairy. The leaves are larger at the bottom of the plant becoming smaller towards the top. The tubular shaped flowers, which appear in August in most regions, occur in clusters at the top of the plant. They range in color from white to pale pink, yellow or red and are sweetly fragrant. There are many varieties of seeds available. A few of the more popular are: Madole, Small Stalk Black Mammoth, Burley, Perique, Havana [there are several Havanas] Kentucky, Mountain, Walker's Broadleaf and the whimsically named Lizard Tail Turtlefoot.

Growing Conditions and Propagation
Tobacco is fertilized by insects and wind, propagates by seed and it is subject to the same diseases and pests as other nightshades such as the tomato and aubergine or eggplant. It makes a handsome and unusual show plant for the home garden. Tobacco will benefit from the same fertilizer used for the other nightshades. It can be grown almost anywhere as long as it has 65 to 70 frost free nights to mature.

The seeds are very tiny [roughly 300,000 per ounce] so they are difficult to manage when it comes to planting. For the home gardener sprinkling a few on the top of prepared potting soil in the garden and thinning the weakest seedlings out later is a good method. Tobacco seeds need both light and air in order to germinate so they should be kept moist but not covered with soil. Germinating seeds in peat pots approximately 50 to 60 days prior to the date of transplant is also a good method, especially in areas where summers are short. The pots should be planted about 6 to 8 inches deep once all danger of any frost is past. Plants need about 3 feet between them for best results.

Generally a 5.8 soil pH is ideal. The plants need full sun and adequate rainfall in soil that is moist but well-drained. Commercial growers cut the flower stalks as soon as they appear, a process called topping, to force larger leaf growth. Any tiny leaves appearing at the base of larger leaves should be pinched off and discarded. The appearance of these little leaves is called suckering and they affect the quantity and the quality of the harvest.

Because tobacco represents such a large market in the world it has been the subject of a significant investment in research all of which is freely available. The temperature, soil, sunlight and water requirements are precisely known for every region of the world.

Harvesting

Tobacco leaves must be both dried and aged or cured before use. At harvest time the whole plant can be cut to the ground and hung to dry, or individual leaves can be cut incrementally as they turn yellow. Individual leaves are strung on twine, not too close together and not too far apart, and hung in a warm, dry space for about 8 weeks to dry. The drying process must be carefully managed. Too low a temperature or too high humidity and the leaves spoil, mildew and rot. Too high a temperature and too dry and the tobacco will be "green" and not have a good aroma or flavor.

Curing or aging of the leaves is a little more challenging. Curing requires temperature ranges of 60 F to 90 F and humidity levels between 65 to 70%. For the home gardener this is difficult to manage without a building that can be opened and closed as needed. Curing is also a matter of individual taste, knowledge of which can only be acquired through experience. Curing takes as long as 5 or 6 years and as little as two months.

Tobacco that is not aged but only dried is harsh and lacks a good flavor. A properly dried and cured or aged leaf should still be pliable but dry to the touch. After curing the central stem of the leaf is cut away and the remainder is ready to be rolled, shredded, pulverized or powdered. Commercial growers age leaves at least a year before processing and use rigidly controlled conditions to maintain heat and humidity at optimum levels. The home grower will find a great many sources of information on curing, aging, flavoring and other handling and preparation methods from which to choose.

Use in the Edgar Cayce Readings

Tobacco is a companion plant in the Cayce system. It is used therapeutically [in pulverized form or as snuff] combined with other materials such as oil of butterfat or tincture of benzoin, oil of turp [Canadian balsam] mentholatum or Atomidine in a highly effective preparation for the treatment of hemorrhoids. Several variations of this formula have been given and the salve can easily be made at home if a commercial brand by the name of "Tim"[106] is not available.

No recommendations were given related to the use of snuff or chewing tobacco and no questions were asked, although in one case [4212-1] the individual is told that excessive use of chewing tobacco has caused a harmful over-stimulation to the salivary glands producing a chain reaction resulting in high blood pressure. In general cigarettes are preferred over cigars or a pipe. Burton's snuff is the only brand name mentioned but several cigarette brands from the 1920's are favorably recommended. Virginia Rounds, Piedmont, Pall Mall and Virginia Ovals are mentioned by name.

Those around Cayce gradually began to refer to the formula below by the letters of the major ingredients, T for tobacco, I for iodine and M for menthol, resulting in TIM. The earliest formula recorded for TIM was first given on May 15, 1924:

106   The Heritage Store 314 Laskin Road, Virginia Beach, Virginia 23451 757-428-0500
http://www.heritagestore.com/

953-9 M 52

2. For the condition as gives trouble in the rectum at the present time, we would use a solution or a salve of this character: Take four ounces of butter [without salt, or fresh butter] just churned, and reduce by application of heat to the oil of butterfat. To this we would add three minims of Mentholatum and six grains of Pulverized Tobacco, with two grains of White Castile Soap. Mix this all well to-gether and use as a lotion. [GD's note: This was an early simple formula for the hemorrhoid compound which was later referred to in the readings as TIM - See [1800] series for other more complicated descriptions of the formula.]

A second formula for the same condition was given July 29 of 1924:

3818-6 M 39

5. To 1/2 ounces of oil of butterfat, there would be added powdered tobacco sufficient to make a salve. Added to this and mixed well would be 10 minims - [long pause]

6. [Q] Will you please continue with this reading?
[A] We have the conditions here. In this would be added that of Camphor 2 minims. That of the solution 10 minims of - we have it here -

This would be applied to applied to those portions that are affected, this producing an astringent in the system, and with the laxness of the tissue would produce the tautness that would be necessary to relieve permanently the conditions as we find.

Occasionally the formula is altered, tailored to individual needs. In the following buckeye kernel oil is be added.

2711-2 M 58

16. LOCALLY, apply those properties as would be found in a combination of THIS character; using this as an ointment following the stools, or WHEN there is irritation. RESTING, keeping feet up, will also aid these conditions - as well as aid the general HEALTH of body, with the taking of the medicinal properties and the manipulations [which should be had at least ONCE each day]. This salve [Tim], or ointment, would be made in THIS manner:

17. To 1 ounce of OIL of butterfat, add 1 dram of very fine POWDERED tobacco, 2 grains or 2 minims of oil of aloe, and 2 minims of oil of the buckeye kernel. Stir well together and use as an ointment.

Another variation of the tobacco formula given in 1932 includes oil of turp:

340-17 F 44

3. Take the oil of butterfat [fresh butter, not that that's been salted], and reduce same so that there is no water in same, or milk - see? Take one-half ounce of this, see? To this add one-quarter ounce of Burton's powdered tobacco or snuff. Boil this together, or heat together, so that the tobacco is cooked. To this add four drops of Tincture of Iodine and one drop of Oil of Turp [not turpentine, but Oil of Turp, or Canadian Balsam]. Use this as an ointment, mixed thoroughly together while hot - then let congeal, see? [Another simple formula for that called TIM?]

In the following excerpt a specific exercise is required as well as the application of the tobacco formula:

147-34 F 54
4. For those conditions that produce irritation in the eliminating channels [hemorrhoids], with that being applied [the Tim] we would take those exercises which will stretch arms high above the head, bending the body forward, stooping as far forward as the body can. Take this exercise at least three times each day, for three to five minutes each period, see?

In 1924 efforts were begun by those around Edgar Cayce to make some of the remedies available on the open market. At this time an element of standardization entered in to the tobacco formulation as follows:

1800-20 BUSINESS September 13, 1924
19. ...As we find, there are other properties much preferable in the use of same than the old formula. Here's the better formula:

To 1 ounce Oil of Butterfat, add:

> **Tincture of Benzoin...................10 minims,**
> **Atomidine, or atomic iodine...........5 minims, [or**
> **iodine, though atomic iodine is that with the poison**
> **out - but plain iodine is not as expensive as the**
> **Atomidine]**
> **Powdered tobacco or snuff.............3 drams, preferably**
> **the snuff - the powdered.**

Stir well together. Preferable that this never be put in tin, but rather in the porcelain or glass; and should be in an ounce or ounce and a quarter hexagon-shaped jar, preferably. The directions would be to apply as an ointment to affected portions once or twice each day. Rest as much as possible AFTER application, with the feet elevated ABOVE the head. It'll cure it!

Refinements to the formula and an explanation of the action of individual ingredients were recorded on May 6th of 1936. T.B. House was an osteopathic physician, long associated with Edgar Cayce. At one time he was on the staff of the Cayce Hospital:

1800-26 BUSINESS
3. [Q] First: T-I-M, a remedy for hemorrhoids, a jar of which T. B. House holds in his hand. Does this product carry enough Tincture of Benzoin to act as an effective astringent in reducing the surplus skin or sac left by the hemorrhoid after it has been assimilated in the system?
[A] In this particular jar here, not sufficient; though it will act as an astringent. But a small quantity added to same would make it more effective, though in some types more irritating.

4. [Q] Should the amount of Benzoin now being used according to the formula that has been given be increased for general distribution?
[A] Should be increased about one percent.

5. [Q] How many drops to each ounce should it be increased?
[A] In the preparation of this there is a great deal of difference depending upon the time it is added to the solution, see? and in the temperature and in the condition of the oil that is reduced from the butterfat, or the butterfat oil; the condition of this as the base, as well as the quantity of the tobacco that is absorbed by same - or snuff. And when this is added then, to the whole amount we would add - for the ounce - five more drops. Instead of from six then to twelve, add fifteen drops. For in this the proportion is ten.

6. [Q] Please explain the reactions and effect of the Atomidine and the Snuff in this preparation.
[A] The Atomidine being broken up from kelp [carrying an effective activity upon irritation] makes for an activity upon the tobacco, which also is as a preservative as well as a deodorant, as well as an activity that enhances the action of the atomic forces in the iodine, see?

7. [Q] At what temperature of the Butterfat should the Benzoin be added?
[A] Hundred and one degrees.

8. [Q] At what temperature should the Atomidine be added?
[A] At ninety-eight.

9. [Q] Is a sufficient quantity of the Atomidine being used?
[A] Sufficient quantity, provided this same strength is kept.

10. [Q] Is the one percent solution of the Atomidine the proper amount?
[A] There's more than that in this!

11. [Q] What percent solution of Atomidine should be used in this?
[A] The REGULAR solution that is put up for commercial use, which makes it about one and one-half percent of the atomic forces in same.

12. [Q] Is the pack of Tobacco now in the office of the Health Home Remedies Corp. as good to use as Snuff?
[A] No.

13. [Q] Do you recommend any changes in this product for use in internal hemorrhoids?
[A] Necessary that those put in tubes be MORE of the Butterfat and less of the Tobacco.

14. [Q] Just how much should the Tobacco be cut down?
[A] When this is put in the solution, it would be stirred until it is the consistency of soft soap - or in proportion this would be, for each ounce of Butterfat there would be added half and a quarter of the Tobacco, see, or Snuff.

The following statement speaks to the effectiveness of the tobacco preparation:

257-198 M 45
16. [Q] Will Tim cure or dry up these hemorrhoids without any other action?
[A] Consistently used, it will not only remove the cause but remove the hemorrhoids.

To Smoke or Not To Smoke

To smoke or not to smoke is a question as frequently asked during Cayce's time as it is today. While the Cayce system clearly advocates what is described as the "natural leaf" - or unadulterated pure tobacco - smoking in moderation is not said to be harmful, although in two cases he advises against the use of Turkish tobacco and in one case advises against mentholated cigarettes. As remarkable as it seems today smoking was not prohibited by Cayce as can be seen in the following excerpts:

279-2 M 31

5. [Q] Is smoking injurious in my present condition? For instance, one or two cigarettes after meals, or the like?

[A] Not injurious, unless the body thinks so! Having been told this, there come times and periods when they don't taste good - then throw them away! But when desired, smoke! Be careful of the BRAND you smoke and you'll be careful of how and when these react upon the system! Those that carry more of tobacco itself, rather than the COMBINATION of others - as would be in Piedmont, or those of such character. Those that carry any of the Turkish tobacco becomes obnoxious!

2378-4 F 33

8. We would leave off at least half of the smoking, and DO NOT inhale when this is taken. Smoke Virginia Rounds, when you smoke, or the all tobacco brands, and not those carrying a mixture too much with Turkish tobaccos, - these are harmful for such conditions. Do not attempt the mentholated cigarettes, though; for these are not well for this body.

303-23 F 54

17. [Q] Would smoking of cigarettes in any way be beneficial to my body; if so, what brand, and how many a day?

[A] The nicotine for the body would supply a poison that would counterbalance some of the disturbances in the system. Three to five a day would be correct. This does not necessarily mean that these would be inhaled, but the brand that is of the purer tobacco is the better.

18. [Q] Which brands are the pure tobacco?

[A] Virginia Ovals and of such natures.

1131-2 M Adult

19. [Q] Is smoking injurious to the body, if not what brand should be used or would be best for the body?

[A] Smoking in moderation will be helpful to the body. The best brands, we would find, are those that are of the purer tobacco that are not either toasted or mixed with foreign conditions. Those known as or called Piedmonts are the better.

Moderation is defined by limiting the number of cigarettes to between 4 and 6 per day and in one rare case the individual was not to smoke over 20 in one day. One other individual was told they could smoke between 10 and 20 in one day without harm provided they were spaced far enough apart. The most frequently seen recommendation is 5 to 6 cigarettes per day:

5107-1 F 22

17. [Q] Should I smoke cigarettes or are they harmful?

[A] If these are taken in moderation it is not harmful, but don't smoke over six a day.

Cayce suggests it is best not to smoke before meals, but AFTER eating, and in the last transcript does not advocate smoking late at night:

243-24 F 56
11. [Q] Is smoking a detriment to me?
[A] In moderation not harmful. Too much is VERY harmful. DO NOT smoke of mornings BEFORE MEALS!

294-190 M 60
4. And the next - DO NOT SMOKE! only once or the like AFTER meals!

830-4 M 20
19. [Q] Is cigarette smoking injurious to health and growth of this body?
[A] In moderation not injurious. In excess, very injurious. Cigarette smoking before breakfast or after twelve o'clock at night is injurious.

Cayce tells this middle-aged lady to keep quiet before and while smoking or she won't reap the benefits:

303-32 F 55
10. [Q] What is cause and relief for the nervousness, especially after eating or smoking?
[A] Tiredness, lack of resistance in the body. Take time to be quiet before eating. Take time to be quiet before smoking, or when smoking. Don't smoke and talk or carry on at such a rate that the mind is running away with the body. This does not allow ANY stimulant to come from the relaxation that should come in smoking.

As in all things recommended in the Cayce system smoking is an individual matter:

442-2 M 57
25. [Q] Is the inhaling of smoke harmful to the body?
[A] More harmful than would be to some other bodies. Not to excess; but the activity is as this: Nicotine, as indicated from the tobacco upon the system, in most activities is a stimuli. Any stimuli to excess is harmful, but a stimuli that makes for the circulation in that portion of the body may clarify, as it were, the cobwebs, or across from the circulatory activity to the brain, which is by the circulation through the secondary cardiac forces, as indicated disturbances there. Hence moderation. Moderation would mean, for this body, anywhere from three to six to eight smokes a day. Above this will be excessive.

Nicotine is described as a poison which acts upon the nerves in a way which is beneficial to digestion:

2390-4 F 30
33. [Q] Are cigarettes in moderation harmful to me?
[A] Rather in most cases, as well as here, these would be beneficial in moderation. True, they add a poison - but it is of such a character that it is active upon the nerves so as to be beneficial in digestion, as well as in quieting the nerves.
34. [Q] Is alcohol in moderation harmful to me?
All forms of alcohol are HARMFUL; especially anything made with hops!

There are better sources of nicotinic acid if an individual chooses not to smoke:

1158-1 F 46
52. [Q] What is best source of nicotinic acid?
[A] Of course, the greater source is from smoke. But in vegetables, carrots, squash, pumpkin, and especially in what is called the oyster plant.[107] **[Salsify]**

For some individuals it is apparent that trying to stop can cause more trouble than smoking:

2794-2 F 34
13. [Q] If I stopped smoking, would it help my condition?
[A] Not very much - you'd be more irritated by the wanting to smoke.

A straight forward answer is given for a 49 year old male who asked:

462-4 M 49
8. [Q] What kind of tobacco, if any, should this body use?
[A] Pure tobacco is always better than any concoction of the compilation of other things with same. If it's to be used at all, use the Natural Leaf. Then you won't use so much of it either!

Most smokers will find the transition from modern cigarettes to the natural leaf quite a challenge.

It seems only fitting to leave the last word on smoking to Cayce:

391-7 M 22
4. [Q] Would it be advisable for me to stop smoking altogether?
[A] As has been indicated or said about other stations in life, [I Cor. 7:38 in re marriage?] he that smokes doeth well, he that smokes not doeth better. But in moderation, this is not harmful to the body. In excess, harmful to ANY body.

---

107   See Volume II

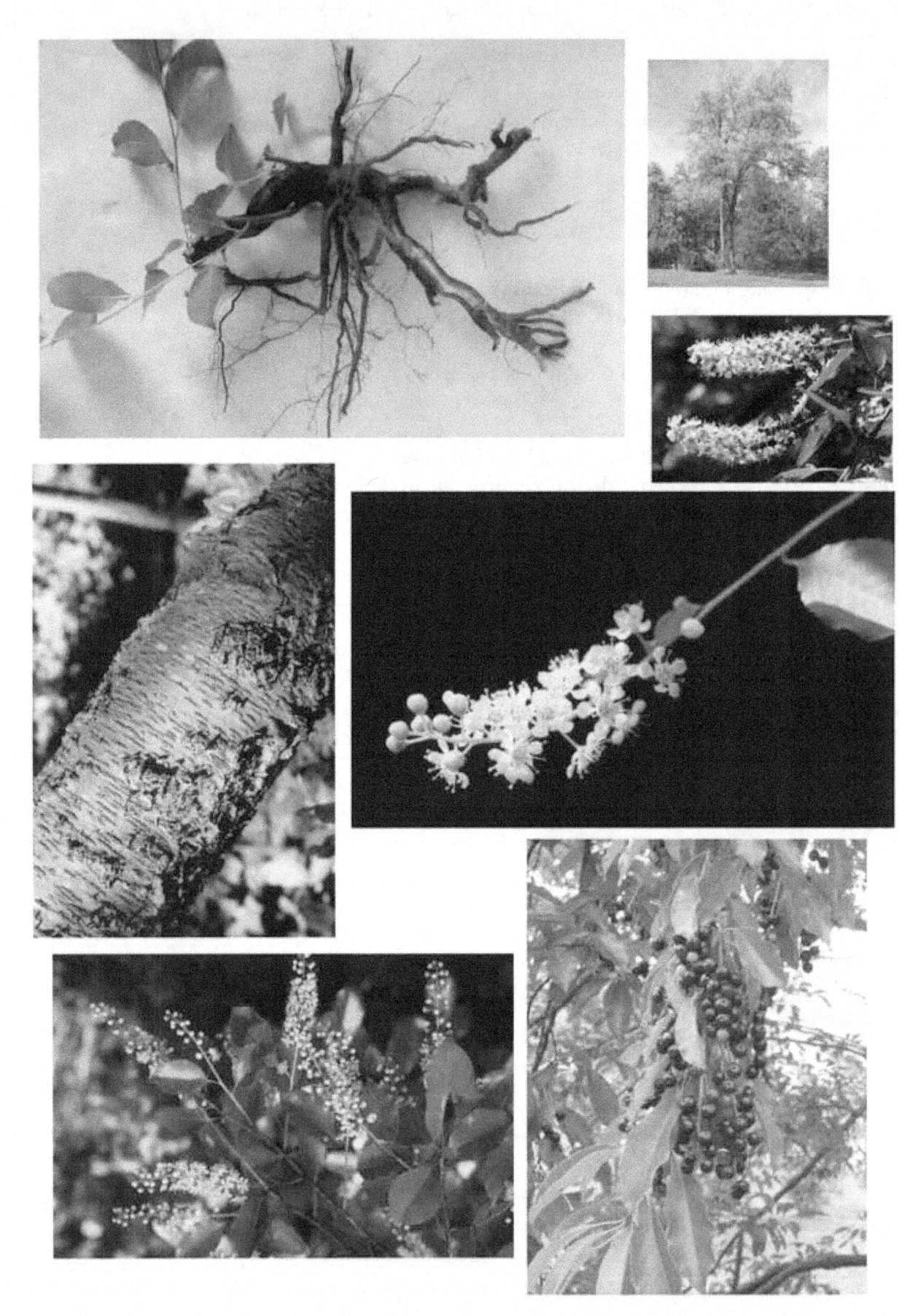

WILD BLACK CHERRY
Prunus serotina, Fam. Rosaceae

Common and Regional Names
Black Cherry, Wild Black Cherry, Virginian Prune, Rum Cherry, Whiskey Cherry, Cabinet Cherry

History and Common Usage
The wild black cherry, originally indigenous to North America, now grows in most all the temperate regions of the world. It is prized for its fine grained and compact wood as a source of hardwood for fine furniture and cabinetry. It is found from Ontario to Florida, in Europe and the Pacific regions of Central America, Columbia and Peru.

Wild black cherry is classified as poisonous with a high toxicity rating due to the presence of what are called "cyanogenic precursors" in the leaves which are released at the time of injury or damage. When the leaves are injured through unseasonable frost, drought or when, for example, the tree is blown down during a storm a chemical called prunasin in the leaves splits off free cyanide [also called prussic acid or hydrocyanic acid]. Browsing animals, when deprived of their normal forage and faced with starvation will eat the leaves. When ingested in any amount by cattle, sheep, goats and deer, the cyanide in the distressed leaves and twigs causes respiratory distress, sometimes followed by respiratory failure and/or cardiac arrest. As the leaves die or dry out the toxic properties degrade and dissipate.

The ripe black or very deep purple berries are safe to eat and were used by early American settlers to flavor rum and in making homemade wine. They have a sweet and slightly astringent taste. The pitted fruit can be eaten raw, used in pies, jelly and juice. It is a tedious but necessary chore to pit the small cherries but the raw pits should not be eaten. The pits of wild cherries as well as their cousins the apricots, peaches, plums and cultivated cherries contain toxic levels of cyanide. While cooking destroys most of this, it is still best not to consume the pits. An easy method of obtaining pit free juice is to cook the cherries in a small amount of water straining the finished juice to separate it from the pits and skins. It can be sweetened with honey or sugar to use as a beverage or cooked until the liquid reaches the syrup stage for jams and jellies.

Wild black cherry bark has an ancient and persistent anecdotal tradition as to its efficacy in the treatment of lung disorders. Indigenous peoples have long made use of it as a cough medicine in cases of cold, congestion and bronchitis. It has also been used for the treatment of diarrhea and for the relief of pain. The Cherokees used it as a pain reliever in the early stages of labor administered as a decoction or tea. The glycosides [more specifically prunasin] in the bark, once broken apart in the body, act on the smooth muscles lining the bronchioles, relaxing them and relieving coughs.

Wild black cherry can often be confused with choke cherry, which is similar in appearance and is sometimes used as an adulterant to the true black cherry bark. The two were often confused in early pharmacopoeias and it was not until the work of Jacob Friedrich Ehrhart[108] [1742-1795] that the choke cherry and wild black cherry were formally distinguished as two different species and *Prunus serotina* was officially named.

---

108   A German botanist, Ehrhart was a pupil and friend of Linnaeus. His body of work is housed at Moscow State University in Moscow, Russia.

The 21ˢᵗ Edition of the United States Dispensatory lists wild black cherry as an official drug plant described as having the effects of simple bitters but used primarily to flavor cough syrup.

Description

Mature specimens have attained heights of 100 feet with a trunk diameter of 4 feet but most are found between 50 and 80 feet high with a trunk between 2 and 3 feet around. The bark on the adult tree is black and rough. The younger, smaller branches are smooth and reddish in color. Bark on younger trees is a deep reddish-brown color. The youngest twigs and young trees are characterized by prominent cross-marks called "freckles" or lenticels. This outer bark separates naturally from the trunk in slender thin strips called laminate.

The leaves are oval to oblong shaped, 3 to 5 inches in length, dark green and shiny alternating on reddish stems. The tree flowers in May in most areas of the United States with a beautiful display of small white flowers born on long structures called racemes, reminiscent somewhat in shape to the wisteria. The fruit ripens in August and September forming first as small dark red berries about the size of an English pea. As they ripen they turn to purplish-black in clusters around 3 to 6 inches in length similar in structure to that of grapes. The cherries are an important food source for birds who obligingly carry the seeds throughout their range.

Wild black cherry can be distinguished from choke cherry by its choice of habitat, the appearance of its trunk and bark, leaves, by the fruit and the odor of the bark. For purposes of Wildcrafting, black cherry is more often to be seen in the true forest setting whereas choke cherry is most often seen around swamps at higher elevations. The young seedlings of both varieties are often found in great numbers along power lines and other structures used by resting birds.

The mature black cherry is a much larger tree than choke cherry. The choke cherry is classified as a tall shrub or small tree not often found over 30 feet tall. The straight trunk of the black cherry in full sun will often grow to 30 feet before putting out limbs. The choke cherry frequently has a twisted or crooked trunk with a narrow and irregular crown.

The outer bark of the black cherry is black, sometimes dark reddish brown to black depending upon the age of the tree, roughly breaking into stiff, thin scales. Choke cherry bark is smooth and does not peel easily. It is a dark reddish-brown to grayish-brown. When scraped the bark of the choke cherry gives off an unpleasant odor whereas the scraped bark of the black gives off an aromatic, medicinal scent. The young branches and stems of the black cherry are reddish in color, freckled by immature lenticels, but in the choke cherry they are smooth and gray.

The leaves of the black cherry are larger and slightly more oval in shape. The choke cherry leaves are a thin, dull green with a greenish, hairy underside. Choke cherry leaves are smoother than the black and their ridge veins slightly less pronounced. The taste of the fruit of both trees is decidedly different and, in addition to the difference in the appearance of the bark, is the definitive factor in identification. The fruit of the black cherry is slightly astringent but palatable whereas the fruit of the choke cherry tastes sweet at first but soon causes a drying and choking sensation in the throat and mouth which takes some time to wear off. The tree is aptly named.

The dried fruit of both trees is an important source of winter forage by both humans and animals. The dried cherries are a great winter favorite of birds.

Growing Conditions and Propagation

Pollinated by insects and wind, propagated most often by birds the wild black cherry is a true deep forest dweller, however, younger specimens can often be found growing in hedge-rows, open woods and along roadsides. In some areas it is so successful it is classified as a noxious invasive. It prefers full sun in good soil that has adequate moisture but should not be subject to standing water for any great length of time. The tree grows very quickly, sometimes putting on between 30 to 36 inches of height in a single growing season.

An area for planting needs some planning and fore-thought as it is a messy tree. If planted over patios, roofs or driveways the fruit has to be swept up because when crushed underfoot they stain wooden patios and concrete a dark reddish purple. Birds are attracted in great numbers to the trees adding their own contribution to the cleanup. Once an appropriate space has been selected, the quickest method of propagation for the homeowner is to transplant a young tree, not over 3 or 4 feet tall from the wild.

For seed collection purposes identify the tree in the spring as it begins to flower and mark the trunk with spray paint or a brightly colored ribbon. Visit the area frequently during the growing season. Watch the fruit as it matures in August and September subjecting it to a taste test when the fruit is fully ripened. Collect the seeds when they are withered and leathery. Always take more than needed and always plant more than needed. Plant seeds 1 to 1 ½ inch deep in prepared soil in full sun. Watch the area for seedlings the following spring and thin accordingly. If planted for use as a medicinal the new plants should be spaced 3 to 4 feet apart and allowed to grow until needed.

Harvesting

The root bark is considered the most desirable part of the tree for medicinal purposes; however, bark is taken from all parts of the tree. The age of the tree is a factor. Bark is collected only from the roots, branches or trunks of young trees or from the youngest or newest growth of larger older trees. The bark is at its best when collected in the fall of the year.

The outer layer or cork is peeled away or scraped off with a sharp knife and the inner bark, slightly reddish in color, is cut into appropriate lengths and dried. A heat source such as a home oven is ideal although the bark can be cut, tied into bundles if necessary, placed in a warm area away from the light and protected from rain and moisture during the drying process. When the bark is completely dry, it can be chopped into pieces for use as a decoction or tea. The usual dosage is 1 teaspoonful of the dried bark infused in boiling water for 10 to 15 minutes and then drunk. The remaining bark can be pulverized or powdered by grinding. Very small amounts of very dry bark can then be processed in a home blender or food processor.

Dried bark is carefully stored in airtight containers and labeled as to contents and date. It cannot be kept longer than 12 months as it deteriorates with age.

Use in the Edgar Cayce Readings

As a true companion plant wild black cherry is mentioned over 300 times in a great variety of physical conditions ranging from adhesions to arthritis, from coughs to debilitation and in cases of edema, hypertension and rheumatism. It is used as syrup, an essence, a pectoral,[109] a fluid extract, an elixir and as a tincture.

---

109   Treats the chest.

Wild black cherry is most often used as a carrier, or a base or foundation upon which, in that directive so unique to the Cayce system other ingredients are added *"in the order named."* The living chemical building blocks of all other ingredients are precisely placed in a specific sequence in constructing or compounding the Cayce formula.

The following are only a few of the hundreds of ways wild black cherry is used in the Cayce system:

979-8 F 66 DEBILITATION:GENERAL

5. Then we would begin, after this has acted upon the system, with a stimulant and a tonic and a help for the cough - which may act as a builder-up for an appetite and be a general help for the body throughout. Prepare same in this manner:

6. To 2 ounces of Strained Honey add 2 ounces of Distilled Water. Let this come to a boil. Skim that which arises. Set aside to cool, and as soon as cool add - in the order named:

> Wild Cherry Bark - as an elixir or pectoral,
> you see; as an elixir, not as a syrup but as
> an elixir or as a fusion...............1 ounce,
> Syrup of Horehound......................1 ounce,
> Syrup of Rhubarb.....................1/2 ounce,
> Elixir of Calisaya...................1/2 ounce.
> Sufficient Apple Brandy to make the whole quantity
> come to 8 ounces.

Shake this together and take about every three hours; of course except at night - teaspoonful every three hours, but do not take it through the evening.

643-1 M Adult Cancer:Tendencies Assimilation:Eliminations:Incoordination

9. We would also prepare a compound to be taken internally to work with the blood supply, and to create an activity with the glands and the assimilating system as to alleviate the conditions; so that not only may there be the overcoming by the releasing of oxygen for the blood supply through the Ash and the electrical forces in same - that give a surcharge, as it were, to the red blood cells themselves - but that the eliminations and assimilations and activity of glands - through this compound of properties - may aid in creating the CORRECT balance for the body. It would be prepared, then, as follows:

10. To 32 ounces of DISTILLED water, we would add [each ingredient to be CRUSHED before adding, but added in the order named]:

> Wild Cherry Bark.................2 ounces,
> Sarsaparilla Root...............1 ounce,
> Wild Ginseng....................1 ounce,
> Indian Turnip.................1/2 ounce,
> Yellow Dock Root................1 ounce,
> Buchu Leaves....................1 dram,
> Mandrake Root.................15 grains.

Reduce this by slow boiling to 16 ounces. Strain while warm and add [while still warm] 3 ounces of grain alcohol with 1 dram Balsam of Tolu cut in same. Shake the solution well together before the dose is taken, which would be a teaspoonful 4 times each day - before the meals and before retiring.

In the following Cayce volunteers a rare explanation of the action of each ingredient in the formula as well as the unusual admonition to collect the bark from the north side of the tree:

2790-1 F 23 HYPOGASTRALGIA

5. To relieve the condition for this body we would keep those forces for the system much as we have at the present time. We would only take those of a stimulation to the body to give the correct vibration through the system with the air and water as is being shown or given in the body, as in this:

6. To one gallon of rain water we would add:

>   Wild Cherry Bark...............4 ounces,
>   preferably from the North
>   side of the tree,
>   Yellow Root...................2 ounces,
>   Red Root......................2 ounces,
>   Prickly Ash Bark..............1 ounce,
>   Elder Flower..................1 ounce.

7. Reduce this by simmering, not boiling, to one quart, strain, while warm add:

>   Balm of Gilead................2 drams,
>   Grain Alcohol.................6 ounces.

8. The dose with this would be teaspoonful four times each day before meals. The effect with this on the system is to give the stimulation to the organs and to the eliminating forces in the system, as in this:

9. The active principle from the Wild Cherry Bark with the other ingredients is a stimulation to the lungs, throat and bronchials and those organs above the diaphragm.

10. The Yellow Root is for the pneumogastric forces and gastric juices of the pyloric end of the stomach itself.

11. The Red Root is a stimulus for the secretions given by the pancrean forces and the spleen in its functioning from the blood cell forces as destroyed there.

12. The Prickly Ash Bark is for the blood supply as acted upon in the emunctory forces of the liver itself proper.

13. The Elder Flower is as that in the functioning of the organs of the pelvis with the action of the kidneys, with the stimulation from the alcohol and Balm of Gilead in these organs.

This simple and effective expectorant is easily made at home:

4. We would ALSO prepare as this, as an expectorant and as an active force in the system, that will give appetite, will give stimulation to the blood supply, will give those proper activities in the system:

5. Take 4 ounces Wild Cherry Bark, put this in 32 ounces of distilled water. Reduce this to 1/2 the quantity. To this we would add:

> Syrup of Horehound......................1/2 ounce,
> COMPOUND Syrup of Sarsaparilla........1/2 ounce.

Cut 2 ounces of rock candy in 1/2 pint of Spirits Frumenti, until it is all dissolved, and add to the solution Spirits Frumenti - see - 1/2 pint [4 ounces]. The dose [and this should be shaken together before dose is taken] would be a full teaspoonful at least twice each day, in the morning and in the afternoon - NOT at meal time.

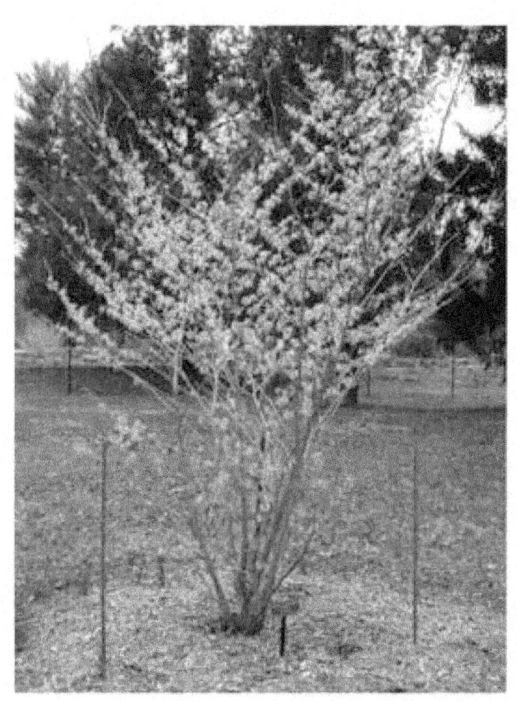
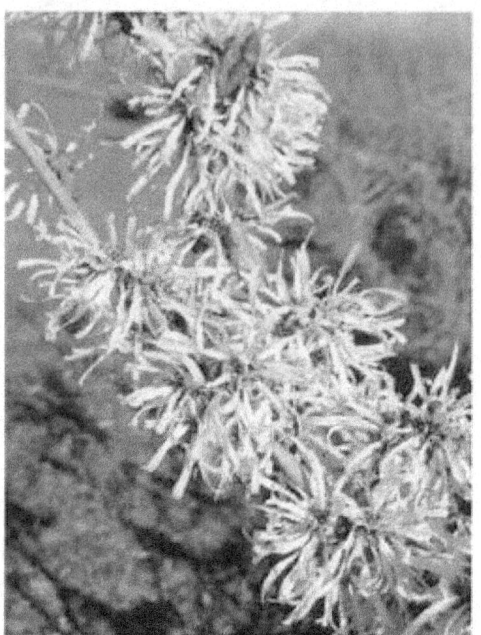
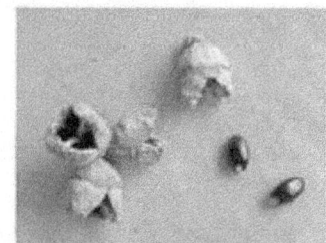
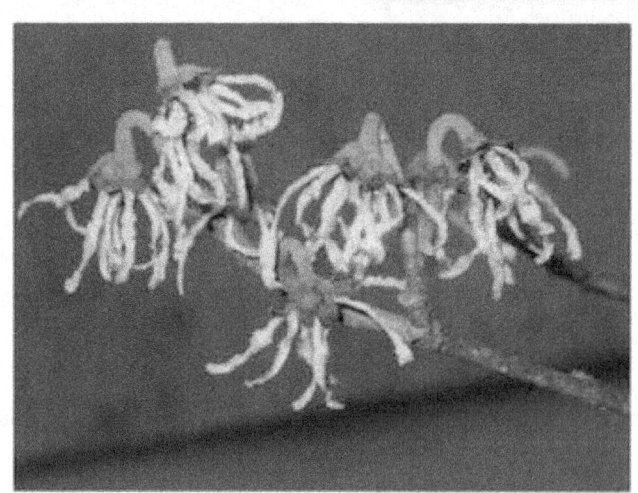

WITCH HAZEL
Hamamelis virginiana, Fam. Hamamelidaceae

Common and Regional Names
Witchhazel, Spotted Hazel, Striped Alder, Winterbloom, Snapping Hazel, Common Witchhazel

History and Common Usage
Witch hazel was brought to the attention of western medicine in the United States during the early settlement period by the Native Americans who used it to stop bleeding, as a sedative, in eye infections, and as a topical application in the treatment of external inflammation and painful tumors. It is often cited as being a native of what is today the state of Arkansas with a modern range extending throughout the Eastern and Central United States.

The properties of both the bark and leaves owe their utility to their action on the muscular fiber of veins, especially in the treatment of bleeding varicose veins, where a moistened pad will stop the bleeding. Diluted witch hazel is also used as eyewash. It is very effective as a topical astringent and antiseptic for burns and scalds in the kitchen, in cases of insect bites, and for the relief of hemorrhoids. A salve is easily made at home by compounding of 2 ½ to 3 grains powdered extract of the bark combined with an ounce or two of pure melted cacao butter. Witch hazel is commercially available today in the form of pads, wipes and ointments for the relief of hemorrhoids and in skin care products, creams and soaps.

The bark and leaves [which are official in the current U.S. Pharmacopoeia] contain tannic and gallic acids. United States and British Pharmacopeias during the time the Cayce information was being given cite both the dried bark and the fresh and dried leaves of *Hamamelis virginiana* as an official preparation as a local astringent and a haemostatic and for other conditions *"in which tannin is used."*

Description
Witch hazel is a perennial shrub which can also be found as a small tree. It grows anywhere from 5 to 30 feet tall. Shrubs can spread to a circumference as wide as 25 feet with many trunks. The leaves are fairly large and upright, dark green and veined, 3 to 6 inches in length and scalloped at the edges. Bright yellow flowers appear in the fall from October to December and can often be seen under snow. The thread-like, long-lived blossoms can last up to a month, closing up when it becomes too cold and re-opening in the sun. They can often be seen on the same branch with the brilliant gold of last years leaves providing both long lived color and their delicate citrus like fragrance to enjoy throughout the fall and early winter months.

Growing Conditions and Propagation
Witch hazel prefers dappled sun. They are usually seen along the lightly shaded areas at the edge of forests. Yet they are also completely adaptable to full sun where they put on great height and circumference with a spectacular showing of their blossoms against a snowy landscape. They prefer moist well-drained acidic soils which are typical of forest settings. Witch hazel makes a very satisfactory choice for the homeowner and is becoming popular in landscape plantings due to their unusual habit of blooming in the late fall and winter months.

Witch hazel is pollinated by insects and wind and propagates by seeds which are ejected violently from the ripe seed pods giving rise to one of the common names, snapping hazelnut. The seeds can be collected in the wild and germinated in prepared seed-beds in their permanent location or in peat pots for easier transplanting to a permanent location. Young bushes can also be transplanted from the wild or purchased from nurseries. Witch hazel is very resistant to insect infestations and disease. It is a slow growing shrub often putting on less than a foot of height per year, and will only need pruning to thin out unwanted twigs, which can be saved for extraction purposes if desired.

Harvesting
The fresh leaves can be bruised, crushed and used as a poultice for infections and inflammations and to check bleeding. Steeped leaves and flowers yield a weak astringent that can be used as a lotion for relief of insect bites and sores.

All parts of the bush are used in distilling the astringent which is then preserved by the addition of grain alcohol. Pruning can yield twigs and leaves for home use, but for serious distillation projects a wild stand is needed. The branches are cut to the ground and cut or chopped into pieces suitable for handling. The roots are left to re-grow a new bush. Without distillation equipment extraction of the astringent properties from witch hazel can be only imperfectly accomplished through maceration and decoction.

Use in the Edgar Cayce Readings
Witch hazel is used alone and as a companion plant. Cited over 300 times it is used more than any other additive in cabinet sweats and steam or fume baths, and occasionally in combination with other tinctures. It is used topically for massage often combined with other oils and as a solution used with the Wet-Cell Appliance,[110] usually alternated with gold, silver and camphor. The following are ways witch hazel is used topically:

Massage
294-181 M 57 Bruises:Strains
2. In the bruises on the chest and arm we would massage equal parts of mutton tallow, turpentine, camphor and Witchhazel - stirred together; then apply HEAT - when the body is ready to rest, you see. This will remove the strains in the muscular forces.

646-4 F Adult Pruritis
11. [Q] What should be done for annoying itching on front of lower part of right leg?
[A] These massages and corrections should relieve this. But should it continue, we would massage same with a small quantity of witchhazel, which will burn for the time being but will alleviate the itching.

2679-1 F 24 Physiotherapy :Massage:Cocoa Butter:Scars
6. And while we would continue the use of the massage with Cocoa Butter, we would alternate this with a massage using three parts Peanut Oil and one part Witchhazel, - which would prevent there being so much scar tissue and less apt for any recurrent conditions from same. While the Peanut Oil and one part Witchhazel do not mix, put them in a container sufficiently large to shake well before being poured out to be massaged, - all about the areas of those injuries and bruises, and where there have been these. It will not only be soothing but, as indicated, will aid in prevention of further disturbances in the future. Alternate these, using the Cocoa Butter one time and the Peanut Oil-Witchhazel combination the next time, see?

---

110   The Heritage Store 314 Laskin Road, Virginia Beach, Virginia 23451 757-428-0500 http://www.heritagestore.com/

In the Cayce model witch hazel is used more frequently than any other additive to fume baths and steam baths. The following two excerpts are examples of recommendations for hydrotherapy:

Cabinet Sweat and Steam or Fume Additive

826-14 M 40 Relaxation

14. Occasionally have not only an exercise that tires the muscles but a perfect relaxation, as with the hydrotherapy treatments, - not merely a steam bath but a fume bath, with witchhazel as the fumes, and the rubdown with oils that may be assimilated for stimulating disturbances to the superficial circulation. In the fume bath use a little dry heat, but MORE the fume from Witchhazel in water that may settle over the body in the cabinet, see? The proportions would be an ounce of the Witchhazel to four ounces of water in a croup cup or the like, or in an open container in the closed cabinet. These will aid the body. Have these with the rubdowns at least once each week. Then have the rubdown with Peanut Oil, - if the body would never have arthritis or neuritic reactions.

2543-4 F 34 Dermatitis

12. The hydrotherapy treatment, now, would be changed from the manner in which this has been given. We do not mean to have a colonic irrigation each week, but do each week have a mild sweat with the Fume Bath. The Fumes should carry Witchhazel; about two teaspoonsful of Witchhazel to a pint of boiling water in croup cup or in an open container that allows the fumes to settle over the body. The hydrotherapy treatments that have been given have been fairly good, but these should now be given a little bit differently. Let there be more of Fume Bath than that of the Dry Cabinet heat, see; preferably an ALL FUME Bath - the heat coming entirely from the boiling water in the cabinet, with the fumes rising from same.

The following excerpts are examples of how witch hazel is used as a solution for the Wet Cell Appliance:

Use With The Wet-Cell Appliance

1128-1 F Adult ADHESIONS TUMORS

6. First we would use the Wet Cell Appliance, carrying Spirits of Camphor one day and the regular strength Witchhazel solution the next day, through the low electrical vibrations. If the anode or lead lead that passes through the solution is CLEANSED each time after using, it may be used for both solutions. However, it would be preferable to prepare two anodes, one to carry the Camphor and the one to carry the Witchhazel - for these would be alternated as indicated.

3553-1 F 10 EARS:DEAFNESS

10. Begin with the use of the Wet Cell Appliance carrying to the body vibratorially, alternately, Gold and Witchhazel.

11. The plates would be a little bit different for this particular disturbance in the body. While the nickel plate would always be attached to the umbilical lacteal duct center, the small copper plate connections would vary.

12. The Witchhazel should be used twice to the Gold once, and the copper plate would be attached at the 1st and 2nd cervical centers, and use it for half an hour at each period two days in succession, the Witchhazel would be used commercial strength and use four ounces.

13. The third day, when using the Gold Solution in the proportions of one grain Chloride of Gold Sodium to each ounce of distilled water - and use three ounces, attach the small plate to the 3rd dorsal center, - between the 2nd and 3rd dorsal center. This would be for thirty minutes, every third day.

14. The Appliance would be made with the regular charge solution.

15. Keep the attachment plates very clean. Disconnect from Appliance when not in use. Connect it at least twenty minutes before they are to be applied to the body. Clean when taking from the body, clean when being applied to the body.

16. The larger plate would always be attached to the umbilical and lacteal duct center which for this body will be the width of two fingers to the right from the navel center, one finger up from that point. This would be the nurse's fingers, not the child's fingers. Change the charging solution every thirty days, also changing the Gold Solution, as well as the Witchhazel.

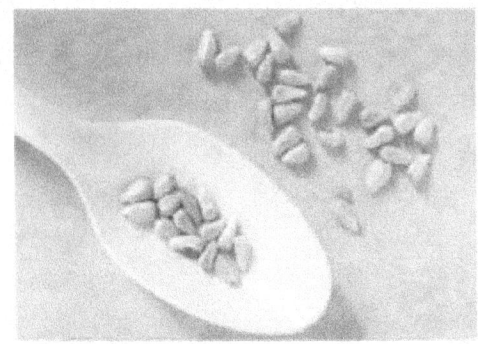

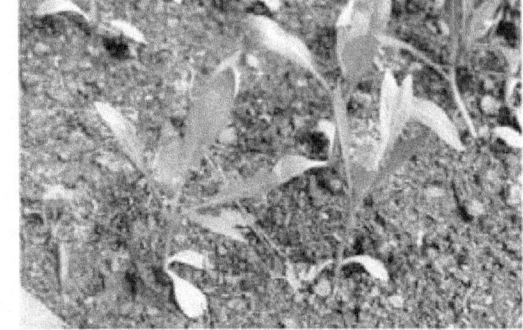

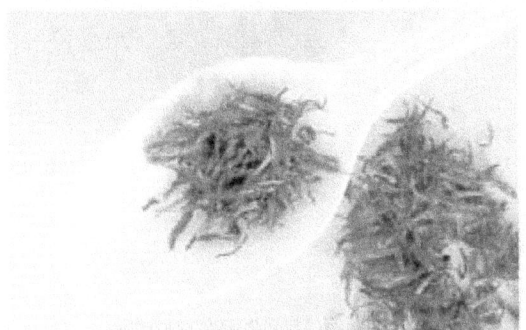

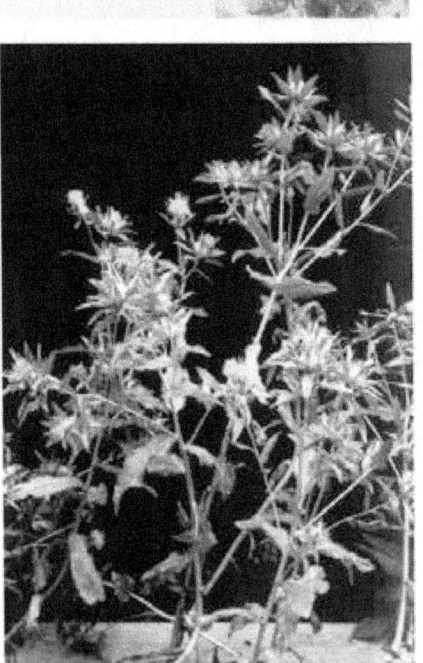

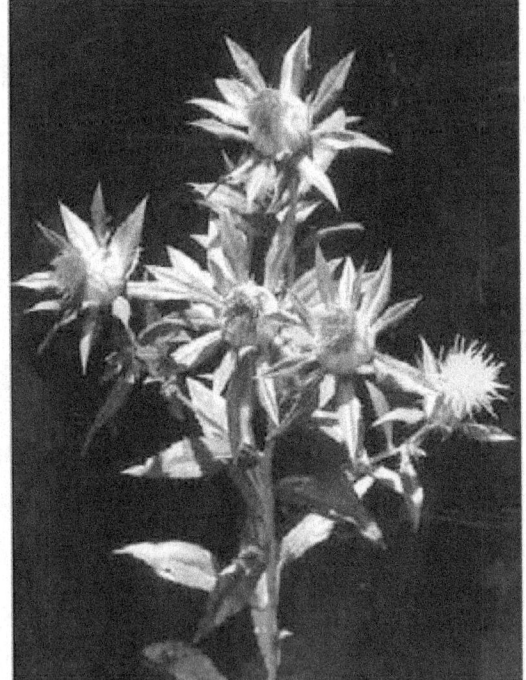

YELLOW AMERICAN SAFFRON
Carthamus tinctorius, Fam. Asteraceae

Common and Regional Names
False saffron, Safflower, African Safflower, Bastard Saffron, Dyers' Saffron, American Saffron, Parrot Seed

History and Common Usage
Yellow american saffron does not command a large presence in traditional herbal medicine. Its historical importance has been mainly as a dye plant. The botanical name *Carthamus* derives from the Arabic verb *kurthum*, or the English word "dye" in reference to the use of safflower flowers as dye. The name saffron comes from the Arabic *zafaran*, which means "yellow." As a source of red dye and because it was so costly[111] it soon made its way to the status of a forbidden colour in the Japanese court during the Heian Period [794-1192 A.D.] where, called kurenai red, only women of the highest rank could wear silk dyed this gentle and elegant color. *Carthamus tinctorius* will also produce yellow, orange and red in linen and cotton. It has long been used in India as a source of brilliant peach, pink and clear yellow colors.

Believed to have originated in southern Asia, the plant is found naturalized in Iran, Kazakhstan, Africa, and from central India to the Nile River, into Ethiopia.

Carthamus tinctorius was not used medicinally by the Egyptians but they used the seeds extensively for oil; the flowers were used in wreaths in both fresh and dried arrangements and extensively as a dye. The seeds have been found in Egyptian tombs dating to 4,000 years ago. Pliny the Elder mentions a plant used by the Egyptians which his translators have identified as the *Carthamus tinctorius* of Linnaeus which is also called bastard saffron. *"The Egyptians have many other plants also, of little note; but they speak in the highest terms of the cnecos; a plant unknown to Italy, and which the Egyptians hold in esteem, not as an article of food, but for the oil it produces, and which is extracted from the seed. The principal varieties are the wild and the cultivated kinds; of the wild variety, again, there are two sorts, one of which is less prickly than the other..."[112]* The Book of Medicines mentions *Carthamus tinctorius* only twice, once in a general way and once in a prescription combined with 9 other ingredients given for jaundice and constipation.

During the Middle Ages *Carthamus tinctorius* began to be cultivated in Italy, France and Spain and during the discovery voyages of the Spanish it was taken to Mexico, Venezuela and Colombia. Commercially introduced into the United States from the Mediterranean region in roughly 1925, the plant is now grown in all temperate zones, concentrated in western Nebraska and eastern Colorado, although California began commercial cultivation in 1949 and can now claim fifty percent of the total American acreage.

The flowers, ground into a fine powder, are used in the cosmetic industry as a tinting additive in facial talc for rouge. The seeds are sold in bulk as bird-seed and are both edible and nutritious. They are usually eaten roasted or fried, and, as in the time of the Egyptians, they are an important source of cooking oil. Saffron oil contains a lower percentage of saturated fatty acids than other edible vegetable seed oils, and for this reason it is used in salad dressings, margarine and is widely available as cooking oil marketed under the brand name Safflower. It is also used in candles, paints and varnish.

---

111   To dye a single pair of silk pants requires two pounds of petals.
112   Chapter 53. – FOUR VARIETIES OF THE CNECOS.

Yellow american saffron is often confused with one of the most expensive spices in the world: *Crocus sativus,* also commonly called saffron crocus, saffron flower, yellow saffron or Spanish saffron. It is expensive because only the 3 stigmas of each flower are used, and each one is picked by hand. Grown commercially in Greece, India, Iran and Spain it can be grown in any area where the crocus grows. It can also be used in place of yellow american saffron if price is no object. Yellow american is also called "false saffron" because it has sometimes been used to adulterate the more expensive true saffron and sadly today many suppliers, especially Indian suppliers, adulterate the true yellow american saffron with marigold petals.

Yellow american saffron was not an official drug plant at the time the Cayce information was being given. It is listed in the 21st edition of the US Pharmacopeia as an unofficial plant, *"used in domestic practice…in measles, scarlatina…to promote the eruption."*

Description

Carthamus tinctorius is a relative of the much larger sunflower. It grows from 1 to 4 feet in height bearing flowers that may be yellow, orange, reddish orange, or upon occasion even white. The plant has a thistle-like appearance, coarse and branching, with a somewhat leggy stem which often requires support. Each plant bears one to five flowers on each stem from which anywhere from 15 to 50 seeds are produced. The flowers range from ½ inch across to the extreme of 2 1/2 inches.

As the plant enters the flower bud stage, stiff spines develop on the edges of the leaves. Because this also makes it moderately uncomfortable to walk through massed plantings, the home gardener might give thought to planting in rows approximately 18 to 24 inches rather than concentrated stands of flowers.

Growing Conditions and Propagation

Yellow american saffron can be easily grown in the home garden. It likes full sun and thrives in the same conditions as wheat, barley and oats. It is pollinated by wind and insects and propagates by seeds. Seeds can be planted in April or May. It is sometimes called a "long day" plant because it requires between 12 to 14 hours of sunlight. It should not be planted later in the season than the middle of May as in most areas the growing season will not be long enough for maturation. It does not easily naturalize except under ideal conditions as other plants can overshadow it before it can become established. Once the plant is well established, it tolerates some shade and a few weeds and requires only adequate soil moisture from planting through flowering to produce an abundant crop of flowers and seeds. It responds well to the same watering and fertilization guidelines as any other garden vegetable or flower.

Seeds can be broadcast by hand for mass plantings, covered lightly with a layer of soil or planted in rows about a ½ inch deep with 18 to 24 inches between rows. Seedlings can be expected to emerge in one to three weeks depending on weather conditions. The flowers are formed in late June and begin to bloom in June to late July. The bloom stage lasts two to three weeks, and the plant goes to seed about four weeks after flowering is completed.

The home gardener should plan on having to provide support for the plants as they grow so that the flowers don't come in contact with the soil. They can be staked or gathered into bunches and loosely held by string or twine. Wire cages such as those used for tomato plants can also be used, gathering a number of plants inside the cage for support.

The plant does well when regular weeding keeps its root territory free from competition, especially critical until young plants are well established. Once established the yellow american saffron can develop a taproot from eight to ten inches long if the soil and moisture conditions are favorable.

Harvesting

Flowers can be harvested over a two to three week period. If they are grown for use as tea the petals are picked only when they have begun to dry on the plant and when they display the reddish/orange color so characteristic of the tea. If picked in the early stages while still bright yellow and dried they will remain bright yellow and the action of the tea will not be the same as those allowed to "ripen" on the plant. The petals should be picked early in the morning when they have begun to wither slightly and darken in color. Continue picking each day until the blooming season has ended. The tiny petals will still be somewhat moist and should be spread thinly and evenly on a clean, dry surface and carefully picked over to remove any other extraneous material. They should be kept out of direct sunlight until dry but still pliable. If powdered saffron is desired, they should be dried to the brittle stage and pulverized for storage.

Drying is completed in 2 or 3 days. The material is sealed in small plastic freezer bags or in small glass jars. Both glass jars and plastic bags should be stored out of the light in the household pantry or even in the freezer, and if kept from moisture the tea will keep for 2 to 3 years.

Yellow american saffron matures in 110 to 150 days from planting and seeds can be collected when the plant has dried completely and turned brown. Since the dried seed pods are very spiny light gloves should be worn. They are shaken over a container and then manually opened to extract the rest of the seeds. Whitish fuzz will be seen around the seed heads, which should be rubbed off and discarded. They are then stored in the usual manner for the next year's planting.

Use in the Edgar Cayce Readings

Yellow american saffron is used alone and as a companion plant. Mentioned in 248 transcripts it is credited as being a "good for everybody" digestive aid. It coats the lining of the stomach and purifies the intestinal tract. It is often alternated with powdered slippery elm bark. A cup of mild yellow american saffron tea is taken in the morning, and a small pinch of powdered slippery elm bark is taken in all drinking water throughout the rest of the day. In one case the two were to be taken three to five hours apart:

4638-1 M Adult
19. [Q] Should the elm water and Saffron be mixed together, or taken alternately?
[A] The elm water taken as drink. The Saffron taken as medicinal properties.

20. [Q] How often?
[A] Three to five hours apart.

If price is no object the "true" or Spanish saffron can be used as shown in the following, but Cayce clearly states the yellow american saffron is "more uniform":

5200-1 F 56 Tumors
8. Also take internally, about 3 times each week, Yellow Saffron Tea, or the Spanish Saffron, though the Yellow American Saffron would be preferable, as it will be more uniform. Take a pinch between

thumb and forefinger, put into a teacup, fill with boiling water. Cover and let stand for thirty to thirty-five minutes, strain, cool and drink.

9. Also, once during each day do take a pinch of Elm Bark. This should be prepared much in the same manner, though this should be let stand for at least an hour and a half, cool and drink.

428-12 F 58 Eliminations
14. [Q] Is the American Saffron alright?
[A] The American Saffron will be found to be most helpful. This is really preferable to the Spanish Saffron, which is much more expensive

Yellow american saffron is recommended for conditions ranging from acne to baby care, from ulcers of the stomach, intestines and mouth to intestinal hemorrhages and on through the alphabetical list of diseases to vertigo. Its special magic, however, is in the treatment of psoriasis. The Cayce system describes psoriasis as a thinning of the intestinal walls causing the body's own waste products to be picked up by the lymph system and carried to the skin:

289-1 M 46
7. [Q] Please give me the cause and cure for the so-called psoriasis with which I am troubled.
[A] The cause is the thinning of the walls of the intestinal system, which allows the escaping of poisons - or the absorption of same by the muco-membranes which surround same, and becomes effective in the irritation through the lymph and emunctory reactions in the body.

2455-2 F 28
20. [Q] Is there an absolute cure for psoriasis?
[A] Most of this is found in diet. There is a cure. It requires patience, persistence - and right thinking also.

Treatment of psoriasis consists of chiropractic or osteopathic treatments and adjustments of the spine, colonic irrigations especially helpful in severe cases, taking powdered slippery elm bark alternated with yellow american saffron tea and dietary changes which must be strictly followed for the duration of the treatment period. The action of yellow american saffron is as follows:

745-1 F Adult Psoriasis
13. First, then, we would change the CHARACTER of water taken by the body. There should be no water taken unless carrying elm bark or Yellow Saffron tea. While these may be in small quantities, the effect of these upon the gastric flow throughout the stomach, throughout the activity of the organs of the system, will so stimulate the walls of the organs themselves as to bring HEALING to those portions that are distressed...

For anyone suffering from Psoriasis it bears repeating that there is no better recommendation than a book mentioned earlier entitled HEALING PSORIASIS: The Natural Alternative, [113] by John O.A. Pagano in which the causes and treatment are so clearly laid out for the reader as to completely de-mystify this troubling disorder. A second valuable book is Dr. John's Healing Psoriasis Cookbook...Plus![114] which is

---

113   Available from John Wiley & Sons. See also the Pagano Organization, Inc., at http://www.psoriasis-healing.com/

114   Available from The Pagano Organizations, Inc., 35 Hudson Terrace, Englewood Cliffs, NJ 07632 (201) 947-0606 and http://www.psoriasis-healing.com/

a collection of over 300 very tasty kitchen-tested recipes compiled to help the psoriasis suffer more easily make the necessary dietary changes.

The following testimony speaks to the efficacy of yellow american saffron:

5016-1 Psoriasis
6/11/76
"When I received the Circulating File on psoriasis I had it over 95% of my body.

"I started chiropractic treatment, putting a castor oil pack with heating pad on my abdomen once each night for an hour and started using saffron tea. I also stopped eating all refined foods.

"What I believe really helped me was the saffron tea. I drink one cup of this strained tea in the morning and one cup at night. All I have left of my psoriasis is a tiny patch on elbow or knee. I can't remember how long it took to clear up so nicely, but I know it didn't take long. I have been in this improved condition for a year and a half now.
"Every time I stop taking the tea for a day or so I immediately start itching all over and pretty soon little patches appear."
A.R.E. Member, Margaret Meyer:

Some individuals learn they are sensitive to certain foods or beverages and from that time on they know what they need to avoid. A few will find they have what might be called a "trigger food" that will even cause a flare up or an allergic reaction. Sometimes this can be quite severe as the following young woman discovered.

R26. 6/3/93 Kim Wagenet's report: "I am 34 year old female, who has had PSORIASIS since the age of 12. I have been through all of the chemical treatments, Stanford's Psoriasis Clinic, and still had psoriasis on some area of my body.

I received from a friend, a Research Bulletin on Psoriasis, from the Edgar Cayce Foundation. I read through the diet & herb list given, along with the mention of … Rochelle Salts…

I followed the diet, as well as I could, eliminating red meats fried foods, sugars – candy – white flours, etc. I included right thinking, meditation & prayer.
Within 3 months, I had no psoriasis anywhere. This lasted for almost 1 year – until chocolate became again.

We are not talking of spots of psoriasis, here or there, I looked like a Armadillo, with cracks & sores, having to cauterize a lot of the cracks so they would heal.

Thank you very much!

[signed] Kim Wagenet
P.S. I'm going away from chocolate!

Yellow American Saffron and Companions

Following are samples of the way yellow american saffron is used internally combined with some of its companion plants.

4368-1 F Adult Debilitation:General

7. To the first, this should be in each capsule:

        Podophyllin.................1/2 grain,
        Leptandrin...............1 1/2 grain,
        Sanguinaria..................1 grain.

8. Make five of these, one taken every other day.

        Cascara Sagrada............1/2 grain,
        Licorice Compound.............1 grain,
        Senna......................1/2 grain,
        Yellow Saffron [powdered]....1 grain.

10. These will make large capsules on account of the Saffron, but would be taken every other evening until five are taken.

3899-3 M Adult Eliminations

10. To correct this condition we must reach higher than has been used in this system. Give to the system this: For one dose –

        Senna..............1 grain,
        Licorice..........1 grain,
        Rhubarb...........1 grain,
        Yellow Saffron....2 grains.

This is one dose in a capsule to be taken twice a day [night and morning for one day]. It is then taken only every fifth day for 20 days. As this is taken well into the system, this is after it has been absorbed, use an exceedingly high enema to cleanse the descending colon, as well as the transverse colon, so that we give the force in the duodenum, and the pancrean juices proper force and incentive to give off enough to prevent this condition again coming into the system.

Bibliography and References

Agard, Walter R., introduction by C.H. Bunting. Medical Greek and Latin at a Glance – 2<u>nd</u> Edition Revised.. Paul B. Hoeber, Inc., Medical Book Department of Harper & Brothers. New York. New York. 1948

American Druggist Pharmacy Handbook. The Official Drugs of Animal and Vegetable Origin. American Druggist. New York, New York. 1938.

American Pharmaceutical Association. The National Formulary on Unofficial Preparations – 3<u>rd</u> Edition. American Pharmaceutical Association. Baltimore, Maryland. 1906.

Anonymous. The Compleat Herbal: Or The Botanical Institutions of Mr. Tournefort, Chief Botanist to the Late French King, Carefully Translated from the Original Latin. Bonwicke, Goodwin, Walthoe, Wotton, Manship, Wilkin, Tooke, Smith and Ward. London, England. 1719.

Arey, Leslie Brainerd, William Burrows, J.P. Greenhill, Richard M. Hewitt, et. al. Dorland's Illustrated Medical Dictionary - 23<u>rd</u> Edition. W.B. Saunders Company. Philadelphia and London. 1957.

Bailey, L.H. and E.Z. Bailey, et al. Hortus Third: A Concise Dictionary of Plants Cultivated in the United States and Canada. New York, McMillan Publishing Company, 1976

Barrett, B. Sc. *The Tropical Crops*. New York. The MacMillan Co. 1928

Bastedo, Walter A., President, et. al. The Pharmacopoeia of the United States – 11<u>th</u> Edition. Mack Printing Company. Easton, Pennsylvania. 1936.

Bastedo, Walter A., President, et. al. The First Supplement To The Pharmacopoeia of the United States of America – 11<u>th</u> Decennial Revision [U.S.P. XI – 1937 Supplement] Mack Printing Company. Easton, Pennsylvania. 1937.

Beers, Mark H. and Robert Berkow, Editors, et al. The Merck Manual of Diagnosis And Therapy – 17<u>th</u> Edition. Merck Research Laboratories. Whitehouse Station, New Jersey. 1999

Bensky, D. and A. Gamble. Chinese Herbal Medicine, 2<u>nd</u> Edition. Eastland Press, Seattle. 1986

Biddle, J. Materia Medica and Therapeutics. P. Blakiston's Son & Co. Philadelphia. 1895.

Blakiston, P. Son and Company. Handbook of Materia Medica, Pharmacy and Therapeutics, Fifth Edition. P. Blakeston & Company of Philadelphia. 1895.

Boen, Dr. A New Mystery in Physick Discovered by During of Fevers and Agues by Quinquina or Jesuits Powder, a translation. London. 1682

Boericke, W. Pocket Manual Of Homeopathic Materia Medica and Repertory – And A Chapter on Rare and Uncommon Remedies. B. Jain Publishers [P] Ltd. New Delhi, India. 1996.

Bradley, P.R., ed. <u>British Herbal Compendium, Volume I.</u> British Herbal Medicine Association. Dorset. 1992

Brock, Arthur J. Greek Medicine – Being Extracts Illustrative of Medical Writers from Hippocrates to Galen. J.M. Dent & Sons, Ltd. London and Toronto. 1929.

Brown, Alice Cooke. <u>Early American Herb Recipes</u>. Bonanza Books, a division of Crown Publishers, Inc. New York, New York. 1966.

Brown, Charles N. <u>The Pharmacopeia and the Physician – The Use of Expectorants.</u> *Journal of the American Medical Association, Vol. 109, pp. 268-271.* American Medical Association. Chicago, Illinois. 1937

Bricklin, Mark, et al. <u>The Practical Encyclopedia of Natural Healing</u>. Rodale Press, Inc. Emmaus, Pennsylvania. 1976.

Bruneton, J. <u>Pharmacognosy, Phytochemistry - Medicinal Plants</u>. Intercept. Ltd. London, England. 1995.

Budge, E.A. Wallis. <u>The Book of Medicines</u>. Kegan Paul. London, New York, Bahrain. 2002

Chang, H.M. and P.P.H. <u>Pharmacology and Applications of Chinese Materia Medica.</u> World Scientific. Philadelphia. 1986.

Christopher, John R. <u>School of Natural Healing</u>. Christopher Publications. Springville, Utah. 1976.

Clarke, A. <u>Oxford Technical Publications, Flavoring Materials – Natural and Synthetic.</u>. Henry Frowde and Hodder & Stroughton. London, England. 1922.

Crellin, J.K. and J. Philpott. <u>Herbal Medicine, Past and Present – Volume II – A Reference Guide to Medicinal Plants</u>. Duke University Press. London. 1990

Crescent Books. <u>Herbs & Other Medicinal Plants</u>. IGDA, Novara. Italy. 1972

Council of the Pharmaceutical Society of Great Britain. The British Pharmaceutical Codex 1934. The Pharmaceutical Press. London. 1934.

Culbreth, David M.R. <u>A Manual of Materia Medica and Pharmacology</u>. Lea & Febiger. Philadelphia, Pennsylvania. 1927

Culpepper, Nicholas. The Complete Herbal. Nicholas Culpepper. London. 1653

Daumas, Francoise. <u>The Civilization of Ancient</u> Egypt. Arthaud, Paris, France. 1993

Dossiers of Archaeology No. 257. Editions Faton. 2000

Douglas, R. Gordon, Chairman et. al. <u>Formulary and Therapeutic Guide</u>. Appleton-Century-Crofts, Inc. USA. 1951

Duke, J.A. <u>CRC Handbook of Medicinal Herbs – 7<u>th</u> printing</u>. CRC Press. Boca Raton. 1989.

Duke, J.A. <u>CRC Handbook of Phytochemical Constituents of GRAS Herbs and Other Economic Plants</u>. CRC Press. Boca Raton. 1992

Duran-Reunals, M.L. The Fever Bark Tree. Doubleday and Company, Inc. New York. 1946.

Dunand, R. and R. Lichtenberg. <u>Mummies and Death in Egypt.</u>. Cornell University. Ithica, New York. 2006

Ebbell, Bendix. Translator. The Ebers Papyrus – The Greatest Egyptian Medical Document. Levin & Munksgaard. Ejnar Munksgaaard. Copenhagen, Denmark. 1937

<u>Encyclopedia Britannica</u>. William Benton Publisher. Chicago, London, Toronto. 1957.

Ellenhorn, M. and D.Barceloux. <u>Medical Toxicology Diagnosis and Treatment of Human Poisoning</u>. Elsevier. New York. 1988

<u>Era Formulary- 5000 Formulas for Druggists</u>. D.O. Haynes & Company. New York, New York. 1893.

Erdmann, E. Value of digitalis. An interview with Professor Dr. Erland Erdmann, Munich. <u>Mediziniche Monatsschrift fur Pharmazeuten</u>. Jan. 9. [2] pages 47-48. 1986.

Feldman, E.G. and D. Davidson. <u>Handbook of Nonprescription Drugs – 8<u>th</u> Edition.</u> American Pharmaceutical Association. Washington, D.C. 1986.

Felter, H.W. and J.U. Lloyd. <u>King's American Dispensatory.</u> The Ohio Valley Company. Cincinnati, Ohio. 1898.

Foster, Steven, ed. <u>Herbs of Commerce.</u> American Herbal Products Association. Austin, Texas. 1992.

Franco, Isabelle. <u>THE RITES AND BELIEFS OF ETERNITY.</u> Edité par PYMALION. France. 1993.

Gathercoal, Edmund N. and Elmer H. Wirth. <u>Pharmacognosy.</u> Lea & Febiger. Philadelphia, Pennsylvania. 1948.

Geiger, Peter, Philom. and Duncan, Sondra, Managing Editor. *The Farmers' Almanac, 2002.* Lewiston. 2002.

Ghalioungui, Paul. The Ebers Papyrus. A New English Translation, Commentaries and Glossaries. Academy of Scientific Research and Technology. Cairo, Egypt. 1987.

Gilman, A.G. et al. <u>Goodman and Gilman's The Pharmacological Basis of Therapeutics – 7th Edition</u>. Macmillan Publishing Company. New York, New York 1985.

Grieve,M. <u>A Modern Herbal</u>. Jonathan Cape. London, England. 1931.

Gupton, Oscar W., and Swope, Fred C. <u>Wildflowers of Tidewater Virginia</u>. University Press of Virginia. Charlottesville, Virginia. 1982.

Hall, Alan. <u>The Wild Food Trailguide – How To Locate and Identify Wild Foods</u>. Holt, Rinehart and Winston. Canada. 1976.

Hansen, Osca. <u>A Text-Book of Materia Medica and Therapeutics of Rare Homeopathic Remedies</u>. The Homeopathic Publishing Company. London, England. 1899

Harborne, J.and H.Baxter. <u>Phytochemical Dictionary</u>. Taylor and Francis. London, England. 1993.

Hardin,J.W. and J.M.Arena. <u>Human Poisoning from Native and Cultivated Plants – 2nd Edition</u>. Duke University Press. Durham, N.C. 1974.

Harshberger, John W. <u>Text-Book of Pastoral and Agricultural Botany – For The Study Of The Injurious And Useful Plants Of Country And Farm</u>. P. Blakiston's Son & Co. Philadelphia, Pennsylvania. 1920.

Hermann, Mathias, text. Engravings by Redoute, Daffinger, et. al. English translation by Grace Jackman. <u>Herbs and Medicinal Flowers</u>. Galahad Books. New York City, New York. 1973

Hechtlinger, Adelaide. The Great Patent Medicine Era or Without Benefit of Doctor. Galahad Books. New York. 1970.

Hoffman, D. <u>The Holistic Herbal</u>. The Findhorn Press. Findhorn, Scotland. 1983.

House, Homer D. <u>Wild Flowers</u>. The Macmillan Company. New York, New York. 1935.

Huff, B.B., ed. <u>Physicians' Desk Reference – 43rd Edition</u>. Medical Economics Company. Oradell, N.J. 1989.

Hylton, William H., ed., <u>Rodale Herb Book</u>. Rodale Press. Pennsylvania. 1974

Kartesz,J.T. A Synonymized Checklist of the Vascular Flora of the United States, Canada and Greenland, - 2nd Edition. Rimber Press. Portland, Oregon. 1994.

Kingzett, C.T. Chemical Encyclopaedia. D. Van Nostrand Company. New York, New York. 1932

Kirk, G.S., Raven, J.E.and Schofield, M. <u>The Presocratic Philosophers</u>. Cambridge University Press. Cambridge, England. 1957.

Kloss, Jethro. Back to Eden. Longview Publishing House. Tennessee. 1939.

Kourennoff, Paul M., English translation by George St. George. Russian Folk Medicine. Pyramid Books. New York, New York. 1971.

Krutch, Joseph Wood. HERBAL. David R. Godine. Boston, Massachusettes. 1976.

LaWall, Charles H. Four Thousand Years of Pharmacy – An Outline History of Pharmacy And The Allied Sciences. J.B. Lippincott Company. Philadelphia and London. 1927.

Lambert, A.B. An Illustration of Cinchona. Lost Cause Press. Louisville, Kentucky. 1980.

Lampe, K.F.and M.A.McCann. AMA Handbook of Poisonous and Injurious Plants. AMA. Chicago, Illinois. 1985.

Leung, A.Y. Encyclopedia of Common Natural Ingredients Used in Food, Drugs and Cosmetics. John Wiley & Sons. New York, New York. 1980.

Lewis, Walter H. Medical Botany – Plants Affecting Man's Health. John Wiley & Sons, Inc. New York, London, Sydney, Toronto. 1977

Lloyd, G.E.R., ed. Hippocratic Writings. Penguin Books Ltd. London, England. 1983.

Loustalot, Arnaud J, Winters, Harold F., Childers, Norman F. Influence of High, Medium and Low Soil Moisture on Growth and Alkaloid Content of Cinchona Ledgeriana. United States Department of Agriculture. Mayaguez, Puerto Rica. July 5, 1947.

Lust, John B. The Herb Book. Bantam Books. New York, Toronto, London, Sydney, Auckland. 1974

Lyman, Rufus A., James M. Dille, Andrew DuMez, Glenn Jenkins, Rudolph Kuever, Hugh Muldoon, Howard C. Newton, et. al. American Pharmacy – Fundamental Principles and Practices – Pharmaceutical Preparations – Biologicals. J.B. Lippincott Company. Philadelphia, London, Montreal. 1945

Macalister, Sir Donald, President of the General Council, et. al. The British Pharmacopoeia. Constable & Co. Ltd. London, England. 1914

McGrath, William R. God-Given Herbs For The Healing Of Mankind. Privately Printed in Costa Rica by the Author, William R. McGrath. 1970.

Majno, Guido. The Healing Hand:Man and Wound in the Ancient World. Harvard University Press, Cambridge 1975.

Manniche, Lise. An Ancient Egyptian Herbal. British Museum Press. London. 1999

Markham, C.R. Travels in Peru and India. John Murray Albemarle Street. London. 1862

Martindale, The Extra Pharmacopoeia, 22nd Edition. Pharmaceutical Press. London, England. 1941

Martindale, The Extra Pharmacopeia, 25th Edition. Pharmaceutical Society of Great Britian. London, England. 1967.

McGuffin, Michael; Hobbs, Christopher; Upton, Roy; Goldbert, Alicia. Botanical Safety Handbook by theAmerican Herbal Products Association. CRC Press. Boca Raton, Boston, London, New York. Washington, D.C. 1997.

Merck & Company. Merck's Index – 4th Edition. Merck & Company, Inc. Rahway, N.J. 1930

Merck & Company. Merck's Index – 11th Edition. Merck & Company, Inc. Rahway, N.J. 1989

Miller, J. et al. Toxicity of some essential plant oils. Clinical and experimental study. *Clinical Toxicology*. 18 [12]: 1485-98. 1981.

Milspaugh, C.F. American Medicinal Plants. Broericke & Tafel. New York, New York. 1887.

Mitchell, H.W. et al. British Herbal Pharmacopoeia – 4th Impression. British Herbal Medicine Association. Bournemouth, U.K. 1991

Morris, Henry. Essentials of Materia Medica, Therapeutics, and Prescription-Writing. W.B. Saunders Co., Philadelphia, London. 191

Muenscher, W.C. Poisonous Plants of the United States. Macmillan Company. New York, New York. 1951.

Muse, Maude B. Materia Medica Pharmacology and Therapeutics. W.B. Saunders Company. Philadelphia and London. 1933.

National Formulary – 5th Edition. American Pharmaceutical Association. Baltimore, Maryland. 1926.

Niering, William A., original author; Thieret; John W. revising author, National Audubon Society. Field Guide to Wildflowers – Eastern Region. A Borzoi Book, published by Alfred A.Knopf, Inc. New York, Hong Kong. 2001

National Formulary – 7th Edition. American Pharmaceutical Association. Washington, D.C. 1942.

Osol, Arthur and George E. Farrar. The Dispensatory of the United States of America - 24th Edition. J.B. Lippincott Company, Philadelphia. 1947.

Osol, Arthur and G.E. Farrar. The Dispensatory of the United States of America – 25th Edition. J.B. Lippincott Company. Philadelphia, Pennsylvania. 1955.

Palmer, E.Laurence. Fieldbook of Natural History. Whittlesey House, McGraw-Hill Book Company, Inc. New York, Toronto. 1949

Peattie, Donald Culross. Flowering Earth. G.P. Putnam's Sons. New York, New York. 1939.

Pharmaceutical Formulas – The Chemists' Recipe Book – Tenth Edition. The Chemist and Druggist. London, England. 1946.

Pharmaceutical Formulas. – Volume I – Eleventh Edition. The Chemist and Druggist. London, Great Britain. 1944.

Phillips, Charles D.F. Materia Medica and Therapeutics -Inorganic Substances -Volume I. William Wood & Company. New York. 1882.

Phillips, Charles D.F. Materia Medica and Therapeutics-Inorganic Substances-Volume II. William Wood & Company. New York, New York. 1882.

Phillips, J.H. The Hippocratic Physician and Astronomie.Actes due Ve Colloque International Hippocratique. Lausanne,Switzerland. 1981.

Pizzorno J.L. and M.T. Murray. A Textbook of Natural Medicine. John Bastyr Publications. Seattle, Washington. 1992.

Potter, Sam'l O.L. Handbook of Materia Medica, Pharmacy and Therapeutics. P. Blakiston, Son & Co. Philadelphia, Pennsylvania. 1895

Potter, Sam'l O.A. Quiz-Compends - A Compend of Materia Medica Therapeutics and Prescription Writing. P. Blakiston's Son & Co. Philadelphia, Pennsylvania. 1898.

Powell, Eric F. The Modern Botanic Prescriber. L.N. Fowler & Co. Ltd. London, England. 1965.

Prevention Magazine. Herbs For Health. Rodale Press, Inc. Emmaus, Pennsylvania. 1976.

Remington, Joseph P. The Practice of Pharmacy – A Treatise – Sixth Edition. J.B. Lippincott Company. Philadelphia and London. 1917.

Remington's Practice of Pharmacy 9th Edition. Mack Publishing Company. Pennsylvania. 1948.

Remington's Pharmaceutical Sciences – 14th Edition. Mack Publishing Company. Pennsylvania. 1970.

Remington:The Science and Practice of Pharmacy – 19th Edition – Volume I and II. Mack Publishing Company. Pennsylvania. 1995.

Riddle, J.M. Dioscorides on Pharmacy and Medicine. University of Texas Press. Austin, Texas. 1985.

Ross,M. and K. Brain. An Introduction to Phytopharmacy. Pitman Medical Press. Bath, U.K. 1977.

Sarton, George, Ead, Hamed A., ed. Introduction To The History of Science - History of Islamic Science 2 ProQuestUMI. 1990

Saunders'Question Compends-Essentials of Materia Medica and Therapeutics and Prescription Writing. W.B.Saunders and Company. Philadelphia and London. 1912.

Sayre, Lucius E. Saunders' Question-Compends No. 18 - Essentials of Practice of Pharmacy. W.B. Saunders. Philadelphia, Pennsylvania. 1894.

Schneider, Albert. Powdered Vegetable Drugs. Calumet Publishing Company. Pittsburgh, Pennsylvania. 1902.

Schoch, Robert, Ph.D. and Robert Aquinas McNally. Voices of the Rocks – A Scientist Looks at Catastrophies and Ancient Civilizations. Harmony Books. New York, New York. 1999.

Schultes,R.E.and R.F.Raffauf. The Healing Forest. Dioscorides Press. Portland, Oregon. 1990.

Science and Technology Department of the Carnegie Library of Pittsburgh. The Handy Science Answer Book. Visible Ink Press. Detroit, Michigan. 1994.

Shealy, C. Norman. The Illustrated Encyclopedia of Healing Remedies. Element Books Limited –A Division of Houghton Mifflin. New York, Boston. 1998

Sievers, A.F. *The Herb Hunters Guide.* Misc. Publ. No. 77. USDA, Washington DC. 1930.

Simon, J.E., A.F. Chadwick and L.E. Craker. 1984. Herbs: An Indexed Bibliography. 1971-1980

Scientific Literature on Selected Herbs, and Aromatic and Medicinal Plants of the Temperate Zone. Archon Books, 770 pp., Hamden, CT.

Shook, Edward E. Advanced Treatise in Herbology. Trinity Center Press and CSA Press. Lakemont, Georgia. 1978.

Solis-Cohen,S. andT.Githens. Pharmacotherapeutics Materia Medica and Drug Action. D. Appleton & Company. New York, New York. 1928.

Squire, Peter Wyatt. Squire's Companion to the British Pharmacopoeia – 19th Edition. J. & A. Churchill. London, England. 1916.

Stuart, Malcolm. The Encyclopedia of Herbs and Herbalism. Crescent Books – Crown Publishers, Inc. of Orbis Publishing, Limited. London. 1979

Taylor, Norman. A Guide To The Wild Flowers East of the Mississippi and North of Virginia. Greenberg Publisher, Inc.,Garden City Publishing Company. Garden City, New York. 1928.

The Druggists Circular. <u>The Druggists Circular Formula Book</u>. The Druggists Circular. New York, New York. 1915

The Garden Club of American. <u>Pronunciation of Plant Names</u>. National Process Company, New York City, New York 1932.

The Pharmaceutical Era. <u>The Era Key to the United States Pharmacopoeia – 10th Revision and The National Formulary [5th Revision]</u>. D.O. Haynes & Co. New York, New York. 1926.

Therapeutic Research Facility. <u>Natural Medicines Comprehensive Database – 3rd Edition</u>. Stockton,California. 2000

Thomas, Joseph. <u>Thomas' Complete Pronouncing Medical Dictionary</u>. J.B. Lippincott Company. London – Philadelphia. 1889.

Thompson, C.J.S. <u>The Mystery and Art of The Apothecary</u>. J.B. Lippincott Company. Philadelphia, Pennsylvania. 1929

Trease,G.E. and W.C. Evans. <u>Pharmacognosy. – 11th Edition</u>. Bailliere Tindall. London, England. 1978.

Tu, G., ed. <u>Pharmacopoeia of the People's Republic of China</u>. [English Edition 1988]. People's Medicinal Publishing House. Beijing, China. 1988.

United States Department of Agriculture. <u>Miscellaneous Publication No. 77</u>. Reprinted by Trinity Center Press. California. 1975

United States Pharmacopoeia Convention. <u>United States Pharmacopoeia – 1st Edition</u>. Wells & Lilly. Boston, Mass. 1820.

United States Pharmacopoeia Convention. <u>United States Pharmacopoeia – 19th Edition</u>. United States Pharmacopoeia Convention. Rockville, MD. 1974.

University of Virginia. <u>Antiqua Medicina:Hipocrates</u>. UVA Medical School, Charlottesville, Virginia. 2001.

Wagner, H. <u>Plant Drug Analysis</u>. Springer-Verlag. Berlin, Germany. 1984.

Walker, Winifred. <u>All The Plant Of The Bible</u>. Harper & Row, Publishers. New York, Evanston and London. 1957

Williams, Francis H. <u>A Text-Book of Pharmacology, Therapeutics and Materia Medica</u>. Lea Brothers & Co. Philadelphia, Pennsylvania. 1888.

Wood, Horatio C. and A.Osol. <u>The United States Dispensatory, 21st Edition</u>. J.B. Lippincott and

Company. Philadelphia. 1926.

Wood, H.C. and A. Osol. The Dispensatory of the United States of America – 23rd Edition. J.B. Lippincott Company. Philadelphia. 1943

Woolf, Henry Bosley, et al. Webster's New Collegiate Dictionary. G. &. C. Merriam Company. Springfield, Massachusettes. 1974.

World Health Organization. World Health Statistics Annual. Geneveve. 1979

Wren, R.C. Revised by E.M.Williamson and F.J. Evans. Potter's New Cyclopaedia of Botanical Drugs and Preparations. C.W.Daniel Co. Ltd. Essex, England. 1988.

Wright, Harold H. and Mildred Montag. A Textbook of Materia Medica Pharmacology and Therapeutics – 3rd Edition. W.B.Saunders Company. Philadelphia and London. 1945

Yen, K.Y. The Illustrated Chinese Materia Medica. SMC Publishing, Inc. Taipei, Taiwan. 1992.

Youngken, H.W. A Textbook of Pharmacognosy. Blakiston's Son & Co. Philadelphia, Pennsylvania. 1921.

Youngken, Heber W. Pharmaceutical Botany – 7th Edition. The Blakiston Company. Philadelphia, Toronto. 1951

Zimmerman, D.R. The Essential Guide to Nonprescription Drugs. Harper & Row, Publishers, Inc. New York, New York. 1983.